Handbook of
OPHTHALMOLOGY

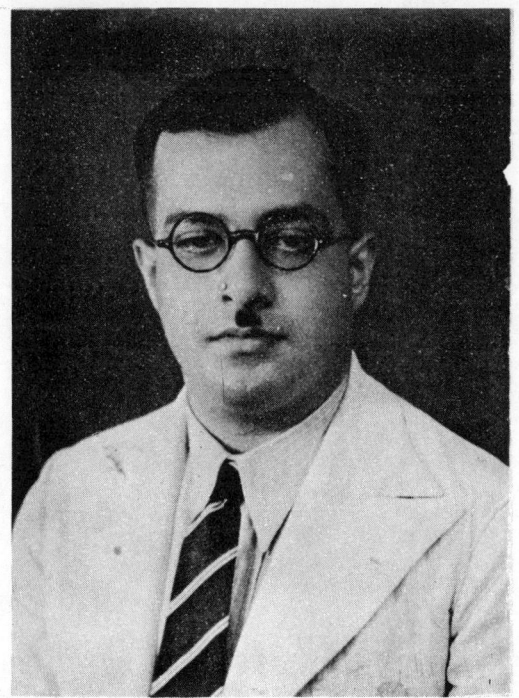

Late Dr. B.M. Chatterjee

Message :

This is the only original edition of Late Dr. B.M. Chatterjee
which carries his photograph and signature also.

B.M.CHATTERJEE'S

Handbook of
OPHTHALMOLOGY

(FOR STUDENTS & PRACTITIONERS)

6th Edition Revised & Enlarged

Updated with the addition of fresh material on special investigations, psychosomatic disorders, use of lasers in ophthalmology, therapeutics and a separate chapter on ophthalmic prescriptions

With 200 illustrations, 4 plates, and 42 colour photographs, and also description of eye instruments and operations

Edited by

Prof. (Dr.) Lalit P. Agarwal

MBBS (Luck.), DOMS, R.C.P. & S. (Eng.), D.O. (Oxon),
M.S. (Luck.), F.A.M.S. (India), F.O.R.C.E. (India), F.S.E.S. (USA)
Formerly :
Director : All India Institute of Medical Sciences, New Delhi
Founder & Chief Organiser : Dr. Rajendra Prasad Centre for
Ophthalmic Sciences, A.I.I.M.S., New Delhi
Chief and Principal Eye Surgeon : A.I.I.M.S., New Delhi
Adviser Ophthalmology : Government of India

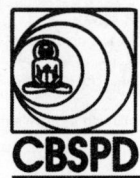

CBSPD

CBS Publishers & Distributors Pvt Ltd

New Delhi • Bengaluru • Chennai • Kochi • Kolkata • Lucknow • Mumbai
Hyderabad • Jharkhand • Nagpur • Patna • Pune • Uttarakhand

BM Chatterjee's
Handbook of
OPHTHALMOLOGY
(*for students and practitioners*)
6th Edition Revised and Enlarged

ISBN-13: 978-81-239-0682-9
ISBN-10: 81-239-0682-0

Copyright © Publisher

Sixth Edition: 1997
Reprint: 1998, 1999, 2002, 2003, 2004, 2006, 2007, 2008, 2010, 2011, 2013, 2014, 2015, 2016, 2017, 2018, 2019, 2021, **2024**

Published by **Satish Kumar Jain** and produced by **Varun Jain** for

CBS Publishers & Distributors Pvt Ltd
4819/XI Prahlad Street, 24 Ansari Road, Daryaganj, New Delhi 110 002, India.
Ph: 011-23266838, 23289259   Website: www.cbspd.com
                                e-mail: delhi@cbspd.com

Corporate Office: 204 FIE, Industrial Area, Patparganj, Delhi 110 092
Ph: 011-4934 4934   Fax: 011-4934 4935
                           e-mail: publishing@cbspd.com; publicity@cbspd.com

Branches

- **Bengaluru:** Seema House 2975, 17th Cross, KR Road, Banasankari 2nd Stage, Bengaluru 560 070, Karnataka, India
  Ph: +91-80-26771678/79   Fax: +91-80-26771680   e-mail: bangalore@cbspd.com
- **Chennai:** 7, Subbaraya Street, Shenoy Nagar, Chennai 600 030, Tamil Nadu, India
  Ph: +91-44-26680620, 26681266   Fax: +91-44-42032115   e-mail: chennai@cbspd.com
- **Kochi:** 42/1325, 1326, Power House Road, Opp KSEB, Power House, Ernakulum Kochi 682 018, Kerala, India
  Ph: +91-484-4059061-65,67   Fax: +91-484-4059065   e-mail: kochi@cbspd.com
- **Kolkata:** 147, Hind Ceramics Compound, 1st Floor, Nilgunj Road, Belghoria, Kolkata-700056, West Bengal, India
  Ph: +033-25633055, 033-25633056   e-mail: kolkata@cbspd.com
- **Lucknow:** Basement, Khushnuma Complex, 7 Meerabai Marg (Behind Jawahar Bhawan), Lucknow-226001, UP, India
  Ph: +0522-4000032   e-mail: tiwari.lucknow@cbspd.com
- **Mumbai:** PWD Shed, Gala no 25/26, Ramchandra Bhatt Marg, Next to JJ Hospital Gate no. 2, Opp. Union Bank of India, Noorbaug, Mumbai-400009, Maharashtra, India
  Ph: 022-66661880/89   e-mail: mumbai@cbspd.com

Representatives

- Hyderabad   0-9885175004
- Patna   0-9334159340
- Jharkhand   0-9811541605
- Pune   0-9664372571
- Nagpur   0-8692091830
- Uttarakhand   0-9716462459

Printed at Mudrak, Noida, UP, India

PREFACE TO THE SIXTH EDITION

The 6th edition of the book is being brought out with the sole objective of providing the students and practitioners of ophthalmology with easy to read and perceive material useful for them. While retaining the previous material, new chapters have been added. Chapter on psychosomatic disorders has been added keeping in view that more and more stress-related pathologies are seen which simulate organic diseases. Lasers have been described to acquaint the reader with the latest therapeutic tool. A chapter on special investigations dealing with ultrasound, automatic perimetry, ophthalmodynamometry and fluorescein angiography has been added to keep in tune with the rising needs of investigative procedures and the newer tools available for such investigations. The chapter on ocular therapeutics has been revised and split into two, separating the ophthalmic prescriptions to enable one to easily reference to them in day to day practice. Many newer therapeutic drugs have deliberately not been added because of their still not being established and too dangerous to use like cytotoxic and immunosuppressive drugs in the management of uveitis.

The book has tried to keep clear of various aetiological, clinical, therapeutic and surgical controversies.

The book, like its previous editions, carries the traditional style in presenting the material in essential form without delving into great details and fineries in the sub-specialities of ophthalmology which cannot be covered in a textbook of this size.

An attempt has been made to keep the comprehensive outline of the whole subject intact. The index has been revised in consonance with the added material.

As far as possible the diseases have been described under the following headings :

- Definition
- Aetiology
- Pathology
- Clinical picture
- Differential diagnosis
- Treatment
- Complications

Some chapters and material have been included from my books "Agarwal's Eye Diseases, 2nd ed.", and "Essentials of Ophthalmology, 1st ed." being published by the same publishers. They have been accorded permission by me to include this material.

It is hoped that the book will serve the day to day needs of students and ophthalmologists. It is contemplated to completely revise the book in about 3 years time from now to enter into the 7th edition by which time many controversial problems in ophthalmology will be solved.

Editor

PREFACE : FIRST EDITION

As a teacher, it has all along been my feeling that Ophthalmology is rather neglected in the under-graduate course, although there is a prescribed course for the subject in the university curriculum. Keeping this fact in mind, this is an endeavour to present the more important and common aspects of this highly specialized subject in a concise and compact form, so that it may not be a time consuming affair to go through the book. In order to build up a liking and a basis for Ophthalmology, particular emphasis has been placed on clinical methods of examination of an eye case avoiding at the same time introduction of highly specialized instruments to which the students have no access.

Considering the requirements of the under-graduate candidates for the purpose of examination, the common eye diseases have only been described in proportionate details including at the same time a short anatomy of individual parts of the eye.

A chapter on common ophthalmic operations and eye instruments used for the operations also has been introduced.

Acknowledgements—It is my pleasure to express my indebtedness to the following works from which I have gathered ideas and illustrations—Parsons' Diseases of the Eye, May and Worth's Diseases of the Eye, Goulden's Refraction of the Eye, Wolff's Anatomy of the Eye and Orbit, Lyle and Jackson's Practical Orthoptics in the Treatment of Squint, Duke-Elder's Text Book of Ophthalmology, volumes 1 to 6, Duke-Elder's System of Ophthalmology, volume 2 and Davson's Physiology of the Eye.

Calcutta
May, 1973

B. M. CHATTERJEE

CONTENTS

PLATE I

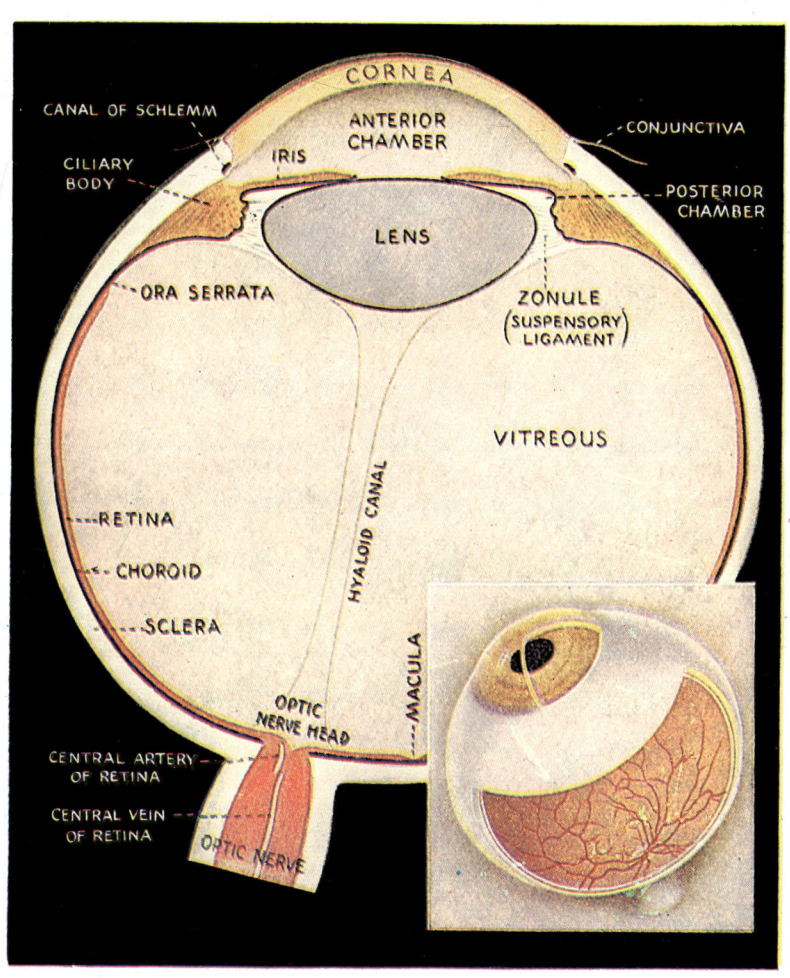

Horizontal Section of the Eyeball (May and Worth)

CHAPTER IA

SPECIAL INVESTIGATIONS OF THE EYE

COMPUTERIZED AUTOMATIC PERIMETERS

Computerized perimeters by and large use the inside of a sphere or bowl as a testing apparatus. They are like Goldmann's bowl used for static perimetry though they differ in details as outlined later. The computerized perimeters are of two types—one those display the targets by fixed LED displays (light emitting diodes and fibre optic) or projected image devices.

The projected devices use a single light source, tiltable mirrors, shutters, filters and stepping motors (Humphrey or Octopus perimeters). The stimulus can be placed at any location on the bowl by projection devices. The perimeter is thus adaptable to any method of analysis.

The testing coordinates or loci can be chosen by the perimeters computerized software and the locations can be as near as 1° or as far as 15° from each other. The accuracy of evaluation is the function of the distance between coordinates (loci) or delivery of points, and the measurement of sensitivity at each retinal location.

The computer can process all information and patient response during the test and convert them into the printed format for simple and easy interpretation. The decibel scale is the most common unit of documentation. If actual thresholding is performed, the computer can rearrange the data into different types of printouts, such as value tables, grey scales or the measurements of the depth of defect from the expected normal values for age related individuals. The information can be stored and used for follow ups on the same patient.

TESTING METHODS AND PARAMETERS

The common parameters that can be varied are fixation position; stimulus size; intensity and colour; fixation monitoring and sensitivity; background illumination; foveal thresholding; fluctuation; test speed; intervals between stimulus presentation; and duration of stimulus. These variables are, however, not available in all machines.

There are two basic testing methods : (a) those involved in screening for an indication of field loss; (b) those for threshold sensitivity of retinal receptors.

Screening procedure

It is a procedure performed by one size and one intensity target. A bright target should be used to evaluate the peripheral isopters and uncover dense scotomas while dim targets will define central isopters and show more subtle scotomas.

Computerized perimetry

The procedures are carried out on perimeters which use the inside of a sphere or bowl as a testing surface. They differ from Goldmann's bowl perimeter dramatically in the depth of the bowl, the ranges of background illumination used for testing and sophistication of the computerized functions performed.

The following conditions need to be fulfilled :

• The room should be light-proof, sound-proof, accoustically tiled or carpeted to decrease sound within, temperature and air controlled, isolated from the general clinical flow, have adequate electrical outlets, have no telephone to cause distractions.

• Room should be dark during testing.

• All programme software should be backed up.

A target is presented statically at one location at a time by fibre optic and light emitting diodes (LED) which is a more common device and the light used is yellow green monochromatic light around 555 nm range.

The second type of parameters have projection devices (Humphrey or octopus) which employ a single light source with tiltable mirrors, shutters, filters, and stepping motors. The major disadvantage of these perimeters is the noise made by filter and mirror changes.

In comparison, the LED perimeters are faster and do not have the distracting noise created by projection perimeters but suffer from the drawback that they do not have the versatility of varying stimulus locations.

Automated perimeters of different types can exploit all types of stimuli as under :

• Friedmann analyser which is a non-computerized test;

• Superthreshold static device (Fieldman's autofield or ocupot);

• Octopus; and

• Baylor visual field programmer which can be attached to standard Goldmann perimeter.

These are all projection devices. LED fibre optic instruments have the drawbacks already enumerated.

Data entry

As in other computerized instruments data is entered in the computer's memory by keyboards, switches or light pens. The light pens are the commonest.

Information is displayed on the monitors. Patient information should be entered in the fields charts in space provided but the same format should be used in every case.

Target presentation

Commonly the testing is done at 6° interval in the central field up to 30° and thereafter 15°. A regular pattern of presenting the targets is not necessary but the testing should be randomized keeping in view that it does not evaluate different isopters. This can, however, be used as a quick screening method to evaluate how the contraction of peripheral field will affect visual efficiency of vocational pursuits like driving.

Multiple level screening

In this method the stimuli are adjusted to the predetermined slope of decreasing peripheral retinal sensitivity expected for the normal eye. As the test object shifts peripherally from fixation, its intensity is adjusted to a value slightly higher than the expected threshold values for each test coordinate. The normal patient should see all test points over the entire tested area.

It may be recalled that the hill of vision was described by Traquair (Figs. 1A.1 and 1A.2). If the vision is tested for normals with a size III aperture on a 31.5 asb background, there are decreases in sensitivity of about 0.3 dBs for each degree of eccentricity from the fovea. Stimulus size affects the hill of vision values. With a size 1 the slope changes 4 dBs per degree whereas for a size V creates only a 2 dBs change for each 10° shift in eccentricity.

It is important to understand that in computerized perimetry a target value is expressed as an arbitrary unit called a decibel (dB) equal to 1/10 of a log unit. The maximum light intensity for a perimeter is assigned a zero decibel value. Decibel numbers do not necessarily have comparable light sensitivity values. Light intensity is expressed as an apostib (asbs) which is an absolute unit of light measurement equal to 0.1 millilamberts (a lambert is a unit of intensity equal to the brightness of a surface which is radiating or reflecting one lumen per square centimetre interval indicated above). Each stimulus should be exposed from 0.1 to 0.4 seconds depending upon the patient's reaction time.

The common parameters used in routine are fixation, size and intensity of stimulus, monitoring and sensitivity, background illumination, colour of the stimulus, threshold of fovea, fluctuation, test speed, intervals between stimulus and the duration of the stimulus. These factors depend upon the versatility of the computerized perimeter available.

The ophthalmologist must decide the purpose for which field assessment is being done. These perimeters are not recommended for routine use. Depending upon what is to be uncovered as fields defect one can use a grid loci in the central 30°; nerve fibre defect pattern in glaucoma fields, macula and disc overlays, point alignments of each side of the 90° meridian, the hill of vision profile, the 30° -60° peripheral ring, temporal crescent arcs, full field maps, arcute scotomas and nasal steps. Any other particular defect that may be relevant to the disease process in an individual case (Figs. 1A.3, 1A.4, 1A.5 and 1A.6).

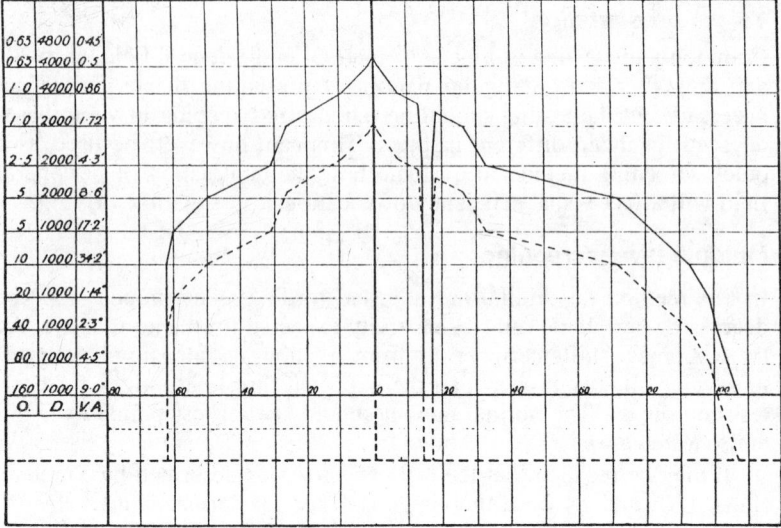

Fig. 1A.1. The field of vision regarded as a hill seen in section. The horizontal meridian is shown. The continuous horizontal base line indicates the extent of the field in degrees; the vertical lines the visual acuity; O, the diameter of the test object in millimetres; D, its distance from the eye in millimetres; and V.A., the visual angle subtended at the nodal point. Beginning with an angle of 9°, the visual angle is halved for each successive isopter of 1 : 2000, and 1 : 4000.

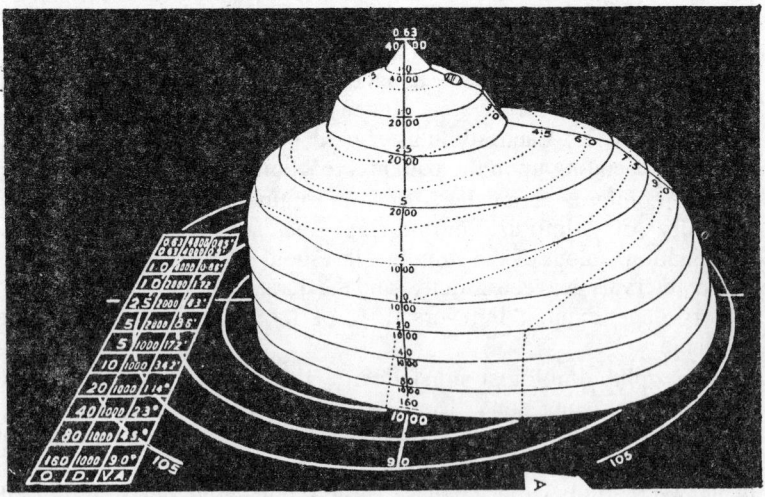

Fig. 1A.2. Model of the field of vision from the measurements given in Fig. 1A.1.

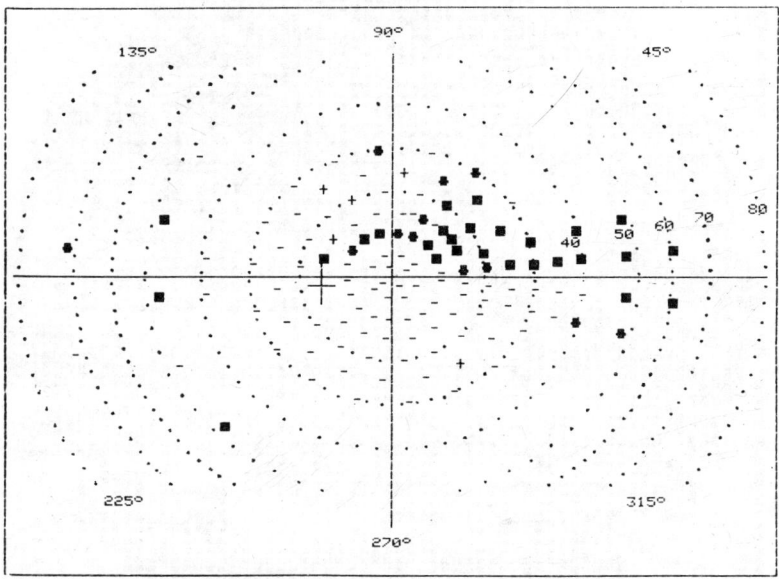

```
ID=                  AGE= 68        28 JAN 1987              12:28 PM
V.A: OD=20/800  OS=20/ 20      TEST RESULTS:            BLINDSPOT RESULTS
P.S: OD=  8.00  OS=  8.00 mm    TOTAL POINTS:      130       -
IOP: OD= 12.00  OS= 28.00 mmHg  ELAPSED TIME:     8:02
                                                          -   +   -
TEST PARAMETERS:    LEFT  EYE  FIXATION-LOSSES=       2
CORRECTION: SC (No)                                      +  +  +

BOWL LUMINANCE:        31.50 Asb  -SEEN POINT         -  - + + +  -
STIMULUS DURATION:     0.40 Sec  +MISSED AT    320  I-3e
STIMULUS INTERVAL:     1.00 Sec  ◆MISSED AT   1000  I-4e     - + +
FIXATION-RATE:        Moderate   ■MISSED AT   3200  II-4e
                                                         -      -
PATTERN: Glaucoma Pattern          DICON    AP-2500
STRATEGY: TWO-ZONE              COOPERVISION              -
FOLLOW-UP                       DIAGNOSTIC IMAGING    860303- 6283-11000
```

Fig. 1A.3. The three-zone test documents state presentation for three different set stimuli as illustrated on the Dicon by the two-zone strategy. This test does not use the patient's hill of vision, and is compatible with doing kinetic perimetry for three different targets on the Goldmann perimeter.

Once the defect has been detected a stepped suprathreshold method is used. The location is tested with an intensity of 0.5 log units higher than the original target. Even if this shows defect the intensity may be further increased by another 0.5 log units.

There are several other methods used and the reader is referred to more comprehensive books on visual field examination.

APPLANATION AND NO-TOUCH TONOMETRY

Applanation tonometry

This tonometer works on the principle of flattening a small standard area

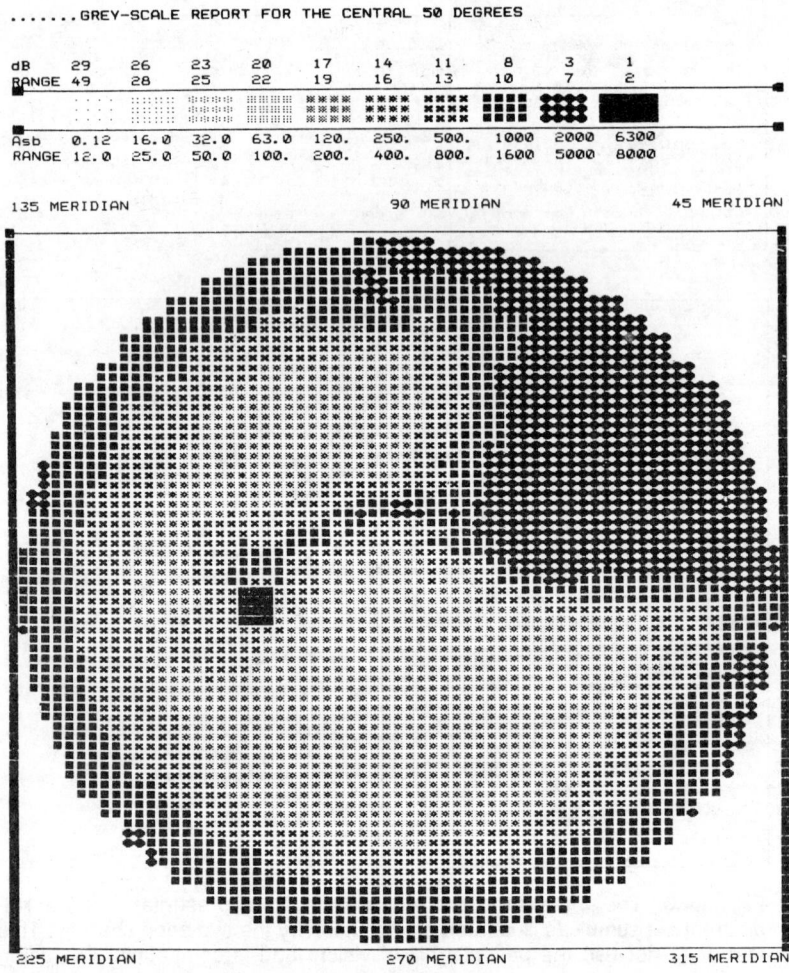

Fig. 1A.4. Grey-scale report for the central 50 degrees.

of the central part of the cornea and measuring the force employed to flatten this part (Fig. 1A.7). It is generally used along with a slit lamp. The most commonly used tonometer is Goldmann's applanation tonometer (Figs. 1A.8 and 1A.9).

Goldmann's applanation tonometer

The Goldmann applanation tonometer determines the force necessary to flatten, i.e., applanate an area of 3.06 mm in diameter of central part of cornea. When cornea is applanated, the force of the tonometer applied is the measure of intraocular pressure. Applanation tonometry displaces only about 0.5 μl of aqueous humour.

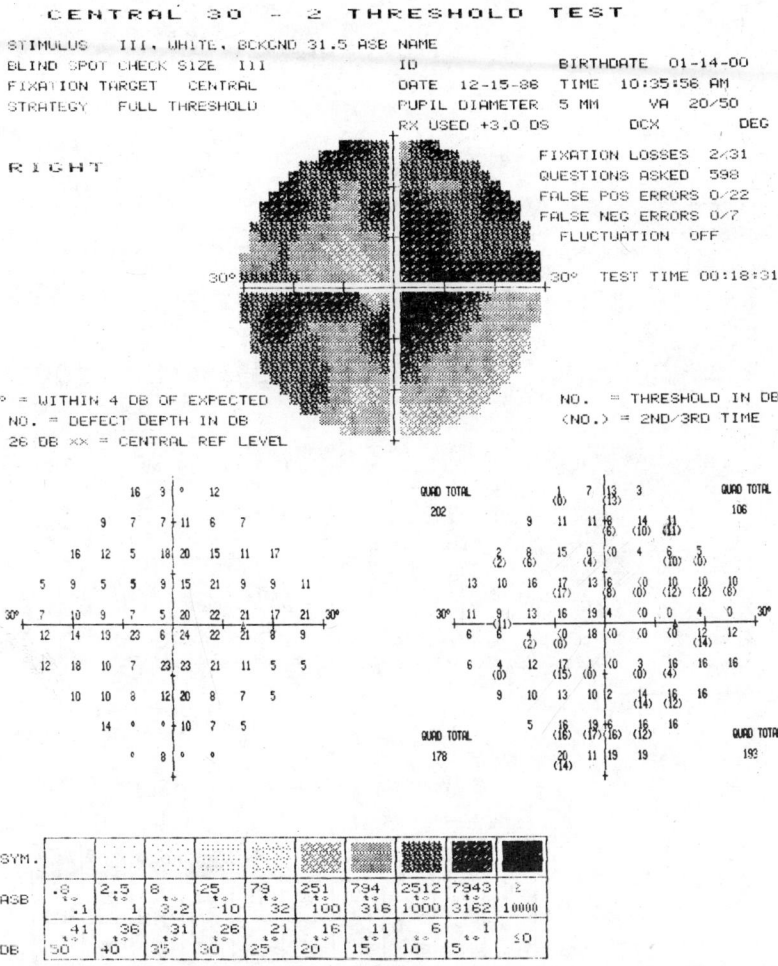

Fig. 1A.5. Threshold testing on the Humphrey field analyzer provides data documentation in three formats; the grey scale, the actual threshold map, and the documentation of defect depth.

The tonometer consists of two parts—a mechanical device which exerts force against the cornea and a contact element indicating the degree of the flattending of cornea. The contact element is a small biprism. The biprism performs two functions (1) splits the field in half and (2) the angle of prism displaces the two half images.

Technique

• Instill a drop of 4% xylocain to anaesthetise the cornea.

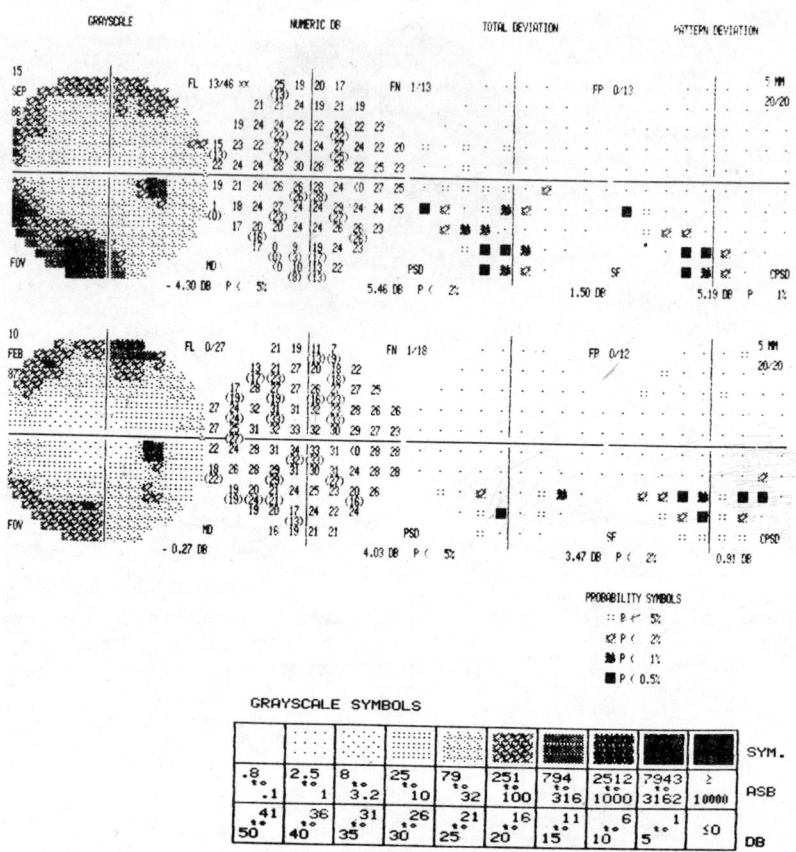

Fig. 1A.6. (*Continued*)

- Touch the moistened area of the cornea with a moistened 2% fluorescein strip.
- The tonometer and the prism are set in correct position on the slit lamp.
- The tension knob is set at 1 g.
- The graduation mark of the prism is set at the white line on the prism holder.
- Cobalt filter is used with the slit beam opened maximally.
- The angle between the illumination and microscope should be approximately 60°.

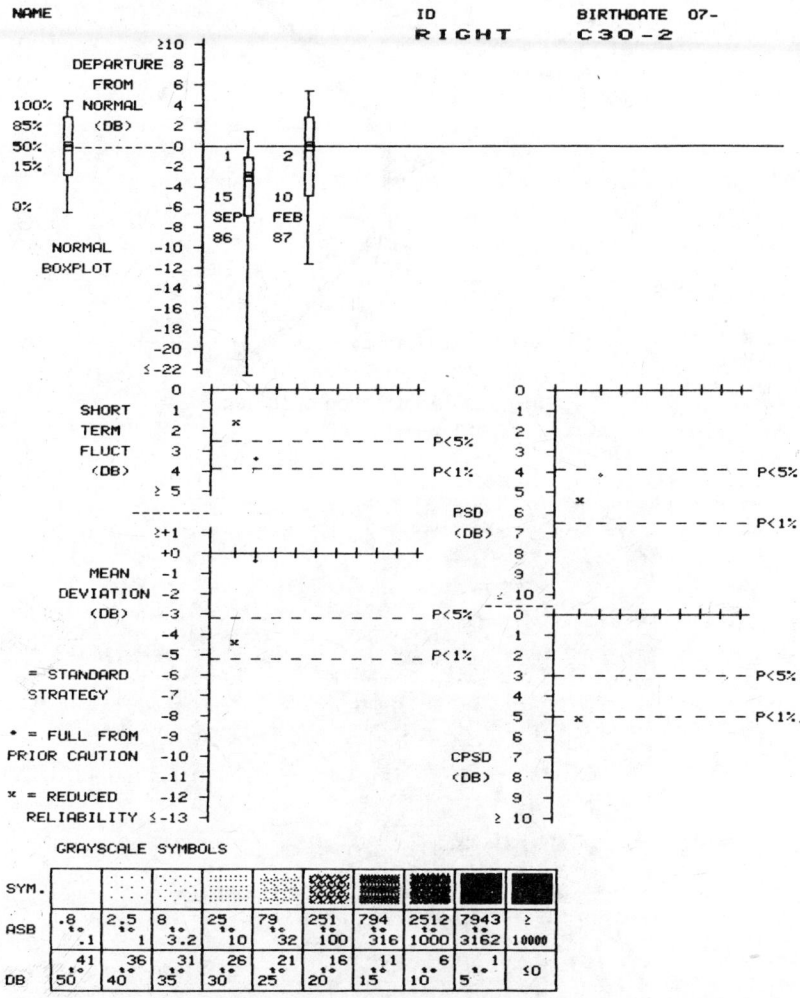

Fig. 1A.6. Threshold testing on the Humphrey field analyzer using the Statpac to include statistical analysis of the field.

- The room should be dark or lowly illuminated.
- The patient sits comfortably, facing the slit lamp. The heights of the patient's chair, the examiner's chair, the slit lamp and the chin rest are adequately adjusted so that a comfortable measurement can be affected.
- The patient's chin is placed on the chin rest and the forehead is supported by the forehead band.
- The operator now sits opposite the patient and looks through the microscope and moves the assembly towards the subject.

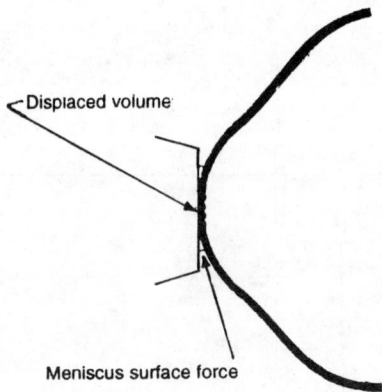

Fig. 1A.7. Applanation of cornea.

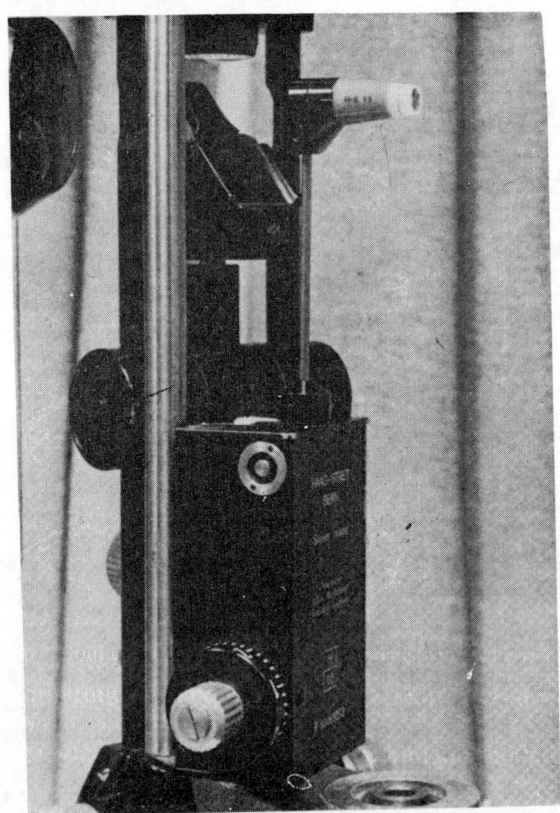

Fig. 1A.8. Goldmann's applanation tonometer

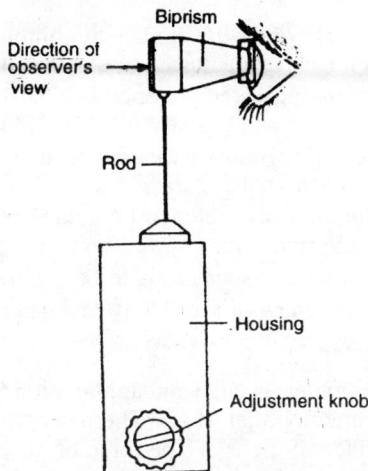

Fig. 1A.9. Optics of applanation tonometry.

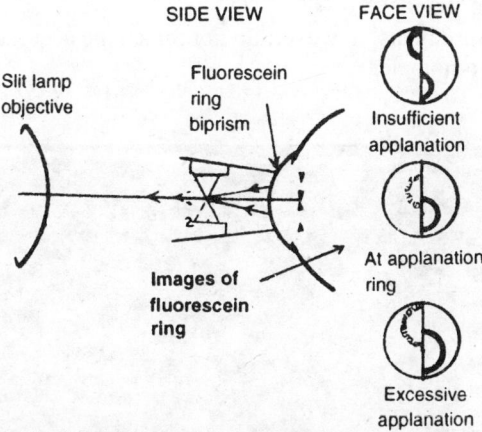

Fig. 1A.10. Optics of applanation tonometry.

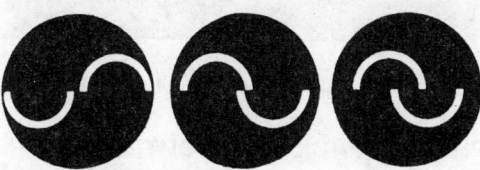

Fig. 1A.11. Schematic representation of rings seen with slit lamp during applanation tonometry. *Right :* rings inside each other indicate too much force is being applied to cornea. *Left :* rings outside each other indicate too little force is being applied. *Center :* inner margins of rings just touching indicate perfect applanation of cornea.

- The clinician now views the applanation through the biprism, the angle of which has been adjusted to displace the two half images.
- The end point is measured by applying the principle of vernier acuity.
- The fluorescein rings must touch each other at the midpoint by rotating the tension knob.
- Many ophthalmologists prefer to take three readings in each eye starting from the right eye.
- The Goldmann's tonometer needs to be calibrated once a month.

The optics is represented in Fig. 1A.10 and end point in Fig. 1A.11.

No-touch tonometer

The no-touch tonometer is also an applanation tonometer but the applanation is affected by a jet of air. There is no contact between the device and the surface of the eye. The force of air jet increases rapidly and linearly with time. The instrument uses a calibrated steadily increasing burst of air to flatten the cornea. The pressure is measured by means of an angulated incidence beam of light that is reflected directly flattened (Fig. 1A.12).

The measurements, however, do not match the accuracy obtained by Goldmann's tonometer.

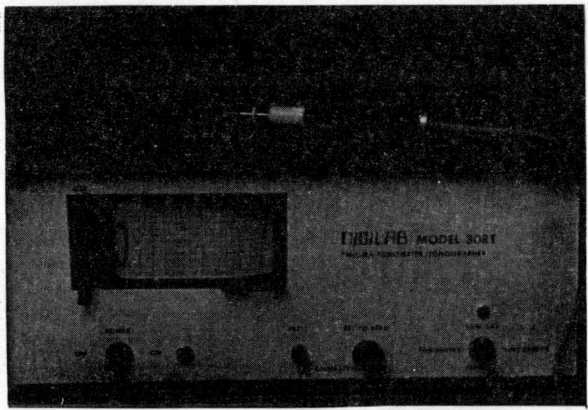

Fig. 1A.12. Pneumatic tonometer.

TONOGRAPHY AND FACILITY OF OUTFLOW

It aims at measuring the intraocular pressure continuously for a period of time and record the tension graphically as a continuous tracing. Though Schiotz's tonometer with weight can be used for the purpose but perhaps Muller's electronic tonometer is more suitable, which is also an indentation tonometer and can be labelled as electrical Schiotz tonometer. The purpose of this test is to estimate the facility of outflow of aqueous humour from the eye. The intraocular pressure is first determined under steady conditions. An electric tonometer or even an ordinary Schiotz tonometer is then placed on the cornea for a few minutes. The weight of the tonometer increases intraocular pressure and also increases the outflow of aqueous humour above its normal rate (Figs. 1A.13 and 1A.14). The tonometer is usually connected to a

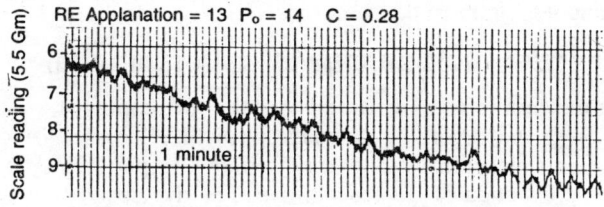

Fig. 1A.13. Tonographic tracing of normal eye.

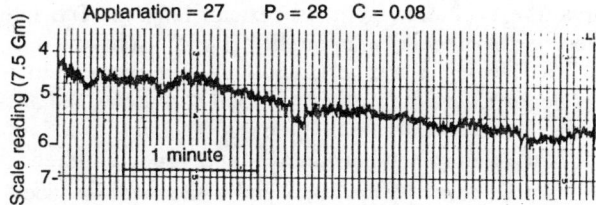

Fig. 1A.14. Tonographic tracing of chronic simple glaucoma.

continuous recording device that measures the subsequent decline of intraocular pressure over time. By comparing the initial and final pressure reading one can calculate the amount of fluid expressed from the eye by using the following formula derived by Grant.

$$C = \frac{\dfrac{\Delta v}{t}}{P_t - P_0}$$

where C is the facility of outflow, $\Delta v/t$ is the rate of fluid outflow, P_0 is the initial intraocular pressure, and P_t an average value of intraocular pressure over the period of test.

This assumes that :

- Aqueous secretion, blood volume and episcleral venous pressure remain unaltered during the period of test.
- All eyes respond with similar distention of the ocular coats to the similar rise in intraocular pressure.

It is now well known that these assumptions are untrue. Besides these there are operator errors, patient errors, instrument errors and reading errors. Several attempts have been made to improve the tonography and make it more reliable. Though tonography and measurement of facility of outflow have to a great extent contributed to the understanding of the aqueous humour outflow mechanism and the glaucomatous processes yet at the present time most ophthalmologists and even experts in glaucoma place almost no or minimal reliance on tonographic values for diagnostic or therapeutic procedures. In view of this, the procedure has been abandoned in most of the clinics.

FLUORESCEIN ANGIOGRAPHY (Figs. 1A.15 to 1A.23)

The fluorescein study is based on the principle of visualising (angioscopy) and recording (angiography) the fluorescence obtained from the intravascular and extravascular compartments following intravenous injection of fluorescein dye. The dye absorbs energy from visible light at a lower wavelength and emits it at a higher wavelength. The fluorescent light from the dye is recorded on a film sensitive to fluorescent light. The emitted light is less intense than the absorbed light.

The fluorescence is produced by a visible light between 420-490 nanometres, the excitation point is best at 425 nm. The intensity of fluorescence is also dependent upon the pH of the solution, the optimum being pH 7.5. The emission is best at 530 nm. The fluorescein molecules are merely deposited on the surface of blood corpuscles and not diffused into the cells. It is well tolerated. The usual dose used is a 5 ml solution of 20%. It is so even in newborn infants and young children.

The films used normally are black and white medium speed one. For colour transparency 64 ASA Kodachrome or Ektachrome film can be used. But coloured angiograms can also be obtained on medium speed colour film.

Method

To get results the following conditions must be satisfied :
- Full mydriasis when using a wide field lens.
- Fully explain the procedure to the patient to elicit his full cooperation.
- Keep an emergency tray for resuscitation ready as sometimes an anaphylactic shock may occur. A test dose may be given first and the patient may need an emergency attendance.
- Warn the patient about temporary discolouration of skin and urine.
- Warn the patient about side effects like nausea, vomiting, skin rash and itching.

The patient is seated in front of the camera with the chin on the chin rest and the forehead firmly against the forehead band. The observer sees through the camera and scans the fundus beginning from the disc, the various peripheral quadrants and finally the central area, in order to select the field where greater attention is required. It is better to take a few exposures of the different parts of fundus to get the fundus photographs without the fluorescein dye. Choroid has auto-fluorescence.

The patient is given 5 ml of 20% fluorescein dye into the anticubital vein rapidly and continuously to achieve a single bolus phenomenon. The dye is followed by normal saline injection to flush it out.

The following sequence takes place. This dye appears in the retina 6-8 seconds after the injection. This time interval is called *arm-retina time*. The time is grossly altered if there is any abnormality in circulation before the blood vessels reach the eye.

The angiogram is divided into various phases :
- Choroidal phase or pre-arterial phase
- Arterial phase
- Arteriovenous phase
- Venous phase
- Late phase

It is better to set the timer in the camera to record the timings of various phases.

Choroidal phase. It is also called pre-arterial phase (Fig. 1A.15) and choroidal circulation starts showing fluorescence but no dye has reached the retinal arteries. Complete filling of the choroid is usually achieved in the arteriovenous phase. If there is a filling defect then it is pathological.

Arterial phase. It starts about 1 second after the pre-arterial phase. The dye starts to enter the retinal artery through the central artery of

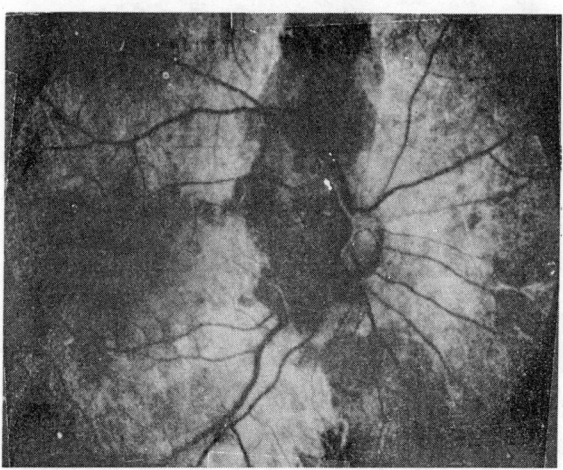

Fig. 1A.15. Choroidal flush in fluorescein angiography.

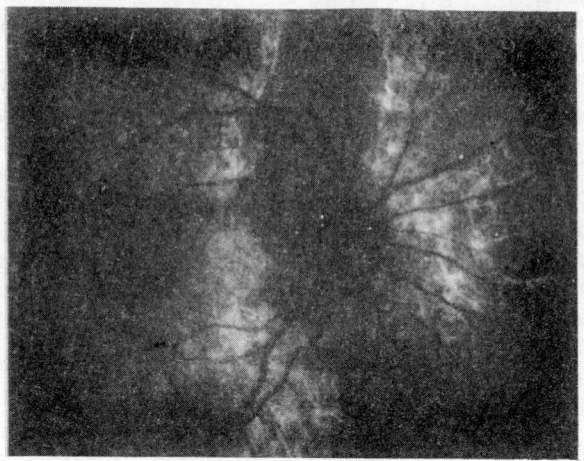

Fig. 1A.16. Pre-arterial phase of fluorescein angiography.

retina (Fig. 1A.16). It fills the inferior and superior divisions of the central artery of retina and displays all the arteries.

Arterio-venous phase. The dye is seen both in the arteries (Fig. 1A.17) and passing through the capillaries into the veins. The retinal capillaries are, however, better visualised alone with veins in the venous phase. There is early lamellar flow in veins.

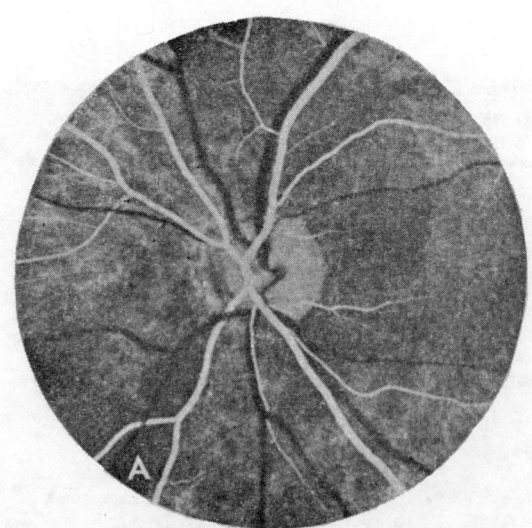

Fig. 1A.17. Retinal arterial phase.

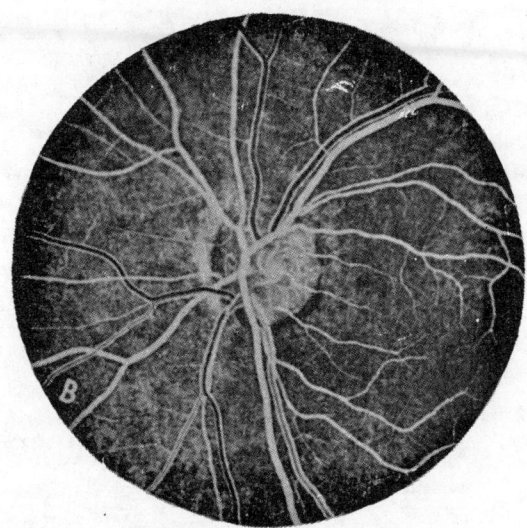

Fig. 1A.18. Early venous phase.

Venous phase. In the venous phase the veins are at first laminated (Fig. 1A.18) and later the whole venous blood column is visible though intensity becomes less.

Late phase. If the blood-retinal barrier has been broken the dye leaks out and (1) stains the abnormal vessels or (2) pools as a collection of fluid (Fig. 1A.18) or (3) can be seen on the disc.

The macular area, as can be seen in fluorescein angiography, is depicted in Fig. 1A.22.

The fluorescein angiograms should be interpreted on the basis of hypo- and hyper-fluorescent areas as given in Table 1A.1.

OPHTHALMODYNAMOMETRY

Ophthalmodynamometry is a simple and harmless procedure but of little clinical value as far as clinical diagnosis is concerned except in the diagnosis of occlusions of the proximal carotid system and in assessing the effect of surgical ligation of carotid artery. It has also been used, though unconvincingly, in general hypertension, intracranial hypertension, toxaemias of pregnancy, simple glaucoma, etc., both for diagnosis and prognosis.

The ophthalmodynamometer is a spring gauge calibrated to reflect pressure applied to the eye (Fig. 1A.24). The instrument was devised to measure the pressure in central retinal artery but the compression of central retinal artery to collapse only measure the lateral pressure in the ophthalmic artery.

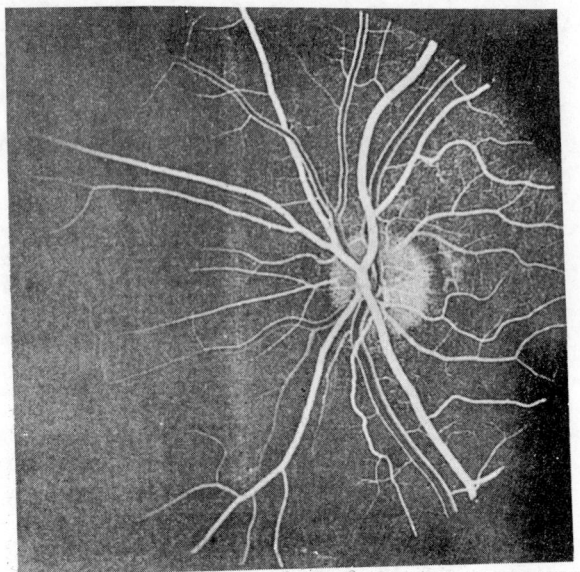

Fig. 1A.19. Early capillary phase.

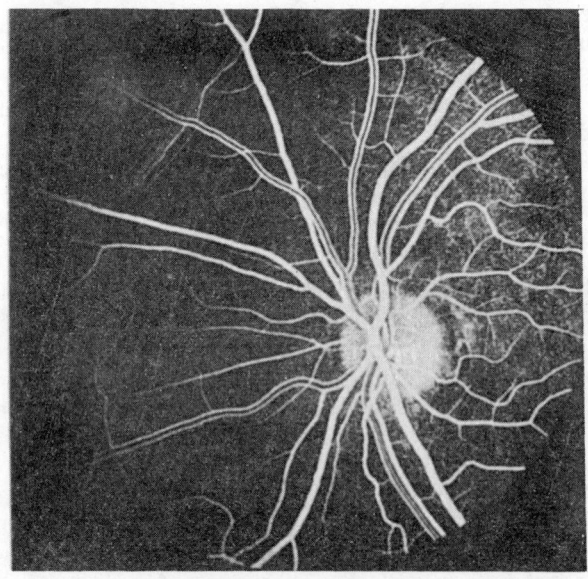

Fig. 1A.20. Arterio-venous phase.

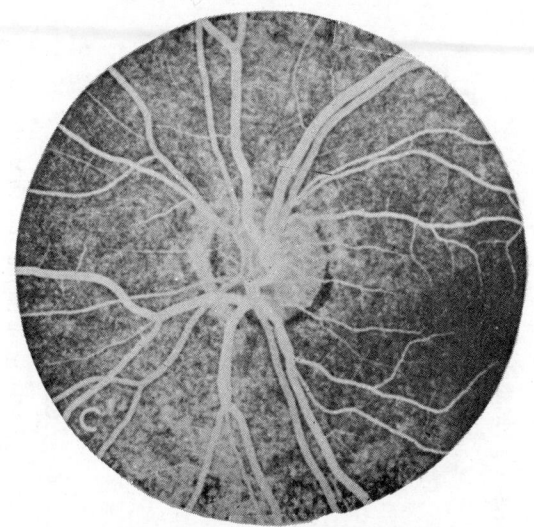

Fig. 1A.21. Late venous phase.

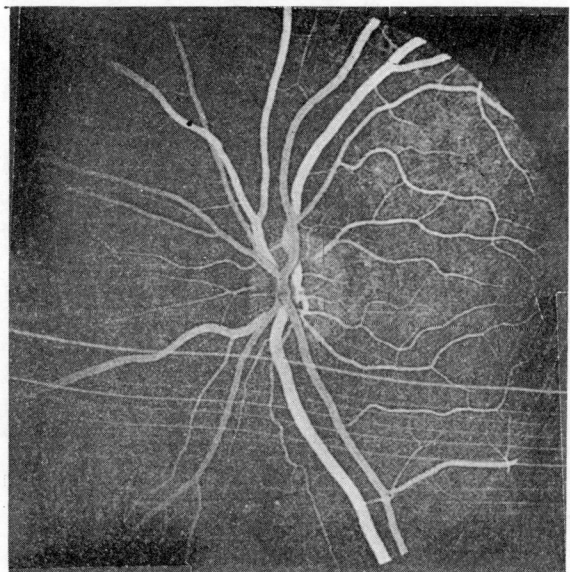

Fig. 1A.22. Dye passing out (late phase of angiogram).

The foot plate is directed radially on the side of the eye on the sclera and directed towards the centre. The observer sees to the disc and the central artery of the retina. He increases the pressure on the eye and as

Table 1A.1. Hyper- and hypofluorescent areas

Hypofluorescence

- Masking
  - Pigment
    - Melanin — e.g. Choroidal naevus, racial characters, RPE hypertrophy
    - Lipofuscin — e.g. Malignant melanomas
    - Blood — e.g. Choroidal haemorrhage, retinal haemorrhage, subhyaloid haemorrhage
    - Xanthophil — e.g. Macular pigment
    - Dark fundus — e.g. Some macular dystrophies
  - Serous fluid in between interphase — e.g. CSR, retinal detachment, disciform degeneration
- Lack of dye
  - Choroid — e.g. Choroidal infarct
  - Retinal — e.g. Vascular occlusions
- Lack of pigment — e.g. Albino, RPE atrophy (window defect)

Hyperfluorescence

- Abnormal vessels
  - New vessels — e.g. Diabetes, vein occlusions, disciform degeneration
  - Retinal telangiectasia — e.g. Coat's disease
  - Tumour vessels — e.g. Malignant melanoma, choroidal haemangioma
- Leakage — Pooling of dye — e.g. CSR, retinal detachment, disciform degeneration
- Staining — e.g. Soft exudate, drusen, scar tissue

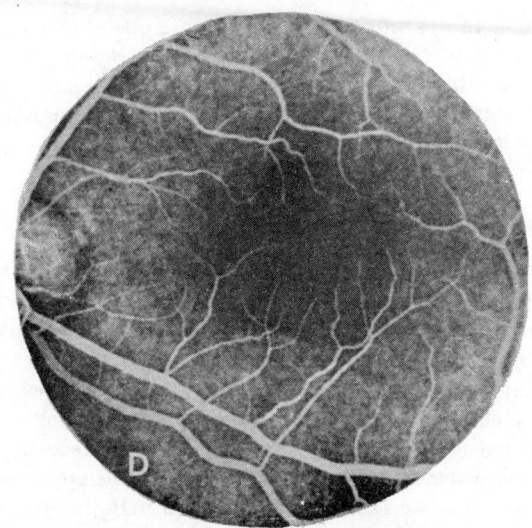

Fig. 1A.23. Capillary network around macula.

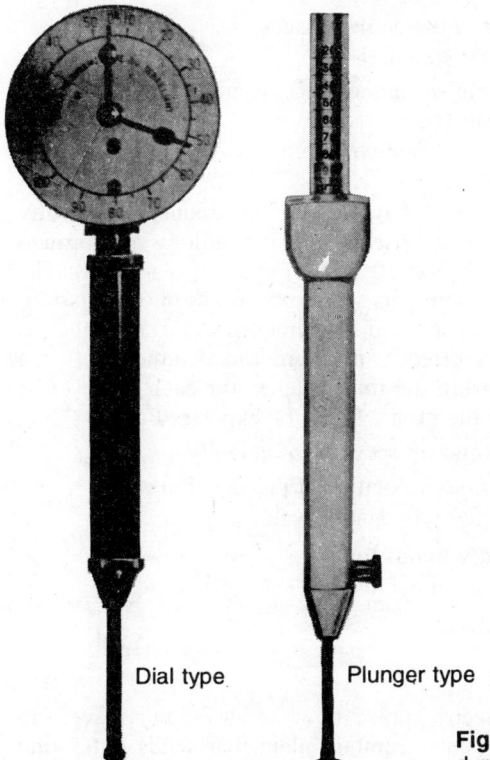

Dial type   Plunger type

Fig. 1A.24. Bailliart ophthalmodynamometer.

the central artery of the retina begins to pulsate, the reading on the dial of the instrument is read. This is the diastolic blood pressure. The pressure is continuously increased till the central artery of retina collapses and does not pulsate at all. This is the systolic pressure. Some instruments give direct reading while others give conversion tables for the readings obtained.

ULTRASONOGRAPHY OR ECHOGRAPHY

Since this method is being increasingly employed, it is being dealt with in some detail.

Ultrasound means ultra high frequency sound waves and which are above the audible level of the human ear.

The method aims at making an image using sound waves. The ultrasound probe sends out a sound beam which is very small and can be precisely directed towards ocular structure. They bounce back off the interfaces of the surfaces, reflecting back some of the energy—some of the energy is absorbed and some of it passes through. In ophthalmology we use ultrasounds as diagnostic ultrasounds whose wave frequencies are measured in cycles per second or hertz (Hz). The ocular diagnostic ultrasound

- does not generate heat in the ocular tissues,
- does not use high power sound energy
- its frequency is much higher, in the range of millions of cycles per second (MHz) or megahertz.

It is, therefore, a safe and effective method of generating ocular images for all types of patients.

Sound waves like light waves have amplitude, frequency, velocity and resolution. The sound waves used in ophthalmology are through probes of a frequency of 10 MHz (10 million cycles per second). The higher the frequency the less deeply its sound penetrates into the tissues. The velocity represents the speed and it is important to know that as ultrasound systems do not directly measure the distance between structures, they merely measure the time it takes for each wave to be returned from a structure to the probe. It can be expressed as :

$$Distance = time \ (in \ seconds) \times velocity$$

It is better to use the term as velocities of propagation.

The following are the usual propagation values :

1532 m/s	Aqueous and vitreous humours
1550 m/s	Average for axial eye length measurement
1620 m/s	Cornea
1641 m/s	Crystalline lens

The instruments use electric pulse to generate sound waves. In modern instruments it is a small ceramic plate that sends out sound waves when energized by electric pulse (transducer probe). Piezoelectric transducer (probe) converts electricity to sound waves and sound waves to electricity thereby making it possible for diagnostic ultrasound to be performed. This ceramic plate sometimes comes into direct contact with the eye (solid tipped A-scan probe) other times it is recessed inside a fluid filled probe which is larger and motorized and is used for B-scan. The scheme is represented in Figs. 1A.25 and 1A.26.

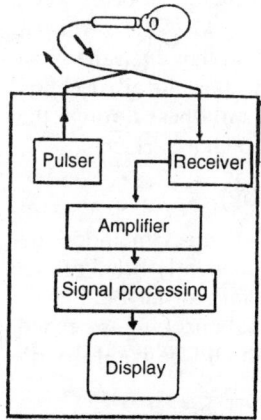

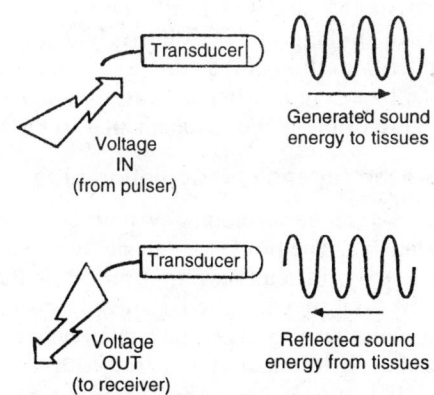

Fig. 1A.25. Transducer voltage in (from pulser) generated sound energy to tissues transducer voltage out (to receiver) reflected sound energy from tissues.

Fig. 1A.26. Schematic diagram of ultrasound system.

Yet another mechanism is that featured is an electronic amplification of a sound wave signal that ' received by the transducer. This factor is a decibel dB (Fig. 1A.27) and is termed as gain. When gain is turned up A-scan echoes get taller and B-scan echoes get brighter. Adjusting the gain allows the observer to vary the resolution, i.e., how close the two things may appear and still allow the observer to determine both objects.

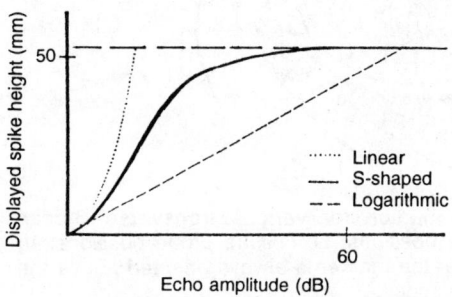

Fig. 1A.27. Amplification curves for linear S-shaped and logarithmic amplifiers.

A-scan (time amplitude ultrasonography)

The standardized A-scan unit is set at tissue sensitivity. The eye is given local anaesthetic drops. The probe is placed directly on the conjunctiva and the probe is angled so as to ensure that it is perpendicular to opposite fundus. It is better to take at least two positions one bypassing the lens opposite the suspected site of lesion and the other through the lens (Fig. 1A.28). More than one sites can be chosen by shifting the probe between the limbus and the fornix in various quadrants. Once the fornix is reached, the probe is extensively angled forward so that even the most anterior portion of the vitreous and the fundus as well as the ciliary body can be examined. In each case the sound wave should pass through the centre of the globe perpendicular to the opposite ocular surface.

B-scan (intensity modulation ultrasonography)

In B-scan ultrasonography both water-bath and contact methods are available. The probe that the author prefers is permanently filled probe. The only difficulty with all probes is the appearance of air bubbles— more so if they have to be filled every time. Careful checking is needed to avoid artifacts (i.e., unwanted echoes). One should be careful with probes. If it falls it may be ruined.

It is always better to examine the patient in supine position on a couch. If he is sitting in a wheel chair he can be examined in a sitting position while infants be examined in the arms of their parents in a supine position. The machine is set for ocular examination by turning the depth control to 0 to 3 cm setting. With 1% methyl cellulose applied to the surface of the probe gentle contact is made against the closed lids. It is better, however, to perform echography by open eye contact system as the echographer always knows exactly what part of the globe is being examined.

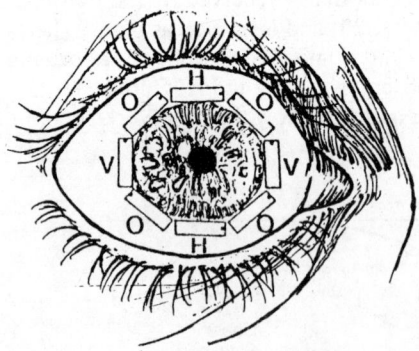

Fig. 1A.28. Probe marker orientation for various transverse B-scan approaches. H, horizontal probe positions; O, oblique probe positions; V, vertical probe positions. Note that the marker is always oriented above the horizontal for vertical and oblique scans.

The open eye technique is contraindicated in :
- Recent trauma or surgery
- Infants and children
- One-eyed patients
- Hesitancy or reluctance of the echographer due to fear of injuring the eye.

By convention horizontal transverse scans, i.e., the transverse scans (12 o'clock and 6 o'clock meridians) are performed with the marker oriented towards the patient's nose. Therefore, the upper part of the echogram always represents the nasal portion of the globe. On the other hand vertical transverse scans (i.e., transverse scans of the 3 o'clock and 9 o'clock meridians) are performed with the marker directed superiorly so the top of the echogram represents the upper portion of the globe. Oblique transverse scans are performed with markers towards the upper portion of the globe (Fig. 1A.28).

There is yet another mode of scanning, i.e., the longitudinal scans (Fig. 1A.29). The probe face is rotated 90° from the position used for the transverse scan. The longest diameter is placed perpendicular to the limbus. The markers point towards the centre of the cornea. This produces an ultrasonogram with the optic disc and posterior fundus

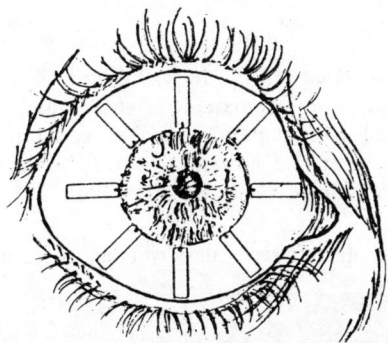

Fig. 1A.29. Probe marker orientation for various longitudinal B-scan approaches. Note that the probe marker is always oriented toward the centre of the cornea as well as the meridian being scanned.

displayed on the lower portion of the screen. It gives the echogram of the meridian which is examined, i.e., if the probe is placed at 6 o'clock position the sound beam sweeps along the 12 o'clock meridian. The probe can be shifted from the limbus to be fornix in the same direction and thus it is possible to scan either the more anterior or the more posterior view of the meridian that is being examined. When it is placed overlapping the limbus it allows better evaluation of peripapillary region. When the probe is placed close to the fornix it displays the periphery of the fundus and often the posterior part of the ciliary body.

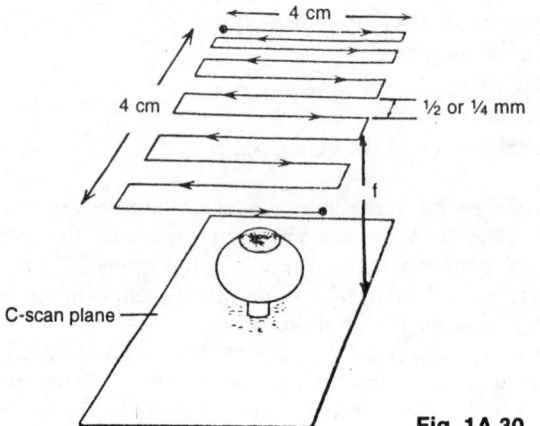

Fig. 1A.30. C-scan technique.

C-scan (Fig. 1A.30)

A transducer is strongly focused and it mechanically scans an aperture of 4 cm square in which the eye is centralised. The focal plane of the probe is arranged to lie in the plane of the area to be examined and echoes only from this plane are recorded.

EXOPHTHALMOMETRY

This procedure is carried out by the use of special mechanical devices, the exophthalmometers. The patient is seated and the surgeon stands behind him and holds the patient's head in such a manner that he looks straight down the nose. The surgeon then rotates the head of the patient backwards until he can just see the other cornea that eye is relatively proptosed.

Simple exophthalmometer (Luedde) is a simple device (Fig. 1A.31)

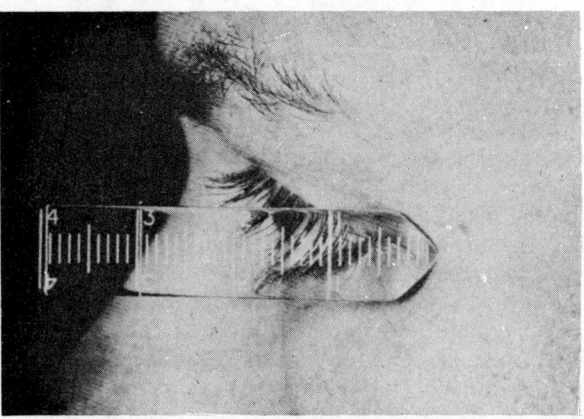

Fig. 1A.31. Luedde's exophthalmometer.

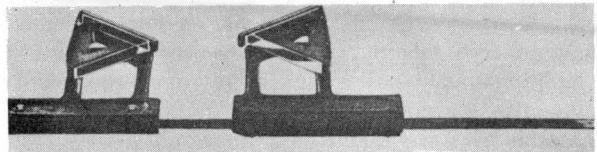

Fig. 1A.32. Hertel's exophthalmometer.

made of transparent plastic with a groove which fits into the outer bony margin of the orbit. The scale is engraved on both sides of the solid bar of the plastic.

The observing eye is aligned to read off the level of the apex of the cornea so that the scales are on either side of the bar.

The observer, standing at the side of the patient whose gaze is directed forwards, sights the apex of the cornea through the transparent plastic ruler and then records the forward protrusion of one eye at a time in millimetres.

Hertel exophthalmometer (Fig. 1A.32) : This instrument consists of a horizontal calibrated bar with movable carriers at each side. Each carrier consists of mirrors inclined at 45 degrees to reflect both the scale reading and the apex of the cornea of profile. Notches on the side carriers are placed on the bony lateral orbital margins of the patient. The patient is then asked to fixate on a point on the examiner's forehead. The apex of the cornea of each eye is superimposed on the millimetre scale reading by the inclined mirrors. The measurement of each eye is recorded by the examiner, alternately viewing with the right and left eye. The distance along the horizontal bar also is recorded as the base figure so that the carriers will be set at the same base for comparison at subsequent readings. This instrument provides a reliable comparison of the forward protrusion of each eye in relation to the bony orbit.

ELECTRO-RETINOGRAM, ELECTRO-OCULOGRAM AND VISUALLY EVOKED RESPONSE (ERG, EOG & VER)

The function of the retina can be assessed by changes in the electrical equilibrium produced by a light stimulus. The methods available are electro-retinography (ERG), electro-oculography (EOG) and visually evoked response (VER) in order to study visual function from retina to the cortex of the brain.

Electro-retinography (ERG)

ERG dates back to more than a century, the first human ERG being recorded in 1877. Clinical ERG began with the introduction of contact lens electrodes discovered by Riggs and his colleagues and Karpe.

The ERG is a mass response of the retina and special efforts are required to differentiate the cone-mediated (photopic, i.e., light-adapted) response from the rod-mediated (scotopic, i.e., dark-adapted) response. There are many variable factors which can affect the resultant ERG record. These are related to the stimulus (intensity, duration, frequency and colour), electrode (type and position), recorder and the subject (adaptation, pupillary dilatation, ocular movement and disease status of retina). The human eye has a subjective range of sensitivity of approximately 10^{10} log units. The ERG range is approximately 1 log unit less than this. At low stimulus intensities only b-wave response is seen while a-wave is seen when light is 2-3 log units brighter.

The form of ERG

The basic features of the ERG are shown in Fig. 1A.33. After a short latent period there is a negative a-wave followed by a positive b-wave, the height of which depends on the stimulus intensity. With weak stimuli a plateau follows the b-wave but with higher intensities a positive c-wave is seen. On stopping the stimulus there is an "off-effect" which is the d-wave. The increasing stimulus intensity increases the amplitude of the a- and b-wave but this is not a simple relationship. Most laboratories use increasing stimulus intensity and then measure amplitudes to develop normal versus abnormal ranges. Nowadays retinal neurophysiologists prefer to use a fixed amount of light to obtain threshold response, i.e., constant amplitude response. The cone-mediated (photopic) and rod-mediated (scotopic) systems give distinct components to the a-wave and b-wave termed as a-photopic (ap), a-scotopic (as), b-photopic (bp), and b-scotopic (bs). Flickering stimuli tend to accentuate the photopic component and if a computer averager is used it can extract small signals from the background interference.

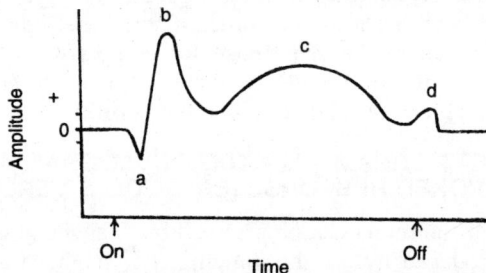

Fig. 1A.33. Basic features of ERG

Interpretation of ERG

Because of its difficulty in interpretation its clinical use is limited. No spatial analysis of retina can be made. The a- and b-wave from the photoceptors and the b-wave from the Müller cells, the c-wave originates in pigment epithelium. The ganglion cells do not contribute to the ERG, and so it can be recorded in the absence of ganglion cells and their axons (including the optic nerve) as is seen in many retinal diseases. The b-waves with a potential less than 0.19 mV or more than 0.54 mV are considered abnormal. Four types of abnormality are seen in the ERG recording (Fig. 1A.34).

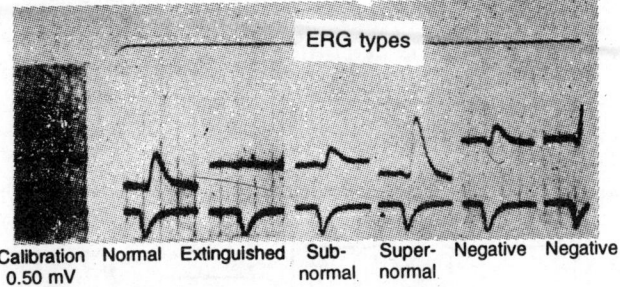

Calibration Normal Extinguished Sub-   Super-   Negative Negative
0.50 mV   normal   normal

Fig. 1A.34. Interpretation of ERG.

1. Supernormal, when the potential is above normal limits as seen in subtotal circulatory disturbance of retina.
2. Subnormal, when potential is less than 0.8 mV.
3. Negative, when a large *a*-wave is seen; a negative + where an abnormal *a*-wave is followed by a *b*-wave and a negative – where an abnormal *a*-wave is followed by a small *b*-wave or absent *b*-wave.
4. Extinguished, wherein there is complete absence of response.

A normal ERG record does not necessarily indicate normal retinal function. Advanced glaucoma, optic atrophy, Tay-Sachs's disease and macular disease may give normal responses.

Clinical applications

The most obvious application is in the study of hereditary and constitutional disorders of the retina including colour blindness.

An extinguished response is seen in retinitis pigmentosa. Choroiretinal degenerations or inflammation, e.g., choroideraemia, Spielmayer-Vogt disease, luetic chorioretinitis, Leber's congenital amaurosis. It is not diagnostic of a particular condition and cannot help to differentiate between these conditions. Retinal ischaemia due to arteriosclerosis, gaint cell arteritis, central retinal artery or vein occlusion can cause a small *b*-wave and a large *a*-wave. Siderosis produces supernormal responses in early stages which is not so in chalcosis. Drugs like chloroquine and quinine as also retinal detachment produce subnormal ERG response. Systemic diseases like vitamin A deficiency (reversible change) mucopolysaccharidosis, hypothyroidism and anaemia can produce subnormal ERG. A normal ERG is seen in cortical blindness, dyslexia and hysteria and may prove of diagnostic value.

Electro-oculography (EOG)

This is based on the standing potential of the eye. The cornea being positive with respect to the posterior aspects of the eye, the eye acts as a dipole. Eye movements are recorded by electrodes arranged in pairs

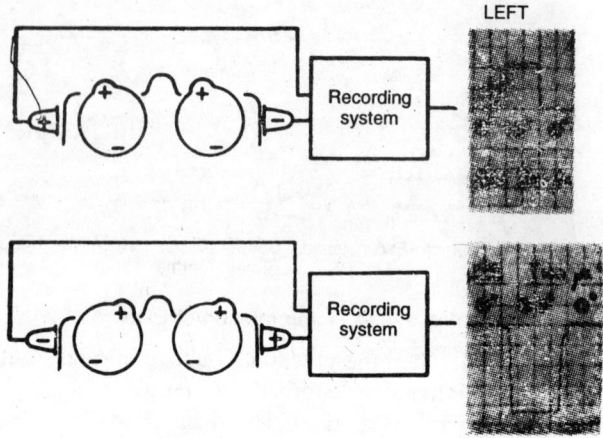

Fig. 1A.35. Recording of EOG.

on the skin near the canthi (Fig. 1A.35). Adaptation affects EOG in a manner opposite to that of ERG. Dark adaptation decreases the amplitude and light adaptation increases the amplitude. The maximum amplitude in light adaptation compared to the minimum amplitude in dark adaptation gives the EOG ratio (Ardin ratio).

Ranges for EOG ratio are :

0	Normal	> 2.00
1	Probably normal	1.80-2.00
2	Probably abnormal	1.60-1.79
3	Abnormal	1.20-1.59
4	Flat	< 1.20

Being a ratio it is unaffected by variables.

Clinical applications

The EOG decreases in most retinal degenerations and parallels the ERG response. The exceptions are Best's disease (vitelliform macular degeneration) where EOG is abnormal even in carriers whereas ERG is normal. In retinopathies due to chloroquine and other anti-malarial drugs EOG shows earlier abnormalities than ERG. Supernormal EOG reflects metabolic activity in retinal pigment epithelium and neural retina and hence is complementary of ERG.

Visually evoked response (VER)

The visually evoked response (VER) or visually evoked potential (VEP) is produced by electrical activity of the visual cortex in response to light or pattern stimulation of the eye. The response is a complex and a gross electrical signal, but by computer averaging techniques it is possible to record VER. The entire visual cortex (area 17, 18 and 19) contributes to

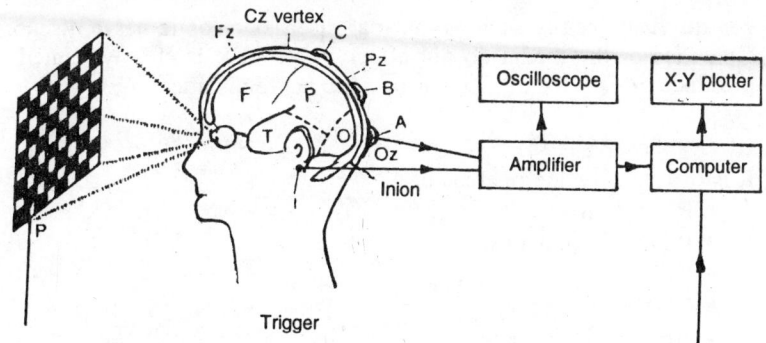

Fig. 1A.36. Recording of VER

the VER but the portion of importance to the ophthalmologist is the primary evoked response attributed to area 17. Since a disproportionately large cortical area represents the central retina as compared to peripheral retina the VER primarily represents central visual function especially visual acuity.

The recording is done by scalp electrodes (Fig. 1A.36) over the occipital cortex. The tiny 5 mV response to flash or patterned stimuli are buried in the background electrical noise which is always present. Therefore repeated stimuli are given and "time locked" responses are obtained which are stored, and averaged electrically in a signal averager. The responses are then recorded.

When both eyes are stimulated the VER responses are larger. The larger amplitude components are related to activity in visual association areas of the brain. Delayed nerve conduction produces long latencies.

The part of the VER response closely relates to visual acuity, the primary evoked response occurs 80 to 100 m. sec after stimulation. This component is enhanced by stimuli delivered at a rate of 10 Hz. The primary evoked response is seen as a smaller wave in a doubled peaked response (Fig. 1A.37). The smaller wave is altered by lesions affecting

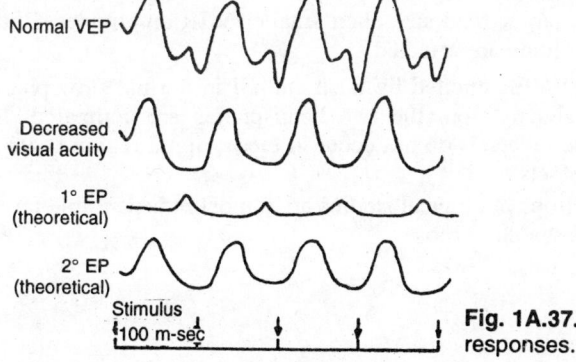

Fig. 1A.37. Primary evoked responses.

central visual acuity such as macular diseases or optic nerve diseases. Opacities of the media do not affect VER. VER is closely related to presence or absence of macular or optic nerve disorders.

Clinical applications

It is of special value in areas of :
- Refraction
- Infant visual acuity
- Diseases of optic nerve
- Colour blindness
- Amblyopia
- Field defects

Refraction : The refractive error can be determined by measuring VER amplitude with changes in power of trial lenses. Retinoscopy can easily assess refractive error but it can only tell us the optical correction necessary whereas VER is directly related to vision. It tells whether the visual system is processing well focused images. Thus it is complementary to retinoscopy.

Infant acuity : It is an objective method for testing visual acuity (V.A.) in non-verbal patients. Peak VER amplitude in adults occurs for checks between 10 and 20 minutes of arc and this corresponds to a visual acuity of 6/5. Using this bridge between subjective acuity and objective VER the infant's visual processes can be studied. However in this regard normal data have to be established.

Optic nerve diseases : VER can detect optic neuritis. The latency period is prolonged and amplitude reduced. Often in the absence of all clinical signs VER is positive.

Colour blindness : Chromatic pattern stimuli offer means of electro-physiologically separating red, green and blue colour channels, hence detecting colour defects.

Amblyopia : It is a means of studying electrophysiological mechanisms underlying amblyopia and also an objective method for early detection. Smaller field size of stimuli elicit larger response in amblyopes while larger field size elicit smaller VER amplitudes. Both laterncy and amplitude are affected.

Field defects : VER elicited by flash stimuli in normal slow phase reversals when signals from the two hemispheres are compared. In hemianopia phase reversals do not occur in the occipital region contra-lateral to field defects.

Thus the electrophysiological studies are almost indispensable tools for clinical and research purposes.

CHAPTER I

EXAMINATION OF AN EYE CASE

History :

History taking is extremely important and the patient should be encouraged to narrate his complaints and the relevant points about the ailments. Enquiries should be made about certain complaints and definite questions are to be put as indicated below :

1. Age, Sex, Occupation

2. Any dimness of Vision—
   a) mode of onset
   b) duration
   c) any glasses used before
   d) dimness for distance or near
   e) any double vision

3. Any pain in the eyeball—
   a) mode of onset and severity
   b) time of the day when worse
   c) relation to close work
   d) any associated nausea. vomiting or fall of vision

4. Headache—
   a) location
   b) time of the day when worse
   c) severity
   d) frequency
   e) any relation to close work
   f) any associated nausea, vomiting or fall of vision

5. Watering of the Eyes—
   a) duration
   b) constant or intermittent
   c) relation to close work, travelling in fast vehicle and after cinema show
   d) any associated redness

6. Discharge of the Eyes—

Any stickiness of the lids

7. Photophobia —i.e. dislike for light

8. Any history of injury—

a) Direct or indirect, including foreign body
b) any dimness of vision associated with it.

9. Past history—

a) redness of the eyes
b) treatment or operations of the eyes
c) general illness, like diabetes, hypertension, thyroid dysfunctions etc. need special enquiry.

Examination of the eye :

A preliminary inspection of the head, face and eyes from a short distance should be done before the closer examination of the eye is performed.

Following points should be noted in the preliminary examination.

1. The head—

a) its configuration
b) its position—i.e. head tilt or head turn.

2. The face—

a) any asymmetry
b) any sign of paralysis
c) any obvious skin change

3. The eye-brows—

a) any loss of hair or depigmentation
b) any elevation from hyperaction of frontalis muscle.

4. The palpebral fissure—wide or narrow.

5. The lids—

a) drooping or retracted in the upper lid
b) lagging in the lower lid.

6. The eyeball—

 a) Size—small as in microphthalmos, shrunken as in phthisis bulbi, big as in buphthalmos.

 b) Position—protruded (exophthalmos), sunken inside the shocket (enophthalmos), deviated from the normal position (squint), spontaneously oscillating (nystagmus) or pulsating.

 c) Congestion or any other discolouration.

7. Orbits—any deformity, or any fullness in any part of the orbit.

Closer examination of the lids and different parts of the eyeball should now be done with a loupe and torch. The loupe works like a magnifying lens.

Examination of the lids—

1. Position of the lid margins in relation to the cornea.

2. Thickness of the lids.

3. Redness, oedema, localised swelling, any pigmentation or depigmentation.

4. Conditions of the lashes—

 a) any misdirection of the lashes as in trichiasis
 b) any scantiness of lashes (madarosis)
 c) any white colouration of lashes (vitiligo)
 d) any nits or parasites adhered to the lashes
 e) any matting of the lashes with conjunctival discharge

5. Lid margin proper

 (a) any entropion (in rolling) or ectropion (out rolling)
 (b) any crust or ulcers
 (c) any thickness of margins (tylosis)·
 (d) any redness of margins (milphosis)
 (e) any defect of the lacrimal puncta i.e.eversion, stenosis or absence, any discharge.

Normal openings of the ducts of meibomian glands are visible as a series of white dots in front of the posterior sharp edge of the lid margin.

Examination of lacrimal sac.
The following points are to be noted—
(a) any redness or swelling over the sac area
(b) any fistula on the skin over the sac
(c) any regurgitation of watery, mucoid or purulent matter through the puncta on pressure over the sac area.

Patency of nasolacrimal passage is tested by introducing a lacrmial canula through the lower punctum and by pushing a coloured fluid like mercurochrome solution or normal saline, if the passage is blocked, the fluid regurgitates through the upper punctum, if the passage is patent then the patient will feel it in the throat via the nose.

Examination of conjunctiva—
1. Bulbar conjunctiva—
   (a) whether normal or congested
   (b) any chemosis or oedema
   (c) any sub conjunctival haemorrhage—petechial or in patches
   (d) any pigmentation, nodule or any tumour

2. Upper tarsal conjunctiva—The lid is everted by a gentle pull on the lashes and a simultaneous pressure over the skin with a glass rod.

   (a) any alteration in the arrangement of normal vascular pattern or any congestion. Normally there are vertical rows of ascending and descending blood vessels meeting at the subtarsal sulcus.
   (b) any follicle or papilla.
   (c) any scarring
   (d) any membrane formation
   (e) any granuloma, tumour mass or foreign body

3. Lower tarsal conjunctiva-
   Only pulling the lower lid downwards exposes the conjunctiva & fornix.
   All the points as in the upper conjunctiva should be noted including any evidence of symblepharon.

4. The conjunctiva of the limbus—
   (a) presence of ciliary or circumcorneal congestion

(b) presence of any nodule
(c) presence of any newly formed tissue

TABLE I
Different between conjunctival congestion & ciliary congestion.

Conjunctival Congestion	Ciliary Congestion
1. Congestion is most marked at the fornix.	1. Congestion is most marked at the limbus.
2. Congestion is bright red in colour	2. Congestion is pinkish red.
3. Vessels are superficial and branching.	3. Vessels are deep and radially arranged.
4. On emptying the vessels by pressure, they fill up from the fornix towards the limbus.	4. On emptying the vessels by pressure, they fill up from the limbus towards the fornix.
5. The vessels concerned for the congestion are the posterior and anterior conjunctival vessels.	5. The vessels are episcleral branches from the perforating branches of anterior ciliary arteries.

Staining of conjunctiva :—
Fluorescine 2% stains any raw area green, Rose Bengal 1% tains conjunctiva pinkish red.
Examination of plica semilunaris and caruncle for any follicle or tumour.
Examination of sclera for any change in colour, pigmetation, protrusion of uveal tissue or any congestion or nodule formation.
Examination of the Cornea-
In case of childern or in the presence of marked blepharospasm, an upper lid retractor like Desmarre's lid retractor may have to be used (see under instruments).
To note the following points –
(a) diameter—normally it is 12-13 mm,
less in microcornea
more in buphthalmos or megalo cornea.
(b) curvature— conical, globular or flat
(c) smoothness of surface—Can be easily detected by window reflex. For accurate examination keratometry and slit lamp study will be necessary.
(d) any opacity—The following aspects of the opacity are to be noted-
(i) density—i.e. nebula, macula or leucoma,
(ii) situation and extent in relation to the pupil,
(iii) any pigmentation of the opacity,
(iv) any iris adhesion.

(e) any pannus or vascularisation
    Fig. 1— A. Superficial vascularisation of cornea.

TABLE II
Difference between Superficial and Deep Vascularization of Cornea.

Superficial Vascularization	Deep Vascularization
i. Vessels are irregular & tortuous.	i. Vessels are regular in arrangement & straight
ii. Rich dendritic branching	ii. Brushform appearance
iii. Vessels are continuous with conjunctival vessels and lie underneath the corneal epithelium.	iii. Vessels are not continuous with the conjunctival vessels and lie deep to Bowman's membrane.

(f) any ulceration or abrasion—
    It is detected as a raw area by absence of distortion of window reflex and by staining with 2% fluorescein solution.

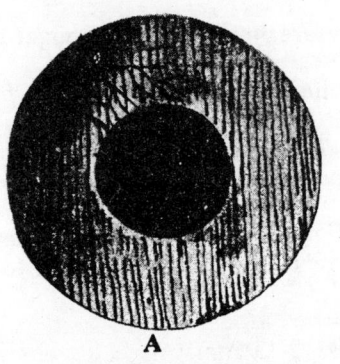
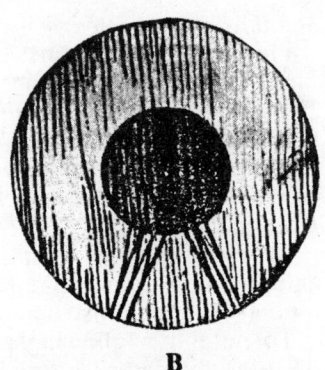

A   B

Fig. 1. A. Superficial Vascularisation of cornea. B. Deep Vascularization of. cornea.

(g) any oedema, vesicles or bullae in the epithelium.
(h) any keratic precipitates—fine, mutton – fat, pigmented, new or old. These are deposits of inflammatory cells on the corneal endothelium.
(i) any change in corneal sensation—elicited by touching the cornea with a wisp of cotton wool.
    Most sensitive part is the central cornea 5 mm in diameter, vertical meridian is less sensitive than horizontal meridian.

PLATE II

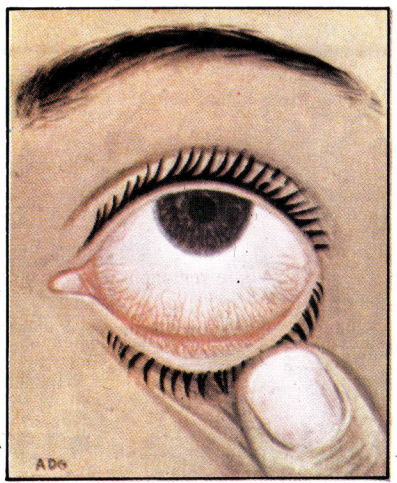

Fig. 1
Conjunctival type of congestion
(May and Worth)

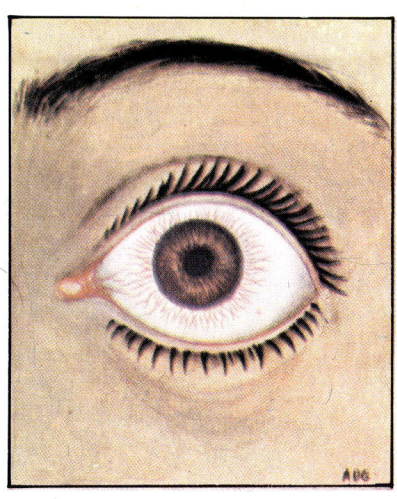

Fig. 2
Circumcorneal or ciliary congestion
(May and Worth)

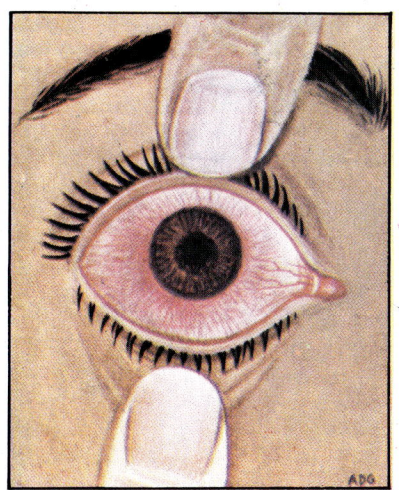

Fig. 3
Ciliary and episcleral Injection
(May and Worth)

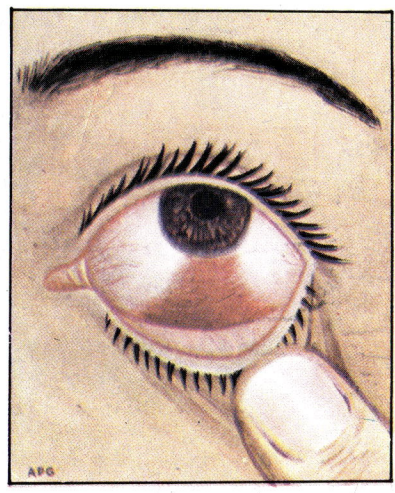

Fig. 4
Subconjunctival Haemorrhage
(May and Worth)

(To face page 6)

Conrea is responsive to pain, temperature & touch, but not to kinaesthetic sensation. That is why a person cannot localise a foreign body in the cornea.

Causes of loss or diminished corneal sensation—
(a) Herpes simplex virus infection i.e., dendritic ulcer
(b) Herpes zoster virus infection
(c) Acute congestive glaucoma
(d) Absolute glaucoma
(e) Tumour pressing on the 5th nerve
(f) Following alcohol injection in the Gasserian ganglion
(g) Leucoma
(h) Leprosy

Staining of the cornea with 2% fluorescein—
(a) Superficial staining—
To detect an abrasion of cornea or an ulcer of cornea a drop of fluorescein is instilled into the conjunctival sac and any excess of the dye is washed off with lotio normal saline. The lesion is stained bright green. The dye does not stain the descemet's membrane and so in case of a deep ulcer only the side of the ulcer is stained.
(b) Deep staining—
If after instilling the dye the lids are kept closed for few minutes then the dye penetrates through the intact epithelium and any infiltrated area in the stroma takes up a grass green colour while defects in the endothelium or K. P. appear as green dots.

Examination of the anterior chamber
Following points are to be noted—
(a) the depth—normal, shallow or deep.
(b) any extraneous matter like pus, blood lens matter etc.

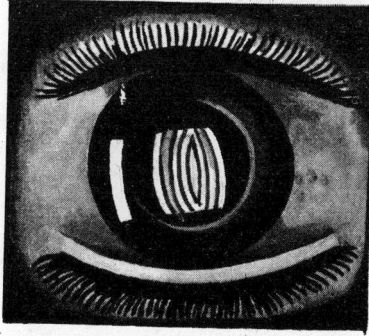

Fig 2. Optical section of the eye with obique slit illumination. Optical sections of cornea and lens are clearly seen. The dark space in between is the anterior chamber.

Examination of the angle of anterior chamber—It is only possible with a gonioscope (see under glaucoma)
Examination of the pupil
Following points are to be noted—
  (a) Size—normally 3—4 mm
  (b) Shape—normally circular. Any irregularity is better noted if the pupil is dilated.
  (c) Position— whether central or eccentric and drawn to one side. Normal position is more or less central.
  (d) Pupillary margin—any adhesion with the lens capsule known as posterior synechia, best elicited after dilatation of the pupil.
  (e) pupillary aperture—clear or occluded.
  (f) pupil reaction—
     i) reaction to light—direct and consensual; direct reaction—when the ipsilateral pupil contracts as soon as light enter the eye; consensual reaction—pupil of the contralateral eye contracts when the light enters in the ipsilateral eye.
     ii) reaction to accommodation and convergence—pupil constricts on looking at a near object.

Examination of the iris.
Following points are to be noted—
  (a) iris pattern—normal or altered,
  (b) colour—normal or any heterochromia,
  (c) new vessels on the iris—normally iris vessels are not visible.
  (d) atrophic patch—usually this area looks worn out and depigmented.
  (e) any gap or hole in the iris—either due to iridectomy usually situated in the upper part or as a congential anomaly known as coloboma usually situated in the lower part. Small holes may be caused by penetrating injuries from sharp objects or intraocular foreign bodies.
  (f) any tremulousness of the iris known as iridodonesis— best elicited by movement of the eyeball particularly in an aphakic eye.
  (g) any iridodialysis i.e. tearing of the iris from its attachment to the ciliary body giving the pupil D shape.
  (h) any adhesion of the iris to the posterior surface of the cornea—known as anterior synechia.

Examination of lens

Thorough examination needs a fully dilated pupil. Following points are to be noted.

(a) Colour ·of lens—grey, brown, white or transparent,

(b) Any opacity—central, peripheral or total,

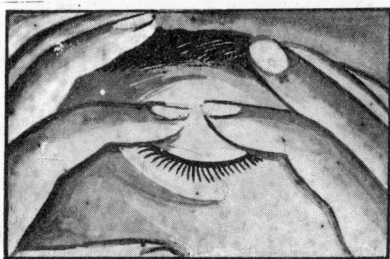

Fig. 3. Digital tonometry.

(c) Any displacement—If partial it is called subluxation. Here some fibres of the suspensory ligament are weak or torn and the lens moves with the movement of the eyeball. If complete it is-called luxation and the lens would be either in the anterior chamber or mostly in the lower part of the vitreous cavity.

(d) presence or absence of the 3rd and 4th Purkinje—Sanson images.

Purkinje Sanson images are elicited as follows :—

When light from strongly illuminated source falls obliquely on the eye, four images are formed by the four reflecting surfaces which are—the anterior surface of cornea, the posterior surface of cornea, the anterior surface of lens and the posterior surface of the lens. The first three surfaces are convex so if the light moves the respective image also moves in the same direction. The images are erect. But as the 4th surface is concave, the image moves in the opposite direction with the movement of .light; moreover the image is inverted. Of these four Purkinje—Sanson images under ordinary circumstances, the first and the fourth images are clearly visible if the pupil is dilated. To see the second and third images, a very strong light and an absolutely dark room are necessary. Presence of the fourth image means that the lens is clear. In an opaque lens the fourth image is absent but the third is present. Similary if the lens is absent as in aphakia, both the third and fourth images are absent.

Examination of intra ocular tension

Two methods are commonly followed—

(a) Digital tonometry, i.e. by palpation of the eyes with fingers. The patient must look down so that the sclera is palpated through the upper lid beyond the tarsal plate. The tension is judged by the amount of fluctuation obtained (Fig-3)

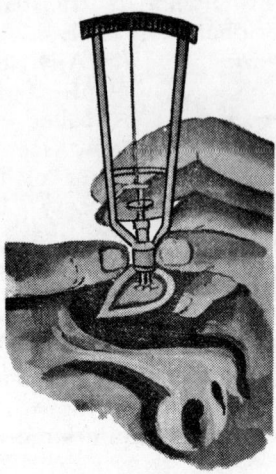

Fig. 4. Schiotz tonometry.

(b) By Schiotz tonometer (Fig-4)

By this instrument, the resistance offered to the different weights used to indent the surface of the cornea is recorded by the movement of the pointer on a scale. After a local anaesthesia the lids are separated with the fingers and the foot plate of the tonometer carrying a weight 5.5 gm is gently placed on the cornea. The deflection can be interpreted in terms of intraocular tension from the chart accompanying the tono-meter. Normal intraocular tension varies from 18—25 mm of mercury.

Examination by palpation
The areas to be palpated are—
1. Orbit—any irregularity of the orbital margin, any mass in the orbit or any tenderness.
2. Regional lymph glands—particularly the pre-auricular glands.
3. Eyeball—for any tenderness and for any pulsation.

Examination of the function of the eye
1. Subjective Examination
This includes
(a) Central or direct vision—(See under visual acuity)
(i) distance vision with Snellen's test types.
(ii) Near vision with Snellen's type, or printer's type of N. Series.
(b) Field of Vision
(i) Peripheral field by confrontation method or by a perimeter.

Confrontation method—Here the patient's field of vision is compared with that of the observer having a normal field of vision. This method is a rough and ready procedure. The surgeon stands facing the patient at a distance of one metre. The patient covers his left eye and fixes his vision on the surgeon's left eye. The surgeon closes his right eye, and moves his hand in from the periphery towards their common line of vision keeping the hand in the plane halfway between him and the patient When he sees it himself, the patient ought to say that he also sees it. The movements of the hand are repeated in various parts of the field—above, below, to the right, to the left and so on.

Perimetry—A perimeter is a metallic semicircle whose radius is $^1/_3$rd of a metre which can be rotated in all meridians. The patient's chin lies on a chinrest placed at the centre of the semicircle, the eye not to be examined is closed by a pad and the eye for examination fixes an object placed at the centre of the metallic arc. A white test object is then moved along the inner surface of the arc from the extreme periphery towards the centre, and the point where the object is first seen is recorded automatically on a chart in degrees. This recording is done in all meridians.

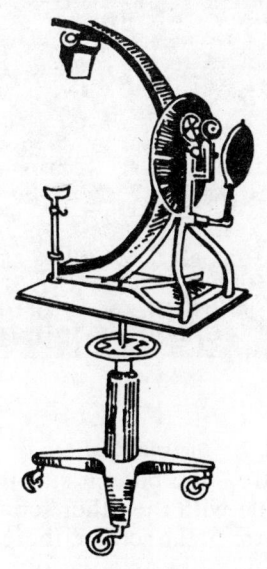

A coloured object may also be used instead of a white object if field of vision for colour is required. The usual size of the white test object is 3mm.

Extent of normal field of vision—(Fig. 6).

On the nasal side—60°.

Above—55° to 60°.

Below—75°

On the temporal side—100°.

A defect in the visual field is called a scotoma. Normal, physiological scotoma is the blind spot corresponding to the optic nerve-head where there is no retina. Scotoma may be positive or negative. When the patient appreciates a dark area in his field of vision, it is a positive scotoma. Negative scotoma is a scotoma which is not perceived by the patient but is only detected when visual field is recorded. The blind spot is a negative scotoma.

Fig-5 Perimeter (Lister)

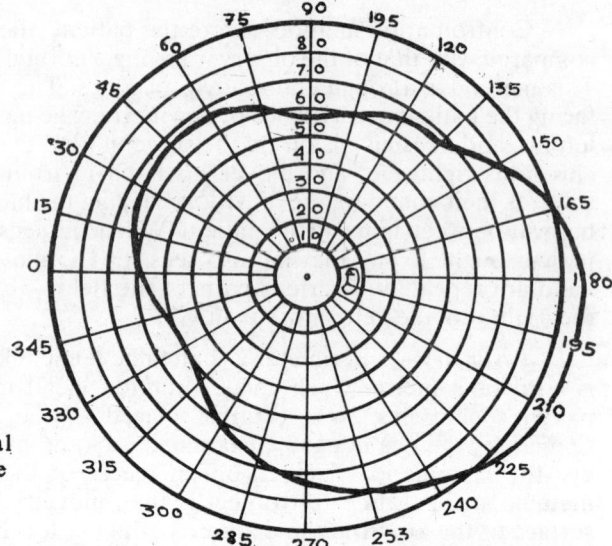

Fig. 6.
Extent of normal
visual field of the
right eye.

(ii) Examination of the central field by scotometry

By this method a minute study of the central field limited to a region within 30° from the fixation point can. be done.

The appliance used is called a Bjerrum's screen (Fig. 7). A Bjerrum's screen consists of a black curtain either 2 meters square

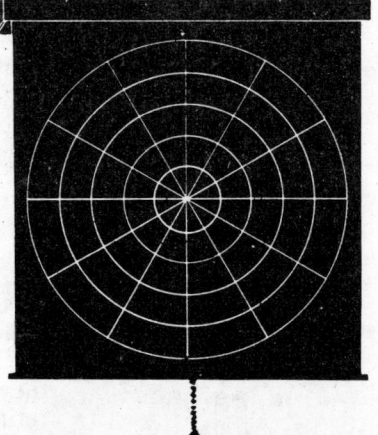

Fig. 7.   Bjerrum's Screen

or 1 metre square. If the screen is 2 metre the patient sits at a distance of 2 metres from the screen, while with the other screen he sits at a distance of 1 metre. On the centre of the screen, there is a white small object for fixation and around the fixation object there are concentric circles of black thread in various degrees—the smallest circle being 5° and the outermost one being of 30°

There are also radial lines radiating from the central object for fixation showing different meridians in degrees. A white disc 1 to 2 mm in diameter mounted on a black rod (Fig 9) is used as a test object. (Fig. 7 Bjerrum's Screen) With one eye covered, the patient sitting in front of the screen at required distance, fixes the test object with the eye for exmination. At first the blind spot is mapped out with a big white object of 10 mm diameter. Then any defect of the central field is found out by moving the small (1 to 2 mm) test object in different meridians.

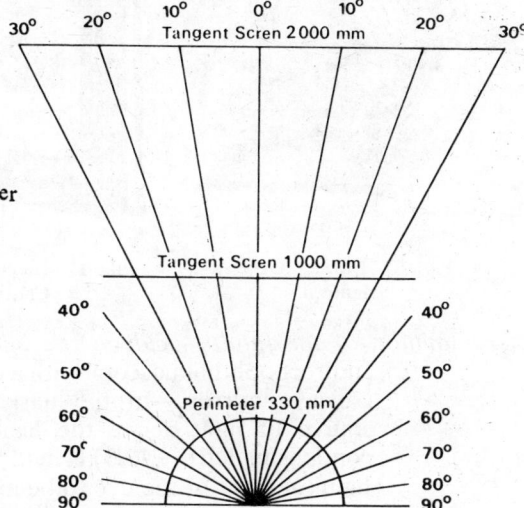

Fig. 8.
Projection on the Perimeter and on Bjerrum's screen at 330, 1000, 2000 mm.

(c) Examination of colour vision—
    (i) By lantern test—
        The usual appliance used is the Edridge—Green's Lantern

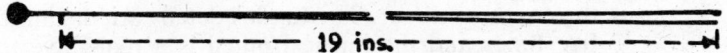

(Fig. 9.) by which various colours are shown to the patient, through a small aperture.
    (ii) By Holmgren's wools-of various colours. The examiner selects a particular colour and asks the patient to pick up the wool whose colour matches with the colour of the selected wool.
    (iii) By Psuedo-isochromatic charts (Fig. 11)
        The most used is the Ishihara's chart. This consists of coloured plates in which bold numbers are shown

in dots of various tints, set amid dots of the same
size but of different tints. A normal person can
easily read the numbers.

2. Objective examination—
Any error of refraction is found out by retinoscopy with a
plain mirror done in a dark room after dilating the pupil.

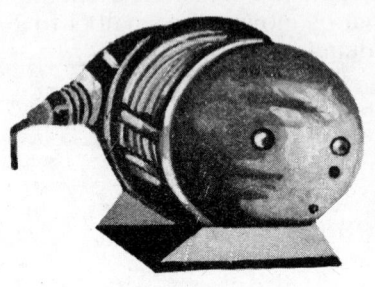

Fig. 10. Edridge-Green's   Fig. 11 Pseudo-isochromatic
         lantern   Charts of Ishihara

Examination of the fundus oculi
  (a) Indirect ophthalmoscopy with a condensing lens and a
      concave mirror.—In the dark room, there lies a
      source of light above the head of the paitent. A
      condensing lens (+13D) is held by the examiner's left
      hand in front of the eye to be examined. The patient
      looks at the opposite ear of the examiner, i.e., if the
      right eye is examined he looks towards the examiner's
      right ear. Then with the right hand the examiner
      throws light on the eye by a concave mirror. An
      image of the fundus is seen in between the lens and
      the concave mirror. The fundus details are magnified
      five times and the image fromed is a real, inverted
      image of the fundus. Binocular Fison type of
      ophthalmoscope is indispensible now a days for the
      retinal examination particularly the periphery.
  (b) By direct ophthalmoscopy with the help of an electric
      opthalmoscope—the fundus details are 10 times
      magnified and the image formed is a virtual, erect
      image of the fundus. During fundus examination the
      following points are to be noted.

1. **Optic disc**—It is a round or oval structure, pale pink in colour, situated at the posterior part of the fundus. It is also known as the optic nerve-head as the optic nerve starts from this point. There is an excavation at the central part known as the physiological cup, whose depth and extent varies in different subjects. The margins of the disc are normally sharp and distinct. So during examination of the fundus the colour, shape of the disc, its margins, the physiological cup, presence of any abnormal vessels or any other abnormality on the disc have to be noted.

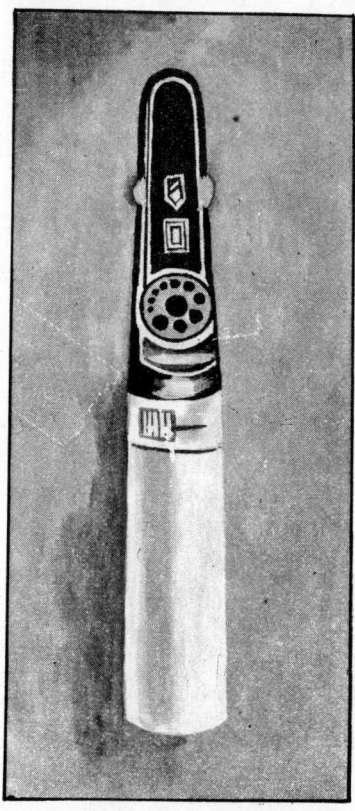

Fig. 12. Direct Ophthalmoscope.

2. **Macular area**—It is a small circular area with a red colour which is deeper than that of the surrounding fundus and it is situated at about 2 to $2^1/_2$ disc diameters on the temporal side of the optic disc, at a level slightly below the centre of the disc. The glistening central point of the macular area is known as the fovea centralis. It is slightly depressed and this depression is known as the foveal pit. During opththalmoscopic examination due to reflection of light, this pit appears as a bright reflex which is known as foveal reflex. Any abnormality in this macular area has to be noted.

3. **Retinal blood vessels**—These consist of arteries which are branches of the central artery of the retina and veins which are branches of the central vein of the retina. These vessels radiate from the optic disc and as they spread over the fundus they divide dichotomously into many branches. The arteries which are in fact arterioles at a short distance from the disc, are narrower than the veins, the ratio of the calibre of an artery to a vein being

2 : 3. The arteries which are endarteries are bright red in colour whereas the veins are purplish red. Normally the walls of the blood vessels are transparent ; so during ophthalmoscopic examination the light gets reflected from the blood column within the vessel. This reflection appears as a light streak on the wall of the vessels which is more marked in case of the arteries. During examination of the fundus, any narrowing, tortuosity or dilatation or sheathing of the vessel, any alteration in the light reflex from the vessel wall and any venous compression at the arterio venous crossings are to be noted. All the blood vessels should be traced up to the periphery.

4. **General appearance of the fundus**— Normally the fundus has a uniform red appearance. But the colour depends on the degree of pigment in the retinal pigment epithelium. Frequently shimmering reflexes are seen on the surface of the fundus during examination with an ophthalmoscope and these are most evident in hypermetropic eyes. The fundus should be examined all round for any abnormality.

5. **Choroidal vessels**— Normally many choroidal vessels are not visible. But if pigmentation of the retinal pigment epithelium is deficient, they are seen in the areas between the retinal vessels. They appear as pinkish flat ribbons which do not show any light reflex. They also anastomose freely. Sclerosed choroidal vessels are whitish in colour and narrow. If the pigment content of the choroid is more than that of the retinal pigment epithelium, deeply pigmented polygonal areas may be seen in between the choroidal vessels. This appearance is know as tessellated or tigroid fundus.

6. **Examination of the fundus with the red-free light**— The ordin– ary white light used for ophthalmiscopy can penetrate the layers of the retina i.e. the retina is transparent to white light. But a light with shorter wave length, like blue light, does not possess this penetrating power and so this type of red–free light gets reflected from the retinal surface. Due to this property of the red–free light minute pathological changes in the retinal nerve fibres or in the macular area are easily detected when red free light is used for ophthalmoscopy.

MEASUREMENT OF LESION IN THE FUNDUS

A lesion in the fundus e.g., a patch of choroiditis or a tumour, swelling of the disc or cupping of the disc or a retinal hole requires measurement as to its exact location, its extent, its depth or its

PLATE III

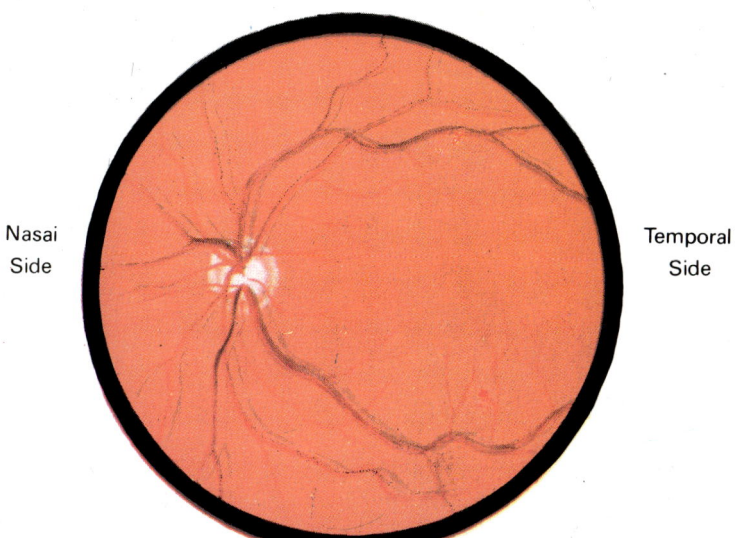

Nasai Side

Temporal Side

Fig. 1 Normal fundus of the left eye as seen by a direct ophthalmoscope. The oval area on the nasal side is the optic disc. The tiny circular area at about 2½ disc diameters on the temporal side of the disc is the fovea centralis. The wider and darker vessels are the retinal veins and the narrower ones are the retinal arteries (Magnification about 15 times)

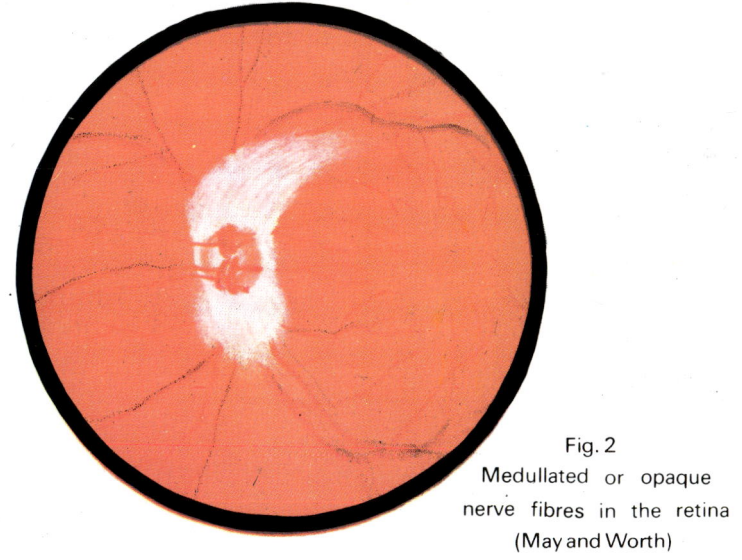

Fig. 2
Medullated or opaque nerve fibres in the retina
(May and Worth)

(To face page 16)

elevation, not only for accurate diagnosis but also for future reference to find out whether the lesion is stationary or progressive. The measurement is usually done in two ways—

1. Linear measurement—This can be done in two ways—

(a) The location and extent of the lesion can be expressed in terms of diameters of the optic disc, e.g., it is situated so many disc diameters on the temporal side from the margin of the disc and it is so many diameters of the optic disc in length and breadth.

(b) A more accurate measurement can be made by incorporating a special scale or graticule in the electric ophthalmoscope which is projected on the fundus during examination.

2. Measurement of depth—To determine at what level a lesion seen on the fundus is situated i.e., to find out whether there is any excavation or elevation the following methods may be employed—

(a) By observing the behaviour of the blood vessels—In a depressed area, as for example, in case of cupping of the optic disc, the blood vessels appear to dip down in the excavated area. In case of a raised area, the blood vessels appear to climb upwards over the area.

(b) With the help of a direct ophthalmoscope—With the help of the lenses incorporated in the ophthalmoscope the top of an elevated area or the floor of an excavated area is focused. During the examination, the ophthalmoscope used should be held at the anterior focal plane of the patient's eye i.e., at 15.7 mm in front of his cornea in the normal case but at 23.27 mm in front of the cornea if the eye is aphakic and the observer must keep his accommodation completely relaxed. In case of a depression concave lenses or minus lenses in the ophthalmoscope have to be used. The power of the plus or minus lens required to focus either the top surface or the floor of a lesion is noted. Then another convenient object in the fundus, as for example a blood vessel, is focused and the difference in the power of lenses required to focus an object in the fundus and the top or floor of the lesion is noted. A difference of focusing of three dioptres between two points on the fundus indicates a difference of level of approximately 1 mm. But in the aphakic, this difference in focusing of dioptres indicates a difference of level of approximately 2 mm. This is a very convenient method of determining the depth of a lesion.

(c) During ophthalmoscopy, if the observer's eye is moved, a point in the fundus at a more superficial level moves in the opposite direction whereas a point in a deeper level moves in the same direction as the observer's eye.

(d) With the help of a slit-lamp—When the sharp band of the light of a slit-lamp is projected on the fundus, its margins become distorted if it falls on a swelling or on a depressed area.

LOCALIZATION OF A LESION IN THE FUNDS

Conditions like a hole in the retina in a case of detachment of the retina or a tumour of the retina e.g., retinoblastoma or a foreign body on the retina, require accurate localization of the lesion in relation to the outer surface of the sclera, because the lesion for the purpose of treatment has to be approached from the scleral surface. The localization must be done in two aspects—(a) the meridian in which the lesion lies and (b) the distance of the lesion in that meridian either from the ora serrata or from the margin of the optic disc.

The meridian is determined by comparing the eye to a face of a clock and describing the situation of the lesion in 5 o'clock, 7 o'clock or at any other position. The distance of the lesion is calculated by the number of disc diameters which separate the lesion either from ora serrata or from the disc margin. The ora serrata, which is the extreme periphery of the retina is situated at a distance of 8 mm from the limbus in an emmetropic eye. But this distance is about 1 mm more in myopic eye as the size of the eyeball is bigger in this case. The diameter of the disc is about 1.5 mm. So from these measurements the lesion can be easily located on the outer surface of the sclera in the correct meridian.

Transillumination of the eyeball

It may be done in two ways—(a) Trans–pupillary transillumination–An intense beam of light is allowed to pass obliquely through dilated pupil in the darkroom. In a normal eye a red glow becomes visible on the scleral surface. But if there is a pigmented tumour in any meridian the glow becomes defective in that meridian.

(b) Trans–scleral transillumination

If a narrow source of light is applied to the sclera over the conjunctiva, the pupil becomes illuminated. This method is known as transillumination through sclera. With a dilated pupil when the source applied on all the meridians, the pupil is equally illuminated. But if there is a disorder anywhere inside the eye, there is defective transillumination in that area.

VISUAL ACUITY

Definition—It is the power of the eye by which objects are distinguished from the other. It is also a measure of the smallest retinal image which can be appreciated regarding its shape and size.

Applies to central vision only.

Standard of visual acuity

Two distinct points can be visible as separate, when the minimum angle subtended by them at the nodal point of the eye is 1 minute.

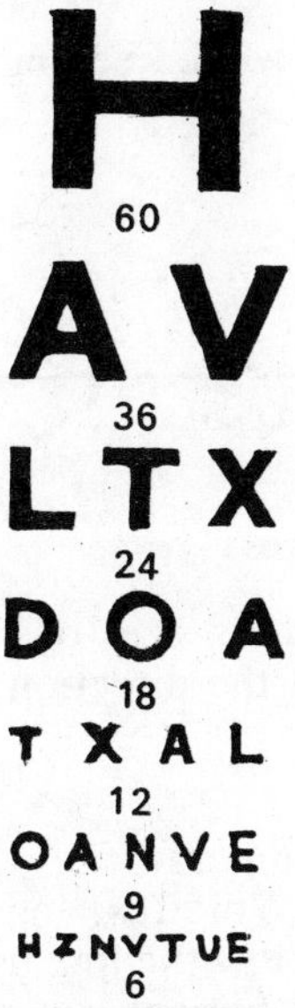

H

60

A V

36

L T X

24

D O A

18

T X A L

12

O A N V E

9

H Z N V T U E

6

Fig. 13. Snellen's test types for distant vision (Parsons).

This is the standard of normal visual acuity. It has to be understood also that although this standard of visual acuity is measured by the minimum angle subtended at the nodal point of the eye, perfect acuity of vision required three other basic factors i.e. the light sense, dissolving power of the eye to distinguish between details of an object and the power to integrate these details into the pattern of an object.

How to record visual acuity or central vision for distance :

1. A chart containing Snellen's test types is essential. These test types are square shaped letters in a Snellen's chart (Fig. 13). In the chart they are gradually diminished in size from above downwards, a numerical number written underneath each line of the test types. Principle of Snellen's test types—Each individual letter subtends an angle of 5 minutes (Fig—14) and each component part of the letter subtends an angle of 1 minute at the nodal point of the eye from the distance in metres shown by the numerical number written under each line of type.This principle is in conformity with the standard of normal visual acuity.

2. Distance at which the Snellen's test types have to be kept. It should be at a distance of 6 metres or 20 feet. The rays of light from that distance·are parallel for practical purposes. Half this

distance may also be utilized, but in that case the test types should be seen reflected through a plain mirror, kept at a distance of 3 metres or 10 feet from the patient.

3. Illumination of the Snellen's test types.—It should not be below 20 footcandles.

4. The test types should be more or less at the eye level of the patient. The test types should be clearly printed in black on white ground with uniform illumination. In Landolts' chart, the gap in the ring subtends an angle of 1 minute at the nodal point of the eye at the prescribed distance.

5. Individual eye must be examined separately while keeping the other eye closed.

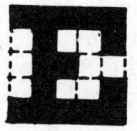 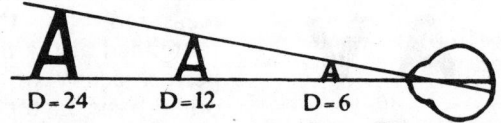

Fig. 14   Principle of Snellen's test types.

6. For illiterate patients a chart containing various sizes of or C can be used. The patient is required to find out the direction the hands of E or the gap of C.

7. Method of recording vision—
The visual acuity is expressed by a fraction, the numerator of which is the distance of the chart from the patient, i.e., 6 metres, and the denominator is the numerical number written below the line up to which the patient can read. For example if the patient can read upto the line under which is written 24, the vision is 6/24 which means that he reads the letters from a distance of 6 metres, which a normal person would have read from a distance of 24 metres.

If the patient fails to read even the biggest letter from a distance of 6 metres, he is brought towards the chart at a distances of 5 metres, 4 metres, 3 metres, and so on until he can decipher the biggest top letter and the vision is recorded as 5/60, 4/60, or 3/60.

How to record near vision

The patient sits with his back towards the light. If he requires glasses for the distance, he must have the same correction when near vision is tested. Snellen's test types for reading or printer's types of the N series is held by the right hand at a distance of 25 to 30 cm. A person with a normal accommodation must read the smallest types, i.e., Sn.5 in Snellen's types or N 6 in printer's types. If he cannot read the smallest types, the types which he can read should be noted by noting the number against the types. Individual eye should be tested separately.

CHAPTER II

GEOMETRICAL OPTICS AND OPTICAL CONSTANTS OF THE EYE

Prism

Definition—A prims is a medium, bounded by two plain refracting surfaces at an angle to each other.
This angle is called the angle of the prism and opposite the angle is the base of the prism.
Refraction through a prism (Fig. 15)—

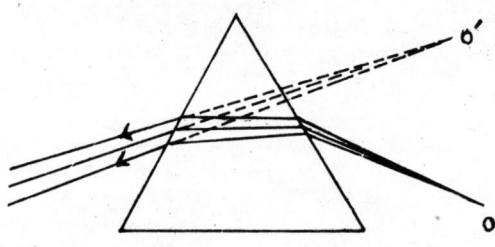

Fig 15. Refraction through a prism

Rays of light from the object O, after refraction through the prism, are deviated towards the base of the prism. These rays of light, when produced backwards, meet at O′ to form a virtual image of O. Thus an observer sees the object shifted towards the apex of the prism.

Use of a prism—For treatment of heterophoria and for convergence insuffieciency and in various instruments.

Spherical lens

Definition of a spherical lens—A spherical lens is a transparent medium bounded by spherical surfaces.

Usually thin lenses are used in ophthalmology.

There are mainly two types of spherical lenses—

1. Convex, converging or plus lens. It may be of three types (Fig. 16)—
   (a) Double convex or biconvex.

(b) Plano-convex.

(c) Concavo-convex or convex meniscus.

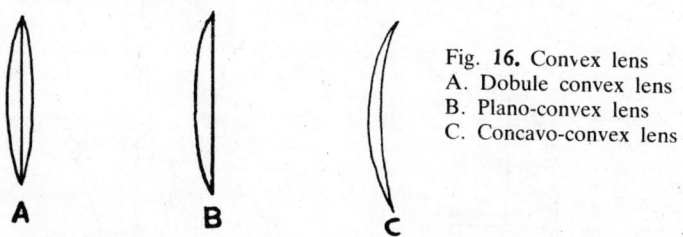

Fig. 16. Convex lens
A. Dobule convex lens
B. Plano-convex lens
C. Concavo-convex lens

2. Concave, diverging or minus lens—(Fig. 17). It may be also of three types—

(a) Double concave or biconcave.

(b) Plano-concave.

(c) Convexo-concave or concave meniscus.

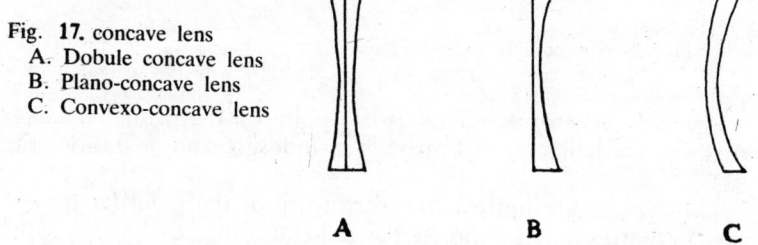

Fig. 17. concave lens
A. Dobule concave lens
B. Plano-concave lens
C. Convexo-concave lens

Structure of convex and concave lenses

(a) A biconvex lens may be considered as a collection of prisms, having their bases towards the principal axis of the lens (Fig. 18).

(b) A biconcave lens may be considered as a collection of prisms having their bases directed away from the principal axis of the lens. (Fig. 19).

Cardinal points of a thin spherical lens

(a) Two principal foci.

(b) An optical centre of the lens corresponding to the nodal point of a thick lens (Fig. 20).

Optical axis of a lens—It is the line joining the centres of curvature of its two surfaces.

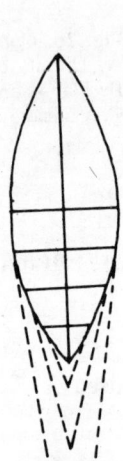

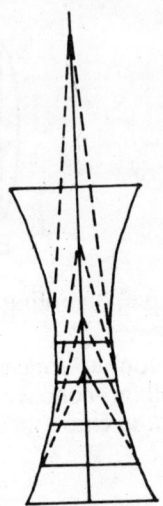

Fig. 18. Structure of
a biconvex lens

Fig. 19. Structure of
a biconcave lens

Optical centre of thin lens—It is a point on the principal axis so that any ray which passes through it undergoes no deviation (Fig. 20).

Dioptre—The dioptre is the reciprocal of the focal length of a lens in metres and is expressed as D. Thus dioptre of a lens with a

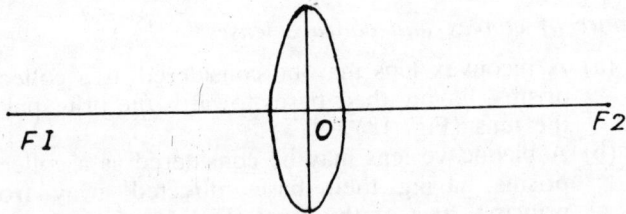

Fig. 20. Optical centre of a lens
F_1 & F_2=Principal foci
O=Optic centre

focal length of 25 cm, i.e., $^1/_4$th metre, is 4D. Numbering of lenses are done according to the dioptric value, i.e., ID, 2D etc.

Image formation by a biconvex spherical lens

(a) If the object is at infinity, the rays are parallel and after passing through the lens, these rays come to a focus on the second principal focus (Fig. 21.)

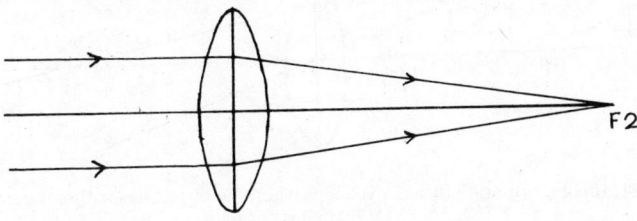

Fig. 21. Convergence of parallel rays by a biconvex lens

(b) If the object is at the first principal focus, the rays, after refraction through the lens, emerge as parallel rays (Fig. 22).

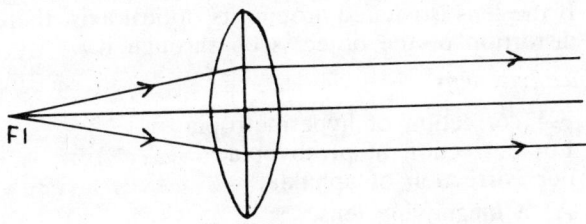

Fig 22. The emergent rays are parallel if the object is placed at the first principal focus of a biconvex lens

(c) If the object is beyond the principal focus, but at a distance less than infinity, a real inverted image is formed (Fig. 23).

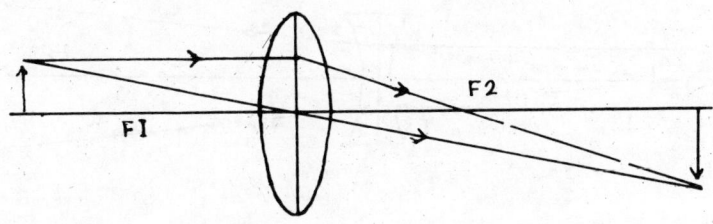

Fig. 23. A real inverted image formation by a biconvex lens

(d) If the object is placed within the principal focus, a virtual, erect and magnified image is formed (Fig. 24).

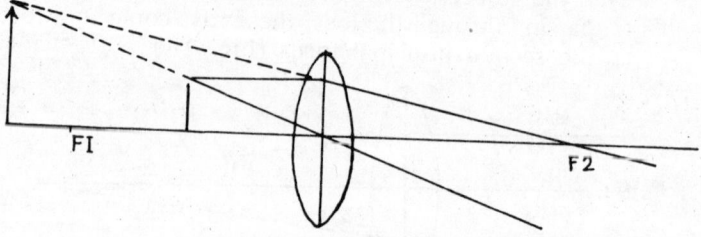

Fig. 24. Image formation by a convex lens when the object lies within the principal focus

Identification of a biconvex or plus lens

(a) If the lens is moved, an object seen through it, moves in the opposite direction as the lens.

(b) An object, if held closed to the lens, appears magnified.

(c) If the lens is rotated around its optical axis, there is no distortion of the object seen through it.

Use of biconvex lens

(a) For correction of hypermetropia.

(b) For correction of presbyopia.

(c) For correction of aphakia.

(d) As a magnifying lens.

Image fromation by a biconcave spherical lens

(a) If the object is at infinity, the parallel rays from the object after refraction diverge, and appear to emanate from the first principal focus (Fig. 25).

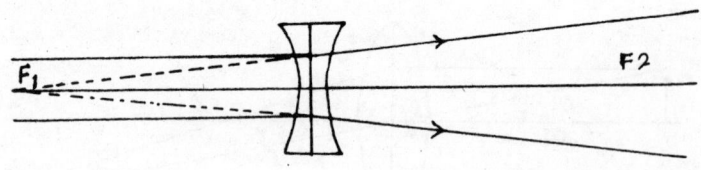

Fig. 25. Divergence of parallel rays after refraction through a biconcave lens

(b) If the object is at a distance less than infinity, a virtual, erect image, and diminished in size is formed (Fig. 26).

Identification of a biconcave spherical lens or minus lens

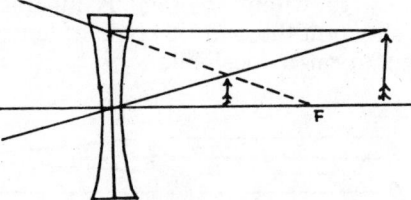

(a) If the lens is moved, an object seen through it, moves in the same direction as the lens.
(b) An object seen through the lens appear diminished in size.

Fig. 26. Virtual erect image by a biconcave lens.

(c) If the lens is rotated around its optical axis, there is no distortion of the object seen through it.

Use of a biconcave lens—For correction of myopia and Hruby lens fundus examination.

Cylindrical lens

Cylindrical lenses are segments of a cylinder of glass cut parallel to its axis. Such a segment forms a convex cylindrical lens, whereas a similar segment forms a mould in which the cylinder was cast, forms a concave cylindrical lens (Goulden) (Fig. 27).

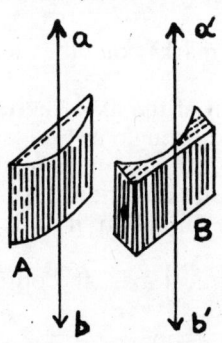

Fig. 27.
A=Convex cylinder,
ab=axis of the cylinder,
B=Concave cylinder,
ab=axis of the cylinder

The axis of a cylindrical lens is parallel to that of the cylinder of which it is a segment, as shown in the illustration (Fig. 27). In the direction of its axis, the cylindrical lens acts as a plain lamina with parallel sides, so that rays of light travelling along the axis pass undeviated. In other words, a cylindrical lens has no power in the direction of its axis. But in the direction, at right angles to the axis, the rays of light meet either a convex surface in case of a convex cylinder or a concave surface in case of a concave cylinder, as shown in the illustration (Fig. 28). Thus the light rays passing through a cylindrical lens, in a direction at right angles to its axis, either converge or diverge, depending on the type of the lens. So it is obvious that a cylindrical lens has power only in a direction at right angles to its axis.

Refraction through a cylindrical lens

As shown in the previous illustration, parallel rays of light after refraction through this type of lens, do not come to a point focus but form a focal line.

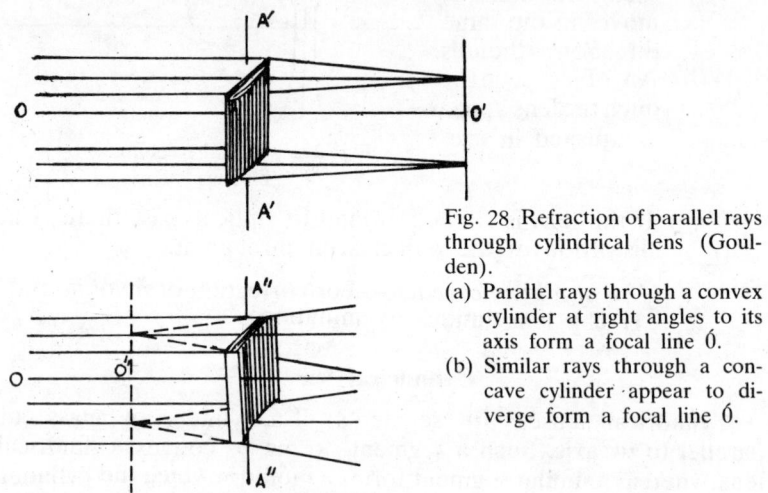

Fig. 28. Refraction of parallel rays through cylindrical lens (Goulden).
(a) Parallel rays through a convex cylinder at right angles to its axis form a focal line Ó.
(b) Similar rays through a concave cylinder appear to diverge form a focal line Ó.

Identification of a cylindrical lens

(a) There are always two scratch marks on the lens indicating the axis.
(b) If the lens is moved in the direction of the axis, there is no movement of the object seen through it.
(c) If the lens is moved in a direction at right angles to the axis, the object moves in the opposite direction if it is a convex cylinder and in the same direction if it is a concave cylinder.
(d) If the lens is rotated around its optical axis, the object seen through it becomes distorted.

Use of a cylindrical lens—For correction of regular astigmatism.

Optical constants of the eye (Gullstrand)

1. Position of the anterior surface of the cornea—0.00 mm.
2. Position of the posterior surface of the cornea—0.5 mm.

3. Position of the anterior surface of the lens—3.6 mm.
4. Position of the posterior surface of the lens—7.2 mm.
5. Radius of curvature of the anterior surface of cornea—7.7 mm.
6. Radius of curvature of the posterior surface of cornea—6.8 mm.
7. Radius of curvature of the anterior surface of lens—10.0 mm.
8. Radius of curvature of the posterior surface of the lens—6.0 mm.

Various refractive indices of the media

Index of refraction of air—1.

1. Index of refraction of cornea—1.37
2. Index of refraction of aqueous humour—1.33.
3. Index of refraction of the cortex of the lens—1.38.
4. Index of refraction of the nucleus of the lens—1.40.
5. Index of refraction of vitreous—1.33.

Schematic eye

The data, regarding the optical constants of the eye, show that refractive indices of the aqueous and vitreous are the same, i.e., 1.33.Cornea has a slightly higher refractive index, but for practical purposes, it can be considered as identical with the refractive index of aqueous and vitreous. Thus the optical system of the eye reduces itself into two elements only (Duke-Elder)—

1. The corneal surface separating air from the common medium, i.e., cornea, aqueous and vitreous.
2. The lens with a higher refractive index immersed in the common medium.

This simplified optical system in the eye was named a schematic eye by Listing.

Cardinal points of the schematic eye

According to Listing and Gauss, for every dioptric system, formed of any number of media, bounded by centred spherical surfaces, there exist three pairs of cardinal points, which are, two principal foci, two principal points and two nodal points, all situated on the principal axis of the system (Goulden).

The first principal focus is the point on the principal axis at which parallel rays emerging from the system intersect. The second principal focus is the point on the principal axis, at which parallel rays entering the system intersect.

The principal points are such, that, an incident ray passing through the first principal point, passes after refraction through the second principal point, but the incident and emergent rays are not necessarily parallel. The two principal points correspond to the conjugate foci of a simple lens.

The nodal points are such, that every ray which before refraction is directed towards the first nodal point, after refraction appears to come from the second nodal point in a direction parallel to the incident ray (Goulden) (Fig. 29).

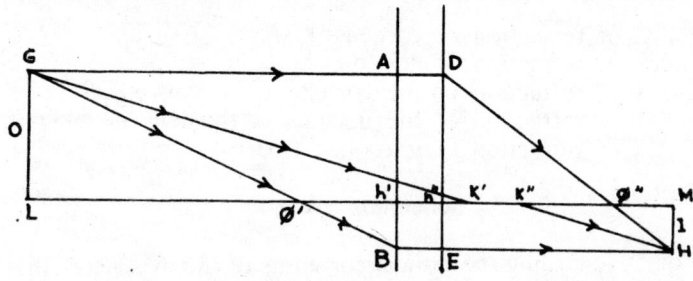

Fig. 29. Listing's cardinal points of a dioptric system (Goulden)
ϕ' and $\phi''=2$ principal foci
h' and h''=2 principal points
K' and k''=2 nodal points
O=object
I=image

Data for cardinal points of the schematic eye (Gullstrand)

Cardinal points.		Distance of the cardinal point from anterior surface of the cornea.
1. First principal point	.	1.35 mm.
2. Second principal point	. .	1.60 mm.
3. First nodal point	. .	7.08 mm.
4. Second nodal point	. .	7.33 mm.
5. First focal point	. .	—15.7 mm.
6. Second focal point	. .	24.4 mm. (Fig. 30)

N.B.—The minus sign is used when the distance is measured in a direction against the direction of incident rays. The second principal focus, 24.4 mm. behind the cornea, coincides with the retina of the normal eye.

From these data the refractive power of the eye has been calculated to be + 58 dioptres, of which cornea contributes + 43 dioptres and the lens + 15 dioptres.

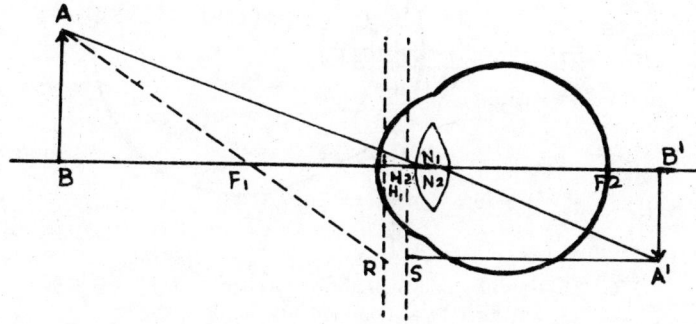

FIG. 30. The cardinal points of the Schematic eye (Davson)
F_1 and F_2=First and Second focal points
H_1 and H_2=First and Second principal points
N_1 and N_2=First and Second nodal points
AB   =Object
A'B'   =Image

Reduced eye

The two principal points and the two nodal points of the schematic eye being so close together, Listing has simplified the data by choosing a single principal point lying midway between the two actual points and a single nodal point, similarly lying between the two real nodal points.

So the simplified data for cardinal points have become as follows (Fig. 31)—

1. Principal point—1.5 mm behind the anterior surface of cornea.
2. Nodal point—7.2 mm behind the anterior surface of cornea.
3. First focal point—17.2 mm from the principal plane, i.e., a vertical plane passing through the principal point.
4. Second focal point—22.9 mm from the principal plane.

According to this simplification of the schematic eye, the eye is considered to have a single refracting surface, which is imaginary and is situated 1.5 mm behind the anterior surface of cornea, with a radius of curvature 7.2−1.5=5.7 mm. Thus the eye has been diminished in size and is now known as reduced eye.

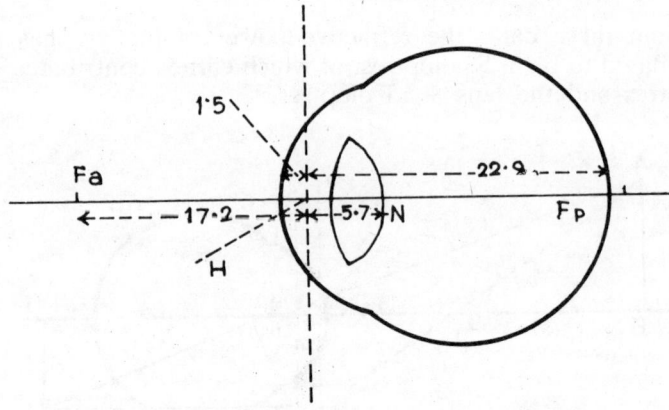

FIG. 31, Cardinal points of the reduced eye (Davson)
Fa=First focal point or anterior focal point
Fp=Second focal point or posterior focal point
H=Principal point
N=Nodal point

Donders' reduced eye

Donders has further simplified the data and has treated the eye
as a single curved surface 2 mm behind the cornea, with a radius of
curvature of 5 mm and anterior and posterior focal lengths of 15
and 20 mm respectively, measured from the imaginary refracting
surface 2 mm behind the cornea. The nodal point in this reduced
eye is 5 mm behind this refracting surface coinciding with the
centre of curvature of the surface. The advantage of this data is
that they are in round figures and so they are easy to remember.
Cardinal points of an aphakic eye (Gullstrand)
   After extraction of the lens, when the eye becomes aphakic,
there is only corneal system for refraction of rays. The cardinal
points of such an eye are as follows—

Cardinal points.	Distance of the cardinal point from anterior surface of the cornea.
1. First principal point	0.04 mm
2. Second principal point	0.05 mm.
3. First nodal point	7.75 mm.
4. Second nodal point	7.75 mm.
5. First focal point	—23.27 mm.
6. Second focal point	30.98 mm.

Refractive power about + 43 D.

CHAPTER III

ERRORS OF REFRACTION, PRESBYOPIA AND ANISOMETROPIA

Errors of refraction

Emmetropia—It is the normal condition when parallel rays of light from infinity come to a focus on the retina (fovea), when accommodation is at rest. Thus in emmetropia, there is no error of refraction.

Ametropia—It is a condition in which due to some refractive error, the parallel rays of light from infinity do not come to a focus on the retina (fovea), when accommodation is at rest.

There are three types of errors of refraction—
1. Myopia or short-sightedness.
2. Hypermetropia or long-sightedness.
3. Astigmatism.

Myopia

Difinition—It is an error of refraction in which the parallel rays of light from infinity come to a focus in front of the retina, when accommodation is at rest (Fig. 32).

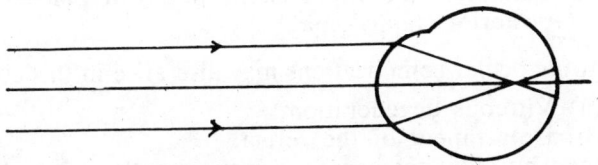

Fig. 32. Myopia.

Depending on the underlying mechanism there are three types of myopia——
- (a) *Axial myopia*—When the antero-posterior length of the eyeball is more than normal.
- (b) *Curvature myopia*—When the curvature of the cornea or the lens is more than normal.
- (c) *Index myopia*—When the refractive index of different media, particularly of the lens is more than normal. The best* and commonest example is lental sclerosis.

Clinical types of myopia
 1. Congenital myopia.
 2. Simple or developmental myopia.
 3. Pathological, degenerative or progressive myopia.

   1. *Congenital myopia*—It is present at birth and may be unilateral or bilateral. Bilateral congenital myopia may be associated with convergent squint.

   2. *Simple or developmental myopia*—This type of myopia is not associated with any degenerative change in the eye. It is the commonest type of myopia. The power of glasses increases usually during the years of study in schools and colleges and then remains steady.

   3. *Pathological myopia*—In this condition the myopia rapidly progresses so that in early adult life there may be myopia of -20 D or more.

   This condition is diagnosed by the following ophthalmoscopic findings—
   (a) Myopic crescent either on the temporal side of the optic disc or surrounding the disc.
   (b) Chorio-retinal atrophy at the periphery.
   (c) Atrophic patches in the macula with sclerosis of choroidal vessels.
   (d) Ectasia of the sclera at the posterior pole—known as posterior staphyloma

   Following ocular complications may also arise in this condition—
   (a) Vitreous degeneration.
   (b) Detachment of the retina.
   (c) Choroidal haemorrhage in the macular region known as Forster—Fuch's spot.
   (d) Nuclear type of cataract.

   Effect of accommodation in myopia—If accommodation is exerted, myopia becomes increased.
   Symptoms of myopia—There is reduced visual acuity for the distance, but near objects are seen clearly. Usually there is no headache. In pathological myopia. the patient may complain of seeing black spots floating in front of the eye, due to vitreous opacities.

PLATE IV

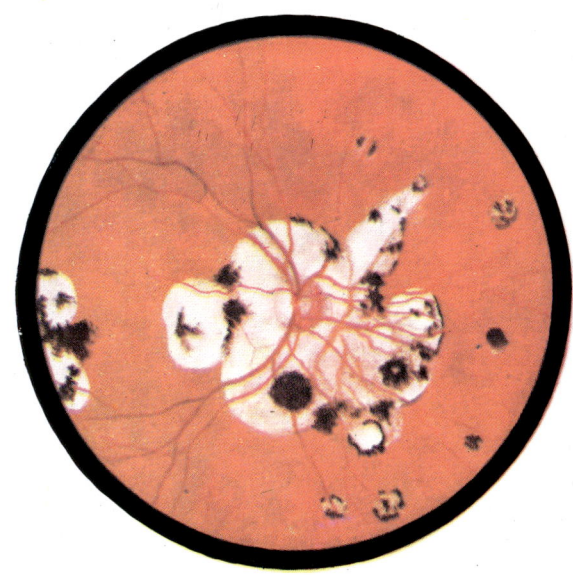

Fig. 1
Myopic degeneration
(Parsons)

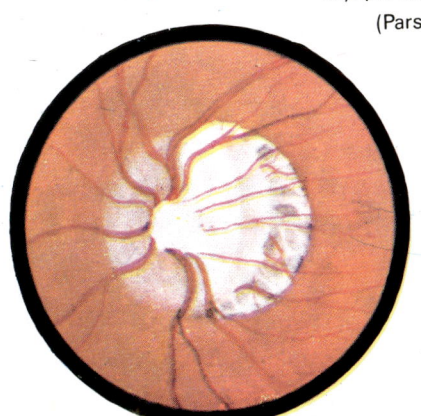

Fig. 2
Myopic retraction
and crescent
(Parsons)

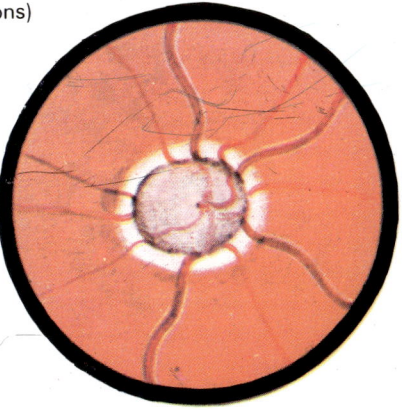

Fig. 3
Glaucomatous cupping
of the optic disc
((Parsons)

(To face page 34)

Diagnosis of myopia—By refraction, followig retinoscopy with the mirror under a mydriatic.

Treatment of myopia—Myopia is corrected by prescribing concave spherical glasses (Fig. 33). The exact power required is determined by retinoscopy. Contact lens is an ideal substitute in high myopia. There is practically no treatment for the pathological changes seen in progressive myopia. Surgery, like radial keratotomy is fast becoming popular.

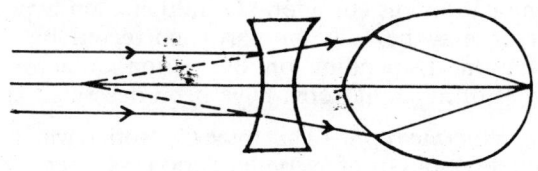

Fig. 33. Correction of myopia with concave spherical lens

Hypermetropia

Definition—It is an error of refraction in which parallel rays of light from infinity come to a focus behind the retina, when accommodation is at rest (Fig. 34).

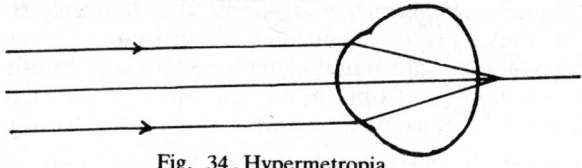

Fig. 34. Hypermetropia

Depending on the underlying mechanism, there are three types of hypermetropia—

    (a) *Axial type*—When the antero-posterior length of the eyeball is shorter than normal.

    (b) *Curvature type*—When the curvature of the cornea or the lens is flatter than normal.

    (c) *Index type*—When the refractive index of the media is less than normal.

Clinical types of hypermetropia

1. *Congenital hypermetropia*—This is rare. It is usually associated with other congenital anomalies of the eyeball, like microphthalmos.

2. *Simple or developmental hypermetropia*—It is the commonest type . A newborn baby is hypermetropic. With growth the eyeball grows in size and the hypermetropia is gradually diminished. But if the growth of the eyeball is retarded, the hypermetropia persists.

3. *Acquired hypermetropia*—This is found in the aphakic condition commonly following extraction of the lens. This hypermetropia is usually high.

Effect of accommodation on hypermetropia

Accommodation has considerable influence on hypermetropia, as this error may be fully or partly corrected by exertion of accommodation. Depending on the action of accommodation, several types of hypermetropia have been described as follows—

1. *Total hypermetropia*—The hypermetropia which is elicited after complete paralysis of accommodation, as after application of atropine.

2. *Latent hypermetropia*—It is the amount of hypermetropia which is corrected normally by the normal tone of the ciliary muscle. It is more in young children than in elderly persons, as the tone of the ciliary muscle is much more in the young than in the adults.

3. *Manifest hypermetropia*—It is the hypermetropia which remains uncorrected in normal circumstances, that is when accommodation is not being actively exerted, or in other words it is the total hypermetropia minus the latent hypermetropia. This manifest hypermetropia is again made of two components—

    (a) Facultative hypermetropia—It is that part of hypermetropia which can be corrected by an effort of accommodation.

    (b) Absolute hypermetropia—It is that part of hypermetropia which cannot be overcome by active exertion of accommodation.

Symptoms of simple hypermetropia—There is not much complaint regarding distant vision, as it can be corrected by exerting accommodation. But there is difficulty in doing close work and the letters become blurred after some time during reading. This effect is due to fatigue of accommodation. Headache is an usual symptom due to constant strain on accommodation.

Diagnosis of hypermetropia—By refraction, following retinoscopy with a plane mirror under the influence of a mydriatic.

Treatment—Treatment of hypermetropia is by prescription of correct convex spherical lens determined by retinoscopy (Fig. 35)

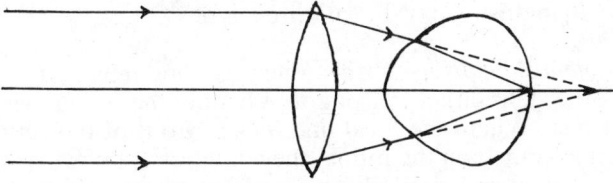

Fig. 35. Crrection of hypermetropia with convex spherical lens

Astigmatism

Definition—It is an error of refraction in which the parallel rays of light from infinity· cannot converge to a point focus due to unequal refraction in different meridians of the optical system of the eye, but form focal lines.

Causes of astigmatism

(a) Unequal curvature of the cornea or lens in different meridians, so that the refracting surfaces are not spherical.

(b) Decentring of the lens due to slight shifting in position or tilting of the lens as occurs in subluxation.

Refraction of parallel rays of light through an astigmatic surface—(Fig. 36)⋆.

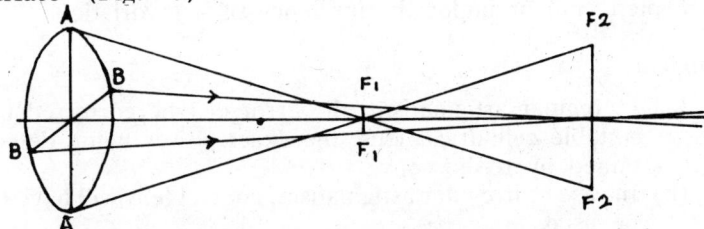

Fig. 36. Refraction through an astigmatic surface—Sturm's Conoid

AA represents one curvature and BB the other. $F_1 F_1$ and $F_2 F_2$ are the two focal lines which are formed instead of two focal points. This configuration of rays is known as Sturm's Conoid.

Types of astigmatism

(a) *Regular astigmatism*—When the refractive power changes uniformly from one meridian to the other.

(b) *Irregular astigmatism*—When the refractive power changes irregularly in different meridians as seen in corneal facets.

Depending on the position occupied by the two focal lines, regular astigmatism may be of three types—

1. *Simple astigmatism*—In this, one focal line falls on the retina and the other falls either in front of or behind the retina, when the eye is at rest. When one focal line falls in front of the retina the other being formed on the retina, the condition is known as simple myopic astigmatism, similarly in simple hypermetropic astigmatism one line is formed behind the retina and the other on the retina.

2. *Compound astigmatism*—In this, both the focal lines are formed either in front of the retina when it is called compound myopic astigmatism of behind the retina when it is called compound hypermetropic astigmatism.

3. *Mixed astigmatism*—In this, one of the focal lines is formed in front of the retina and the other behind that structure.

Symptoms of astigmatism

    (a) Diminished visual acuity.

    (b) Headache due to exertion of accommodation to rectify the defect particularly in hypermetropic astigmatism.

Diagnosis of astigmatism—By refraction, following retinoscopy with a plane mirror under the influence of a mydriatic.

Treatment

    (a) In regular astigmatism, the error can be corrected by suitable cylindrical lens, the exact power being determined by retinoscopy.

    (b) In case of irregular astigmatism, contact lens will have to be used.

Presbyopia

Definition—It is not an error of refraction, but an anomaly of accommodation due to age.

Mechanism—It is a condition, which usually becomes manifest at the age of 40 years, when the least distance of distinct vision recedes beyond 25 cm from the eye, due to loss of plasticity of the lens as a result of aging process. The neuromuscular mechanism of accommodation is not at fault. But on accommodation the lens fails to have the desired convexity.

Symptoms

(a) A person at the age of 40 years complains of blurring of vision while reading books. The vision improves if the book is held further away from the eye.

(b) Appearance of symptoms depends on occupation, i.e., those doing close work feel the symptoms earlier.

(c) Appearance of symptoms also depends on existing error of refraction. In hypermetropes onset of presbyopia is early. In myopes there may not be any presbyopia.

Treatment—Presbyopia is treated by prescribing convex spherical lens, which is added to the glasses, if any, for the distant vision in the following manner.

(a) At the age of 40 years—reading correction is +1D
(b) At the age of 45 years—reading correction is +1.5D
(c) At the age of 50 years—reading correction is +2D
(d) At the age of 55 years—reading correction is +2.5D.

Anisometropia

Definition—It is a condition in which the total refraction of the two eyes are unequal, the difference being more than one dioptre.

Types of anisometropia

(a) One eye emmetropic, the other having an error of refraction.
(b) Both eyes ametropic, but the error is of the same type.
(c) Both eyes ametropic, but the error in one eye is of different type from that in the other.

Causes of anisometropia—(a) Congenital, (b) Acquired—as after uniocular cataract extraction.

Vision in anisometropia

(a) Each 0.25D difference between the refraction of the two eyes causes 0.5% difference in the size of retinal images. So, greater the difference of refraction, greater is the size difference of retinal images. A difference of refraction of 4 dioptres between the eyes, which causes an image size

difference of about 7%, is the maximum limit tolerated.
Any bigger difference causes diplopia.

(b) If one eye is hypermetropic and the other eye myopic,
the vision may be alternating, i.e., the hypermetropic
eye is used for the distance and the myopic eye for the
near.

Diagnosis of anisometropia—By refraction following retinoscopy.

Treatment

(a) For less degrees of anisometropia, i.e., upto refractive
difference of 4 dioptres, proper spectacle lenses should
be prescribed.

(b) For higher degrees of anisometropia, contact lens has to
be used.

CHAPTER IV

ANATOMY AND DISEASES OF THE CONJUNCTIVA

Anatomy of the conjunctiva

Definition—The conjunctiva is a mucous membrane which covers the under surface of the lids and is reflected from the lids to cover the anterior part of the eyeball upto the margin of the cornea.

Different parts of the conjunctiva—

1. Palpebral conjunctiva—consisting of—
   (a) Marginal, (b) Tarsal and (c) Orbital part
Marginal conjunctiva extends from the inter-marginal zone of the lid margin to the subtarsal sulcus underneath the tarsus. The tarsal conjunctiva covers the tarsal plate. The orbital part covers the rest of the eyelid.
2. Conjunctiva of the fornix—
It is the fold of the conjunctiva formed by the reflection of the mucous membrane from the lid to the eyeball.
3. Bulbar conjunctiva—
It covers the anterior part of the eyeball upto the limbus.
4. Conjunctiva of the limbus—
It covers of the limbus around the cornea.
5. Plica semilunaris—
It is a crescentic fold of conjunctiva at the inner canthus, which is the rudiment of the nictitating membrane of lower vertebrates like frog.

Special features of different parts of the conjunctiva—

The marginal and tarsal conjunctiva are firmly fixed to the tarsal plate. The orbital conjunctiva and the conjunctiva of the fornices are loosely attached to the subjacent tissues, showing folds in the fornices and containing accessory lacrimal glands of Krause and Wolfring. The bulbar conjunctiva is also loosely attached to the sclera through episcleral tissue. The conjunctiva of the limbus is firmly fixed.

Histology of the conjunctiva—

Minute structure of the conjunctiva shows two layers—
1. An epithelial layer,

2. A substantia propria consisting of (a) adenoid layer and (b) fibrous layer.

Epithelial layer—
Nature of the epithelium varies in different parts of the conjunctiva as follows—

(a) Marginal conjunctiva—Stratified squamous epithelium with prickle cells.
(b) Tarsal conjunctiva—Two layers of cells—a superficial cylindrical and a deeper layer of flat cells.
    At places there is tendency to form three layers with the appearance of polygonal cells in the intermediate layer.
(c) Fornix and bulbar conjunctiva—Three layers of epithelium, i.e., superficial cylindrical, intermediate polygonal and deep flat cells.
(d) Limbus—Stratified squamous epithelium.
(e) Plica semilunaris—Stratified squamous epithelium.

Moreover the epithelium of the bulbar conjunctiva and that of the fornix and plica contain a large number of mucous secreting goblet cells.

2. Substantia propria—
It is the tissue underneath the epithelium.

Its superficial layer, known as the adenoid layer, consists of a fine network of fibrous tissue infiltrated with lymphocytes. This layer is absent at birth and only develops 2-3 months after birth and extends from the subtarsal sulcus to the limbus. The deeper layer of the substantia propria, known as fibrous layer, consists of collagenous and elastic fibres. It is absent over the tarsal plates and extends from the upper border of the tarsus to the limbus, containing blood vessels and nerves supplying the conjunctiva.

The substantia propria of plica has a similar structure but in addition there are fatty tissue and smooth muscle.

Blood supply of the conjunctiva—

The conjunctiva is supplied by two sets of arteries—

1. The posterior conjunctival arteries derived from the arterial arcades in the lids, formed by the palperbral branches of the nasal and lacrimal arteries of the lids.

2. The anterior conjunctival arteries derived from the anterior ciliary arteries.

The conjunctiva of the limbus is supplied by a pericorneal plexus formed by the branches of the anterior and posterior conjunctival vessels.

Venous drainage of the conjunctiva—

The veins accompany the arteries and drain into the palpebral and ophtHalmic veins.

Lymphatic drainage of the conjunctiva—

Lymphatic vessels in conjunctiva are abundant. Those from the palpebral conjunctiva drain into the lymphatic channels of the skin of the lid, and those from other parts of the conjunctiva pass towards the outer and inner canthus, ultimately joining with lymphatics of skin.

Nerve supply of the conjunctiva—

There are two different sets of nerves—
1. Sensory nerves—
   (a) Branches from the ciliary nerves supplying limbal area.
   (b) Branches from—
      (i) Infratrochlear branch of naso-ciliary nerve.
      (ii) Lacrimal nerve.
      (iii) Supratrochlear and supra-orbital branches of the frontal nerve.
      (iv) Infra-orbital branches of the maxillary nerve.
These nerves supply the entire conjunctiva excluding the limbus.
2. Sympathetic nerves—
These are derived from the sympathetic plexus travelling with the branches of the ophthalmic artery to the conjunctiva.
They supply the blood vessels.

Hyperaemia of the Conjunctiva

It means congestion of conjunctival vessels.

Causes

   (a) Reflexly due to a foreign body in the conjunctival sac.
   (b) Occupation in bad hygienic condition particularly in dusty and smoky atmosphere.
   (c) Error of refraction.
   (d) Reflex irritation from nose.
   (e) General condition like gout.

Symptoms

There is a sense of discomfort in the form of a foreign body sensation or a sensation of grittiness and feeling of irritation in the eyes.

Treatment

    (a) Removal of the cause.

    (b) Astringent drops like zinc sulphate half percent with acid boric one percent drop, three times a day.

Oedema of the conjunctiva (Chemosis)

It is a very common condition, the causes of which are given below. Due to firm attachment of the tarsal conjunctiva, oedema is never manifested markedly in that area. But as the bulbar conjunctiva and the conjunctiva of the fornices are loose, oedema becomes markedly visible in those areas. Due to oedema, the conjunctiva loses its transparency. By chemosis is meant marked oedema of the bulbar conjunctiva, so that this membrane may even bulge out.

Causes of oedema of the conjunctiva—

1. Acute inflammatory conditions of the eye such as a severe corneal ulcer, iridocyclitis, or panophthalmitis.

2. Acute inflammation of the surrounding structures such as external or internal hordeolum, orbital cellulitis, tenonitis or acute dacryocystitis.

3. Marked venous stasis such as in acute congestive glaucoma or due to an orbital tumour.

4. Local application of irritants which cause damage to capillary endothelium.

5. General conditions such as nephritis, heart disease, severe anaemia or angioneurotic oedema.

Bleeding from the conjunctiva (or bloody tears)

It is not a very common condition. Bleeding from the bulbar conjunctiva invariably becomes subconjunctival. But in case of the palpebral conjunctiva, because of its firm attachment to the subconjunctival tissues, any haemorrhage cannot be subconjunctival but it comes out as free bleeding. Thus bleeding from the conjunctiva is invariably palpebral.

Causes of bleeding from the conjunctiva—

1. Any acute conjunctivitis of a severe degree particularly in children.

2. A vascular tumour of the conjunctiva like an angioma.
3. A granuloma of the conjunctiva
4. Blood disease like haemophilia.
5. Jaundice.
6. Vicarious menstruation—in this condition bleeding may occur from many sources such as conjunctiva, nose, ear, stomach etc, during normal menstrual cycle.

Diseases of the Conjunctiva

The commonest disease of the conjunctiva is conjunctivitis. The conjunctiva may be affected by the following methods—

1. Exogenous—In this method the causative agents are introduced in conjunctival sac from outside. These agents may be microorganisms, foreign bodies or chemicals.

2. Endogenous—In this method there may be blood-borne infection or there may be allergic response or there may be conjunctival affection as a result of general metabolic disturbance as in gout.

3. By local spread of lesion from the surrounding structures like skin, lacrimal apparatus, the eye itself from the affection of cornea, sclera or uveal tract or orbit,

Classification of conjunctivitis

A. Infective conjunctivitis—
  1. Conjunctivitis due to bacterial infection
  (a) Acute catarrhal or muco-purulent conjunctivits—
      (i) Acute,
      (ii) Sub-acute,
      (iii) Chronic.
  (b) Membranous conjunctivitis.
  (c) Pseudo-membranous conjunctivitis.
  (d) Purulent conjunctivitis,
      (i) Gonorrhoeal conjunctivitis,
      (ii) Ophthalmia neonatorum.
  (e) Angular conjunctivitis.

  2. Viral conjunctivitis—
  (a) Acute haemorrhagic conjunctivitis
  (b) Follicular conjunctivitis—
      (i) Acute,
      (ii) Chronic.
  (c) Conjunctivitis in measles.

(d) Conjunctivitis in varicella or chicken-pox.
(e) Conjunctivitis in herpes zoster ophthalmicus.
(f) Conjunctivitis in vaccinia.
(g) Conjunctivitis in mumps.
(h) Conjunctivitis in influenza.
(i) Conjunctivitis in yellow-fever and dengue fever.

3. Conjunctivitis due to Bedsonia group of organisms—
(a) Swimming-bath conjunctivitis.
(b) Trachoma.
(c) Inclusion blennorrhoea of the new-born.

4. Conjunctivitis due to specific infections—
(a) Tuberculous conjunctivitis.
(b) Syphilitic conjunctivitis.
(c) Tularensis conjunctivitis.
(d) Conjunctivitis in leprosy.
(e) Parinaud's conjunctivitis.

B. Allergic conjunctivitis—
(a) Simple allergic conjunctivitis.
(b) Phlyctenular conjunctivitis.
(c) Vernal conjunctivitis or spring catarrh.

C. Conjunctivitis following injury.

D. Conjunctivitis associated with skin diseases.

A Infective conjunctivitis

In spite of natural protective mechanism of the conjunctiva in the form of low temperature due to exposure to the air, presence of enzyme in the tears called lysozyme which has a definite anti-bacterial property and the mechanical action of blinking and flushing action of the lacrimal secretion, the conjunctival sac may be infected with pathogenic organism causing infective conjunctivitis.

1. Conjunctivitis due to bacterial infection.

Acute catarrhal or acute muco-purulent conjunctivitis

It is the commonest cause for the "red eye"

Etiology

(a) Age—It can occur in any age.

(b) Sex-No preference for any particular sex.
(c) May occur in association with erruptive fevers like measles.
(d) Bad hygienic conditions and dirty habits help the infection to establish as the disease is highly contagious.
(e) Causative organisms—Any organism which affects the mucous membrane anywhere in the body, can also invade the conjunctiva. According to the frequency the common organisms which affect the conjunctiva are coagulase positive staphylococcus, Koch-Weeks bacillus which is a tiny gram negative bacillus belonging to the haemophilus group and also known as Haemophilus Aegyptius, Pneumococcus and Influenza bacillus. Besides these Adenovirus can also cause conjunctivitis sometiems in epidemic form.

Pathology

(a) Congestion of the blood vessels of the conjunctiva with increased permeability.
(b) Exudation of fibrin and polymorphs and other inflammatory cells in the subtantia propria.
(c) Oedema of the conjunctiva which when marked is known as chemosis of the conjunctiva.
(d) Secretion of mucous by the goblet cells.
(e) Due to looseness of the epithelium particularly of the bulbar conjunctiva and that of the fornix, the exudate containing fibrin and leucocytes comes to the surface in the form of discharge.
(f) The superficial epithelial cells, which form the secondline of defence (first line being formed by the leucocytes), phagocytose the invading agents and are themselves desquamated. The basal layer of the cells proliferates and makes up the deficiency.

Thus the conjunctival discharge. consists of—tears, mucous, epithelial cells, bacteria, leucocytes and fibrin. If the inflammation is very severe particularly in children, diapidesis of R.B.C. may occur and the discharge becomes blood stained.

In mild cases the infection is overcome and the condition is cured within 10 to 15 days ; otherwise it may go to the chronic stage.

If inflammation continues for some time, new vessels are formed particularly in the tarsal conjunctiva in the form of minute tufts of capillaries which run perpendicularly to the plane of the superficial vessels.

Symptoms
  (a) Discomfort and foreign body sensation due to engorgement of blood vessels.
  (b) Photophobia or difficulty to tolerate light, and watering of the eye.
  (c) Mistiness of vision, due to a thin layer of discharge of mucous on the cornea.
  (d) Sticking together of the lid margins during sleep due to the discharge.
  (e) Rainbow halo around the light due to a thin layer of discharge on the corneal surface which breaks white light into its component parts.

Clinical Signs (Fig. 37)

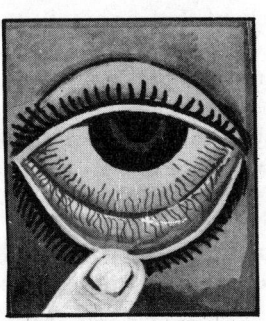

FIG. 37. Acute muco-purulent conjunctivitis

Usually it starts in one eye and then the other eye is affected.
  (a) Conjunctival type of congestion.
  (b) Chemosis of the conjunctiva and mild oedema of the lids if inflammation is severe.
  (c) Petechial subconjunctival haemorrhage particularly when the causative agent is pneumococcus or virus.

Muco-purulent discharge seen accumulated at the inner and outer canthus, lower fornix or at the roots of the eye lashes causing matting of the lashes.

Diagnostic criteria of acute muco-purulent conjunctivitis
  (a) History of sticking together of the eye lids during sleep.
  (b) Conjunctival type of congestion.
  (c) Presence of muco-purulent discharge.

Complications
  (a) The condition may pass on to chronic stage.
  (b) Marginal corneal ulcer due to interference of nutrition following oedema of conjunctiva.
  (c) Blepharitis, i.e., inflammation of the lid margin.

PLATE V

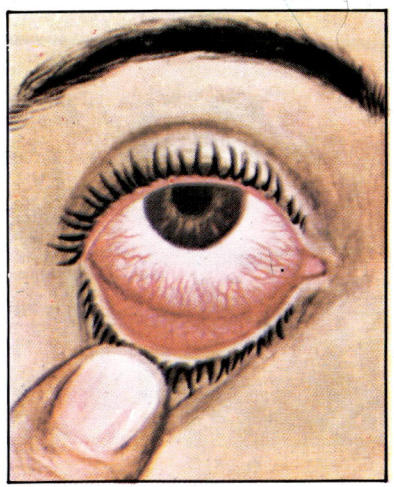

Fig. 1
Acute muco-purulent conjunctivitis
(Parsons)

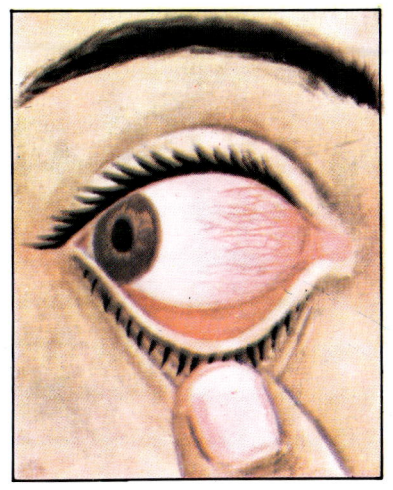

Fig. 2
Angular conjunctivitis
(Parsons)

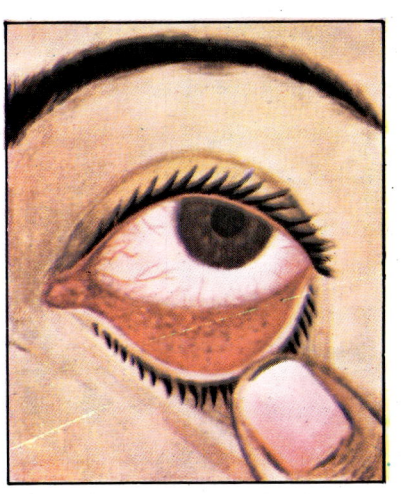

Fig. 3
Follicular conjunctivitis
(Parsons)

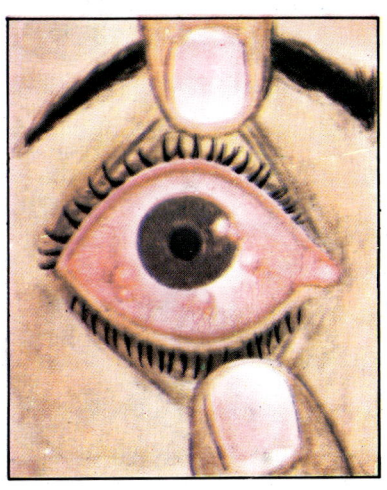

Fig. 4
Phlyctenular conjunctivitis
(Parsons)

(To face page 48)

(d) Rarely chronic dacryocystitis.

Treatment

A. Prophylactic, B. Curative.

A. Prophylactic—

1. Prophylaxis against the good eye, if only one eye is affected—Infection of the good eye may be prevented in two ways—

(a) By not touching the eye with one's own fingure.

(b) By asking the patient to lie on the affected side, so that discharge from the affected eye may not come in contact with the good eye.

2. Prophylaxis against other members of the family—

The personal belongings of the patient like towel, handkerchief, etc., should be kept separate.

B. Curative—

1. The conjunctival sac should be washed with warm normal saline three times a day. The wash helps to remove the discharge and the organisms with it. Frequent eye wash is not desirable, as that dilutes the lysozyme present in the tears, which has definite antibacterial property. Also 1.4 per cent saline which is isotonic with tears may be used for wash.

2. Mild astringent drops like lotio argyrol 5 per cent or lotio protargol 5 per cent may be used three times a day. These organic silver preparations destroy the surface epithelial cells which often contain the organisms.

3. Chemotherapeutic agnets like sulphacetamide 20% drops three to four times a day.

4. Broad spectrum antibiotic in the form of 1% tetracycline or oxytetracycline ointment at bed time, which exerts a prolonged action and prevents the lids from sticking together.

5. If cornea is involved in the form of a marginal ulcer, atropine sulph 1 percent drop twice daily to be used.

6. No pad has ot be used as warmth caused by the pad aggravates the infection. Dark glasses should be used instead.

7. Steriods are contraindicated.

The ideal treatment is of course to take a conjunctival swab for culture, to isolate the organism and to find its sensitivity to any antibiotic and then to use that antibiotic.

Sub-acute Catarrhal Conjunctivitis

Etiology, clinical picture and pathology are the same as acute catarrhal conjunctivitis but the clinical signs are milder.

Chronic Catarrhal Conjunctivitis

Difinition—It is a chronic catarrhal inflammation of the conjunctiva.

Causes

1. As a continuation of acute catarrhal conjunctivitis not treated properly.

2. Continuous irritation to the eyes as due to smoky or dusty atmosphere, abuse of alcohol and error of refraction.

3. Local causes—as misplaced eyelashes, chronic dacryocystitis and chronic rhinitis.

Symptoms

1. Burning sensation in the eyes and a sense of grittiness.

2. Photophobia.

Clinical signs

1. Congestion of the palpebral conjunctiva and the conjunctiva of the fornix.

2. Thin sticky discharge.

Complication—Blepharitis.

Treatment

1. General—Removal of all causes of irritation including correction of error of refraction.

2. Local—

(a) Culture of conjunctival swab and if infection is present corresponding antibiotic to be used.

(b) Stimulating treatment by astringent drop like zinc sulphate with acid boric, which relieves congestion and promotes lymph flow.

(c) In more severe cases, the conjunctival sac has to be painted with 1% solution of silver nitrate.

Memberanous Conjunctivitis

Definition—This disease is rare and is characterized by conjunctivitis with membrane formation on the conjunctiva.

Etiology

1. Age—Usually in Children from 2 to 8 years of age.

2. General ill health following erruptive fevers and unhygienic living condition.

3. Causative agents—

(a) In majority of cases corynebacterium diphtheriae (Klebs-Loeffler bacillus) which are usually associated with staphylococci and pneumococci.

(b) In some cases virulent type of streptococcus haemolyticus.

Mode of infection with diphtheria bacillus

(a) In a case of faucial diphtheria by contamination.

(b) In a case of nasal diphtheria by spread along naso-lacrimal duct.

(c) By infection from a carrier.

Pathology

A virulent strain of the bacillus by invading the conjunctiva produces a severe degree of inflammation. A fibrinous exudate is deposited not only on the surface of the conjunctiva but also within its substance. This exudate forms a membrane in the same way as a membrane is formed in the throat in faucial diphtheria. Usually this membrane is formed on the palpebral conjunctiva, but may also be formed on the bulbar conjunctiva. The membrane is tough in consistency and firmly adherent to the conjunctiva, so that any attempt to remove it leads to bleeding. Along with the membrane formation, there is coagulative necrosis of the conjunctiva. Ultimately the membrane sloughs off and healing takes place by granulation tissue. During healing, symblepharon, i.e., adhesion between palpebral and bulbar conjunctiva or ankyloblepharon, i.e., adhesion between the lid margins may occur and due to contraction of scar tissue entropion or trichiasis may result. As the bacillus can invade normal corneal epithelium, corneal ulcer may develop. This change particularly occurs when the membrane forms on the bulbar conjunctiva.

The clinical course may be mild or very severe. In mild cases there is oedema of the lids and muco-purulent discharge with conjunctival congestion. Pain is moderate. On everting the lid a yellowish white membrane is seen on the palpebral conjunctiva.

In a severe case, the clinical course may be divided into three stages—

(a) Stage of infiltration—It lasts for 5 to 10 days. The lids of the affected eye become red, hot and swollen and hard like a board. Due to this stiffness, it becomes difficult to open the eyes and impossible to evert the lids. There is scanty conjunctival discharge. Pain is severe.

On separating the lids with a lid retractor, if necessary under general anaesthesia, a stiff greyish yellow membrane can be seen, formed either on the palpebral or on bulbar conjunctiva along with marked conjuctival hyperaemia. The pre-auricular glands become palpable (Fig. 38).

(b) Stage of suppuration—Pain is less and the lids become soft. The membrane is sloughed off, leaving a red, raw, granulating surfaces. Discharge is copius.

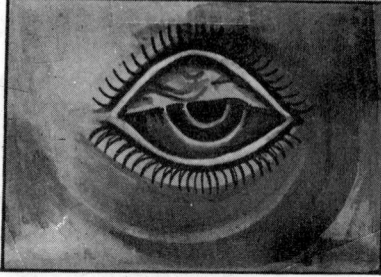

Fig. 38. Membranous conjunctivitis

(c) Stage of cicatrization—During healing the granulating surface becomes covered by epithelium but during the process of healing, the lid may adhere to the eyeball causing symblepharon.

There may be entropion due to contraction of fibrous tissue or even xerosis of conjunctiva due to occlusion of lacrimal ducts and conjunctival glands.

Associated with the eye changes there are systemic signs and symptoms—

(a) The patient is highly toxic and acutely ill.

(b) There is rise of temperature.

(c) Albumen may appear in urine.

Diagnostic criteria

(a) History of diphtheria or contact with a carrier.

(b) Signs of acute conjunctivitis which are very marked.

(c) Tough yellowish white membrane on tarsal conjunctiya which is difficult to remove.

Complications—The most serious complication is the affection of the cornea and formation of corneal ulcer. In severe cases the whole of the cornea may slough out. Later complications are symblepharon, entropion, trichiasis and xerosis of conjunctiva.

Treatment

A. Prophylactic—

     Isolation of the patient.

B. Curative—It is advisable to take a conjunctival swab for culture and smear examination before starting the treatment.

1. Local treatment—

(a) Solution of crystaline penicillin in the strength of 10000 units per c.c. of distilled water to be dropped at frequent intervals, i.e., every half an hour.

(b) Instillation of anti-diphtheritic serum every one hour into the eye.

(c) If cornea becomes ulcerated, atropine sulph ointment 1 percent twice daily to be used.

(d) Broad spectrum antibiotic ointment at bed time.

(e) After the membrane has sloughed off, a glass shell or soft contact lens to cover the eyeball, just to prevent symblepharon formation, has to be used.

2. Systemic treatment—

(a) Intramuscular injection of anti-diphtheritic serum—50 thousand units to be repeated after 12 hours.

(b) Injection of crystaline penicillin 5,00,000 units twice daily.

Pseudo-Membranous Conjunctivitis

This is also a conjunctivitis with the formation of a false membrane.

Etiology

(a) Age—Usually children are affected.

(b) Devitalized condition following erruptive fevers and poor unhygienic condition.

(c) Causative agents—

(i) Organisms like Klebs-Loeffler bacillus of low virulence, streptococcus haemolyticus, staphylococcus aureus, pneumococcus and sometimes Koch-Weeks bacillus.

(ii) Chemical irritants like ammonia, lime, or sliver nitrate.

Pathology

A fibrinous exudation occurs on the surface of the palpebral conjunctiva or on the conjunctiva of the fornix, due to irritation produced by the organisms invading the conjunctiva or by the chemicals. The fibrinous exudate, which forms only on the surface of the conjunctiva and not within its substance, coagulates and forms a pseudo-membrane. This membrane may be easily peeled off, without leaving any bleeding surface.

Symptoms and Clinical signs

The disease starts as a muco-purulent conjunctivitis and the symptoms and signs are similar to this disease. There is soft, painless swelling of the lids and scanty sero-purulent discharge. A membrane appears on the third day. The membrane is yellowish white in colour, either localized on the tarsal conjunctiva or on the conjunctiva of the fornix, but seldom encroaches on the bulbar conjunctiva. It can be easily removed without any bleeding (Fig. 39).

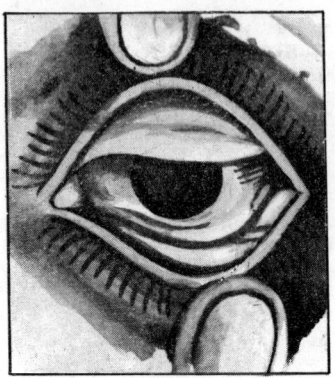

Course—After a period of 10 days to 3 weeks the membrane disappears and the picture of acute catarrhal conjunctivitis persists which gradually subsides.

Diagnostic criteria

   (a) Signs of acute catarrhal conjunctivitis

   (b) Formation of a soft membrane on the tarsal conjunctiva or on the conjunctiva of the fornix which can be removed easily without bleeding.

Fig. 39
Pseudo-membranous conjunctivitis

Treatment

It is similar to that for acute muco-purulent conjunctivitis. The membrane need not be removed.

Acute Purulent Conjunctivitis

This is an acute conjunctivitis where the discharge is frankly purulent. It occurs in two forms—

1. In the adults—mainly as gonococcal conjunctivitis, when the causative agent is Neisseria gonorrhoeae. But sometimes the purulent conjunctivitis may also be caused by B. subtilis, particularly in agricultural areas or by Klebs-Loeffler bacillus and streptococcus haemolyticus, provided the virulence is high and the patient's resistance is low.

2. In the new-born—as ophthalmia neonatorum.

Gonorrhoeal Conjunctivitis

Etiology

1. Age—adults usually with a history of gonorrhoea.

2. Causative agent—gonococcus.

Mode of infection

   (a) From the genitalia by direct contact.

   (b) In case of doctors and nurse, by direct contact with the conjunctival discharge, during examination of the patient.

   (c) Metastatic infection from urethritis.

Pathology

Twenty four hours after infection, (the incubation period may vary from a few hours to 3 days), gonococci form clusters on the surface of the conjunctival epithelial cells and set in a severe inflammatory reaction. Within the next 2 to 3 days, these clusters increase in number. In the meantime, the superficial epithelial cells begin to degenerate. As a result, the organisms penetrate into the deeper layers and may even reach the subepithelial tissues. The superficial cells are then shed off upto the basal layer. There is marked oedema and swelling of the subconjunctival tissues, due to accumulation of inflammatory cells and exudate.

At the end of the first week, the epithelial cells regenerate from the basal layer and these regenerated cells actively phagocytose the organisms. This process of phagocytosis continues until the infection is eliminated. Phagocytosis by leucocytes is less important in gonococcal conjunctivitis.

During these changes in the conjunctiva, gonococcus invades the normal corneal epithelium and corneal ulcer develops. During the process of regeneration of the conjunctival epithelial cells, numerous papillae may be formed, due to the overgrowth of the epithelium. Final healing occurs without any scarring.

Clinical picture

As a rule one eye is affected first, but if the other eye is also affected, the inflammation is not so severe there (Fig. 40).

The clinical picture can be divided into three stages—

1. The condition in the first four to five days is known as the stage of infiltration—

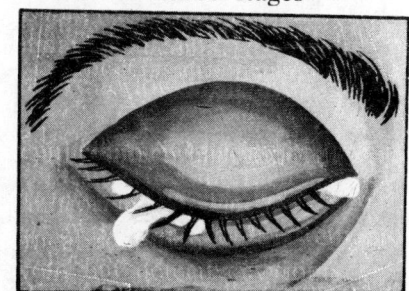

(a) Pain and tenderness of the eyeball is considerable.

(b) Conjunctiva appears bright red and velvety. It may be chemosed.

Fig. 40. Acute purulent conjunctivitis.

(c) Discharge is watery or sanious.

(d) Exudation may coagulate on the surface of the conjunctiva to form a pseudo-membrane.

(e) Lids are tensely swollen.

(f) Pre-auricular glands are enlarged.

2. The next stage is the stage of blenorrhoea. It starts about the fifth day.
   (a) The discharge becomes frankly purulent and abundant and thick, creamy pus drips down the cheeks.
   (b) With the onset of this stage, the tenseness of the lids and the conjunctiva subsides. This stage continues for several weeks.

3. Final stage of slow healing—
   (a) Pain becomes very much less.
   (b) Swelling of the lids subsides.
   (c) Conjunctiva remains red, thick, and velvety. Papillary formation is evident over the tarsal conjunctiva. The bulbar conjunctiva remains hyperaemic for about two months.
   (d) The discharge slowly diminishes, but even at this late stage, virulent gonococci may be present in the discharge.

In the end, resolution is complete and chronic stage is never attained.

Complications

1. Affection of the cornea—
   (a) Oedema of corneal epithelium—a constant feature.
   (b) Ulceration of the cornea, either central or marginal— This occurs, due to actual invasion of corneal epithelium by gonococci, or due to cutting off of nutrition of the cornea from the limbal vessels, as a result of chemosis of the conjunctiva.
   (c) Perforation of the corneal ulcer with all its sequelae.

2. Iritis or iridocyclitis with hypopyon—due to absorption of toxins.

Diagnostic criteria

1. Adult male or female.
2. History of gonococcal infection.
3. Marked inflammation of the lids and the conjunctiva.
4. Copious frankly purulent discharge showing gram-negative intracellular diplococci on smear examination.

Treatment

A. Prophylactic—

To prevent infection of the other eye and eyes of other members of the family—

1. Dressings to be destroyed.

2. Towels and linens used by the patient to be kept separate.

3. In case of an accidental infection of the eye of a doctor or a nurse, silver nitrate solution 1 per cent has to be dropped in the eye followed by broad Spectrum antibiotic.

B. Curative—

1. *Local treatment*—

The treatment should begin with a normal saline wash to wash out the purulent matter as far as possible. As gonococcus is very sensitive to penicillin and as penicillin is effective even in the presence of frank pus, the ideal treatment is frequent drops of penicillin lotion.

A solution of crystalline penicillin in distilled water is prepared in the strength of 10000 units of penicillin in one c.c. of distilled water and is dropped in the eye, at first every one minute for half an hour, and then every 5 minutes for one hour, and then every 15 minutes, half an hour and one hour, until the discharge stops completely. A broad spectrum antibiotic ointment may be applied at bed time. The condition is usually cured within 2—3 days.

If a corneal ulcer develops, atropine sulphate 1 per cent ointment should be applied at bed time.

2. *Systemic treatment*—

If the patient is sufferer of gonorrhoea, the systemic treatment with penicillin injection should be done.

Ophthalmia Neonatorum

Definition—It is a bilateral purulent conjunctivitis occurring in the new born within the first three weeks of life.

Etiology

Causative organisms

(a) Gonococcus.

(b) B. coil, pneumococcus staphylococcus aureus and streptococcus hæmolyticus may be responsible in some cases.

(c) A genital virus present in mother's birth passage—the condition is then known as inclusion blennorrhœa of the new born. Characteristic inclusion bodies are present in the epithelial cells of the conjunctiva of the new born and urethra and vagina of the mother.

Mode of infection

The eye may be infected in three ways—
    (a) Before birth—extremely rare
    (b) During birth, particularly if there is face presentation. This is the commonest.
    (c) After birth—from soiled linen.

Pathology

A few anatomical peculiarities of the new bron sould be kept in mind—
    (a) Absence of tears for 3 weeks to 1 month after birth.
    (b) Conjunctival and corneal epithelium are very thin—only two layers in cornea.
    (c) No adenoid layer in the conjunctiva.
The pathological process is the same as in gonorrhœal conjunctivitis. Papillæ formation is marked in the epithelium. In the sub-epithelial tissue, lymphoid layer is rapidly formed.

Clinical picture

Incubation period for gonococcus is 1 to 3 days, and that for other organisms varies from 1 to 2 weeks. In case of virus, the period is 7 to 9 days.
The condition is bilateral. The clinical sings are the same as in adult, but the whole picture is less virulent and more mild. The conjunctival discharge ceases within 6 to 8 weeks, leaving very little cicatrical changes.

Diagnostic criteria

    (a) Purulent conjunctivitis in the new born.
    (b) Conjunctival smear shows gonococcus.

Complications

In untreated cases, complications usually occur. The cornea is most commonly affected—
    (a) There may be corneal ulcer which may heal leaving an opacity. Due to bilateral corneal opacity, the macula in the retina fails to develop due to obstruction to vision and ultimately nystagmus is developed.

(b) Corneal ulcer may perforate, causing adherent leucoma.

(c) Cornea may slough out, causing anterior staphyloma.

Prognosis

Earlier the treatment better is the prognosis.

Treatment

A. Prophylactic.—
   (a) Thorough antenatal care and examination of the mother for any infection
   (b) Credé's method—
   1% silver nitrate solution is dropped into the eyes of the baby immediately after birth. As a modern method, a solution of crystalline penicillin 10000 units per c.c. of distilled water is dropped with good results.

B. Curative—

Before treatment is started, it is always wise to take a conjunctival swab for smear examination and culture. But treatment must not be delayed. The treatment is the same as in gonococcal conjunctivitis in adults. If cornea is affected atropine sulphate ointment has to be applied.

Angular Conjunctivitis

Etiology

   (a) Age—Usually adults are affected. There may be associated nasal discharge.
   (b) Climate—More common in spring and summer
   (c) Infecting agent—Morax-Axenfeld diplobacillus. They are gram-negative bacilli placed end to end in pair. They are also known as Haemophilus lacunatus.

Mode of infection—Infection is carried by fingers and handkerchiefs. Rarely there may be ascending infection from the nose. Incubation period is four days.

The infection is usually bialteral and highly contagious.

Clinical picutre

Symptoms—There is irritation, itching and smarting sensation in the eyes.

Clinical signs

   (a) Hyperaemia and excoriation of the epithelium of the

intermarginal strip of conjunctiva of the lid margin, both at the inner and outer canthus (Fig. 41).
(b) Excoriation of the skin in the surrounding area near the canthi.
(c) Congestion of the bulbar conjunctiva at the inner and outer angle.
(d) Scanty and muco-purulent discharge.

Course—No tendency to spontaneous cure, but the course is prolonged.

Pathology

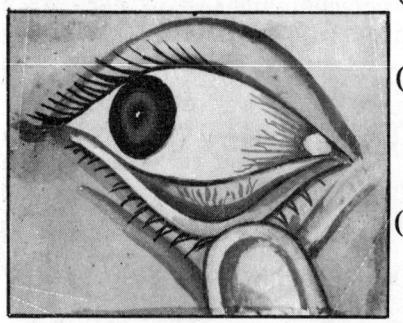

Fig. 41. Angular Conjunctivitis.

(a) Secretion of a proteolytic ferment by the bacilli which macerates the epithelium.
(b) This ferment is inhibited by tears and so the lesions occur, only in those places which are not bathed in tears.
(c) There is accummulation of chronic inflammatory cells, mainly plasma cells, in the subepithelial tissues.
(d) Typical eczematous change occurs in the surrounding skin.

Diagnostic criteria

(a) Typical excoriation and hyperaemia of the conjunctiva of the lid margin, at the inner and outer canthus.
(b) Eczematous condition of the skin in the immediate neighbourhood.
(c) Scraping from the lesions shows the typical diplobacilli.

Complications

Marginal corneal infiltration or corneal ulcer.

Treatment

Zinc sulphate 1% with 2% acid boric drops 3 times a day is specific. The organisms are also susceptible to oxytetracycline, which may be used as 1% ointment at bed time.

2. Viral Conjunctivitis

A several number of viruses can cause conjunctivitis. The conjunctival reactions to virus infection may be variable. Chiefly they are as follows—

(a) Inflammation with follicle formation in the conjunctiva i.e., follicular conjunctivitis. This is the commonest reaction. There may be associated enlargement of the regional lymph glands.

(b) A serious conjunctivitis with oedema of the conjunctiva and minimal conjunctival discharge but copious lacrimation and big patches of sub-conjunctival haemorrhages are seen in epidemic varietes.

(c) A simple hyperaemia of the conjunctiva.

(d) Formation of conjunctival ulcers or membrane.

In case of viral conjunctivitis there is always a tendency for the affection of the cornea so a typical viral lesion is a kerato-conjunctivitis.

Nature of corneal reaction in association with various types of viral conjunctivitis—

(a) Usual initial corneal reaction is the appearance of foci of superficial punctate keratitis.

(b) These foci break down to form superficial erosions of the cornea.

(c) Frequently the underlying corneal stroma is affected either as a result of direct spread of the virus or due to dissemination of a toxic product from the virus or due to an antigen-antibody immune reaction and an opacity of the stroma develops.

(d) Quite often these stromal opacities are transient as in mumps. But sometimes although they may be minute they persist for one or two years as in epidemic kerato-conjunctivitis (S.P.K.)

(e) If necrosis of the stroma occurs on a large-scale as in some cases of herpes, small-pox or vaccinia, permanent opacities are left behind.

Follicular conjunctivitis (in general)

Definition—It is a type of conjunctivitis of an infective nature, characterized by formation of follicles in the conjunctiva.

What is a Follicle ?

A follicle is a localized aggregation of lymphocytes in the sub-epithelial adenoid layer of the conjunctiva, appearing as tiny round translucent swelling.

Conditions in which follicles are formed in the conjunctiva—
(a) Folliculosis.
(b) Follicular conjunctivitis.
(c) Trachoma—stage I and II.
(d) In drug allergy due to local administration of atropine, eserine or pilocarpine.

Folliculosis

The clinical features are as follows—(Fig. 42)

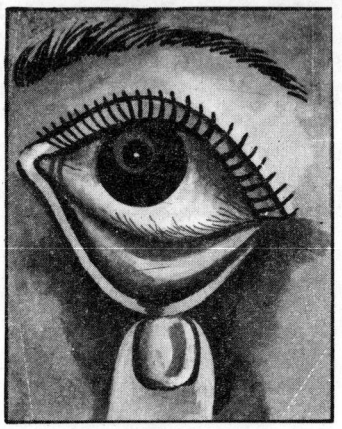

Fig. 42.
Conjunctival; folliculosis.

(a) Formation of discrete follicles mainly in the lower fornix
(b) No sign of inflammation or discharge.
(c) Chronic but benign course, without sequelae.

Etiology

(a) Age—usually children. Rare above 20 years of age.
(b) Unhygienic condition and injudicious diet.
(c) Error of refraction—usually hypermetropia.
(d) Associated with enlarged tonsils and adenoids.

Symptoms—There are no symptoms. The condition is detected during routine examination.

Clinical signs

(a) Follicles arranged in parallel rows in the conjunctiva of the lower fornix mainly, but sometimes in the upper tarsal conjunctiva.
(b) No follicle in the bulbar conjunctiva or on plica semilunaris.
(c) Conjunctiva in between the follicles is normal.
(d) No discharge and no congestion.

Course—The condition perisists for $1^{1}/_{2}$ to 2 years and then subsides without any complication or sequlae.

Treatment

(a) Improvement of general health and removal of enlarged tonsils and adenoids.
(b) Locally no treatment is required, but zinc sulphate 1% with acid boric 2% solution may be used as drops 3 to 4 times a day.

Acute Follicular Conjunctivitis

Definition—This is characterized by follicle formation with signs of acute catarrhal conjunctivitis.

The causative agent is a virus. There are several of this type of conjunctivitis produced by different viruses. They are as follows—

1. Acute herpetic conjunctivitis—

The causative agent is the virus of herpes simplex. It occurs as a primary manifestation of herpes simplex in the young children. The conjunctival follicles are usually large. In the cornea vesicles appear which may merge into a dendritic ulcer. The corneal scarring following vesicle formation tends to be permanent. The preauricular glands are enlarged.

2. Epidemic kerato-conjunctivitis (S.P.K.)—

The causative agent is the type 8 adeno-virus. The disease often occurs in an epidemic form. Clinically it is an acute follicular conjunctivitis with marked inflammation of the conjunctiva, but the discharge is scanty. There is enlargement of the preauricular gland. The corneal complications appear 7 to 10 days later on, first in the form of superficial punctate keratitis and later on as sub-epithelial opacities. The conjunctival condition gradually subsides but the corneal opacity may persist for many months.

3. Pharyngo-conjunctival fever—

The causative agent is again the adeno-virus. There is acute follicular conjunctivitis in association with pharyngitis and fever. It occurs in the children in epidemic form. There may be enlargement of the pre-auricular gland. Superficial punctate keratitis is rare. The disease is acute but subsides quickly.

4. Newcastle conjunctivitis

The causative agent is a myxo-virus, derived from contact with fowls. It is clinically similar to the follicular conjunctivitis associated with the pharyngo-conjunctival fever. The conjunctival secretion may be scanty or profuse. The pre-auricular gland is constantly enlarged. Corneal complications are rare but there may be superficial punctate keratitis.

Treatment : Antiviral drug like Idoxuridine drop or adenine arabinoside (Ara-A) may be helpful.

N.B.   Although inclusion blennorrhoea of the newborn and swimming-bath conjunctivitis (inclusion blennorrhoea of the adult) are other types of acute follicular conjunctivitis, they have not been included in this group, because according to recent conception the causative agents in these cases are not true viruses but Bedsonia group of organisms. So they have been described under the heading conjunctivitis due to Bedsonia group of organisms.

Conjunctivitis in association with other types of virus infection

Conjunctivitis in measles

The causative agent is the exanthematous virus of measles. Before the skin rash appears, the conjunctiva becomes inflammed with a muco-purulent discharge. When the skin erruption commences Koplik's spots may appear on the conjunctiva or even on the caruncle. The conjunctivitis usually subsides when desquamation of the skin begins. In virulent cases corneal complications may appear in the form of superficial punctate keratitis or multiple epithelial erosions.

Conjunctivitis in chicken-pox

The causative agent is the exanthematous virus. The occurrence of vesicles in the conjunctiva is rare. But sometimes phlycten like lesions may appear on the lid margin, the conjunctiva and the limbus. They may undergo resolution or may develop into excavated ulcers. Such a lesion on the limbus may affect the cornea in the form of a marginal infiltration. Frequently, Keratomalacia develops.

Conjunctivitis in herpes zoster ophthalmicus

The causative agent is the herpes zoster virus. The conjunctival lesions are rare. The usual conjunctival reaction is congestion, sometimes with petechial haemorrhages. Rarely a follicular conjunctivitis with regional lymphadenopathy may develop. If the first division of the fifth nerve is involved, small pustules similar to those found in the skin may be observed on the acutely inflamed conjunctiva of the upper tarsus or on the globe.

Conjunctivitis in small-pox

The causative agent is the pox virus. A catarrhal conjunctivitis develops on the fifth day of the disease which easily clears up with treatment. Sub-conjunctival haemorrhages are common in the haemorrhagic type of small-pox. The occurrence of typical pustules is rare. But when they appear they occur usually on the bulbar conjunctiva between the limbus and the outer and the inner canthus rembling phlyctens and sometimes on the tarsal conjuncitva and the caruncle. These lesions rapidly undergo cellular necrosis and membrane formation takes place. This type of lesion is extremely painful. The conjunctiva becomes intensely congested and chemosed and there is profuse discharge. The cornea may be involved in the form of superficial infiltration and ulceration.

Conjunctivitis in mumps

The causative agent is the myxo-virus. A mild conjunctivitis without marked discharge is common. But there may be marked oedema of the bulbar conjunctiva associated with some conjunctival haemorrhage. The corneal involvement is usually in the form of an interstitial keratitis.

Conjunctivitis in influenza

The causative agent is the myxo-virus. At the commencement of the disease a catarrhal conjunctivitis is a constant feature. Occasionally an acute follicular conjunctivitis may occur. Some conjunctival haemorrhage and superficial punctate keratitis have been observed.

Conjunctivitis in yellow fever and dengue fever

The causative agent is the ARBOR virus (Arthropod-borne virus). A very marked conjunctival congestion is the important feature which is most noticeable in the bulbar conjunctiva. There may be subconjunctival haemorrhage.

Treatment—There is no specific type of treatment for the various types of virus conjunctivitis described above. The conditions should be treated on general principles followed for the treatment of acute catarrhal conjunctivitis. Local antibiotics should be used to prevent secondary infection. Atropine must be applied in the form of one percent ointment whenever there is corneal affection.

Conjunctivitis due to vaccination

The causative agent is the pox virus. This type of conjunctival lesion is not due to auto-inoculation, but due to contamination after contact with the vaccination vesicle of another person. In a person who has been previously vaccinated i.e., who has immunity against small-pox the reaction takes place in the form of an acute conjunctivitis with blepharitis with very little chance of corneal affection. But in a non-immune person i.e., who has not been vaccinated previously, the reaction is alarming. Following an incubation period of about three days, there is intense swelling and redness of the lids with purulent conjunctival discharge. On opening the eye, extensive ulceration is seen over the palpebral conjunctiva covered with a thick necrotic membrane. The pre-auricular glands are enlarged. This inflammatory process lasts for seven to ten days. Corneal complications are often very serious. There is keratitis, necrosis of corneal stroma and perforation of the eyeball.

Treatment

1. For the immune persons simple treatment for blepharitis and catarrhal conjunctivitis is all that is necessary.
2. For the non-immune persons concentrated preparation of gammablobulin prepared from the plasma of a recently vaccinated person is highly effective. For local use drops of 250 mg. of gammaglobulin dissolved in 2.5 ml of sterile distilled water may be given at half-hourly intervals during the working hours. For systemic administration 1500 mg. can be administered intramuscularly.

Chronic Follicular conjunctivits

It is the commonest amongst all types of follicular conjunctivitis. It is in fact folliculosis with superadded mild infection.

The causative organism for the infection has never been isolated and probably it is a virus.

Symptoms

Irritation and mild photophobia.

Clinical signs

In addition to the presence of follicles, there is congestion of the conjunctiva of the lower fornix and of the upper tarsal conjunctiva. The discharge is scanty.

Course—Prolonged course for $1\frac{1}{2}$ to 2 years.

Treatment

Mild astringent drop like zinc sulphate 1% with acid boric 2% 3 to 4 times a day is useful.

3. Conjunctivitis due to Bedsonia group of organisms

Bedsonia group of organisms are not true viruses but they occupy an intermediate position between the smaller bacteria and the viruses. Their features are the following—

(a) Size about 250μ to $500\ \mu$.
(b) Visibility under light microscope when properly stained.
(c) Presence of both DNA and RNA in the organism (a true virus contains either DNA or RNA).

(d) Division by binary fission.
(e) Inability to grow in ordinary media.
(f) Sensitivity to tetracycline and sulphonamides.

Types of this group of conjunctivitis—
1. Inclusion blennorrheoa of the newborn (inclusion conjunctivitis)—
The causative agent was formerly called the TRIC agent (TR for trachoma and IC for inclusion conjunctivitis). It is similar to the causative agent for trachoma belonging to the Bedsonia group and is derived from the mother's genital tract. At first there is papillary hypertrophy of the conjunctiva of the lower fornix. After three months of life, when the adenoid layer develops in the conjunctiva, follicles appear in large numbers. Signs of acute conjunctivitis with purulent discharge are also present. It runs a relatively benign course. Spontaneous cure occurs within three to twelve months. As a complication there may be occasional superficial punctate keratitis but there is no scarring of the cornea. The clinical picture resembles that of ophthalmia neonatorum.
2. Swimming-bath conjunctivitis—
It is also known as inclusion blennorrhoea of the adult. It is similar to the inclusion blennorrhoea of the newborn and the causative organism belongs to the Bedsonia group. Infection takes place in the swimming pool from the genital tract and may occur in an epidemic form. There is acute conjunctivitis with follicle formation.

Treatment—The causative agent is susceptible to the sulpha drugs and the broad spectrum antibiotic tetracycline. The condition should be treated as acute conjunctivitis with free local and systemic use of sulpha drugs and tetracycline.

3. Trachoma

Definition—It is a kind of kerato-conjunctivitis, with simultaneous affection of the cornea and conjunctiva, the causative agent being Chlamydia or Bedsonia group of organisms.

Etiology

1. Age—In endemic areas, children are usually affected during the first few years of life. Otherwise there is no age limit.
2. Race—It is very uncommon amongst Negroes, but very common amongst certain races as Jews. In India it is common in Northern India and Punjab.

3. Classes of people affected—
Usually poorer classes are more affected.
4. Climate—Disease is more common in countries with dry and dusty weather.

Causative agent—Trachoma is caused by Chlamydia or Bedsonia organism. The causative agent is not a true virus, but it occupies an intermediate position between a true virus and smaller bacteria. It affects the epithelial cells of the cornea and the conjunctiva and produces inclusion bodies known as Halberstaedter-Prowazek inclusion bodies or in short H.P. bodies. The incubation period is 6 to 12 days.

Mode of infection—The infection spreads by contamination with the conjunctival discharge through fingers, towels or flies.

Symptoms—Usually the onset is gradual, but a massive infection—experimental, accidental or clinical, produces an acute onset. In the absence of secondary infection, symptoms are mild in the form of lacrimation, mild foreign body sensation and slight stickiness of the lids due to scanty mucoid discharge. In the presence of secondary infection, signs and symptoms of acute muco-purulent conjunctivitis develop in addition to those due to trachoma.

Stages of trachoma—Mac Callan has divided trachoma into four stages. Pathology and clinical signs in different stages of trachoma are considered together.

MacCallan's stages I and II show the following changes—

1. Changes in the conjunctiva—
   (a) Marked congestion of the papebral and bullbar conjunctiva.
   (b) Formation of papillae in the upper tarsal conjunctiva and in the fornix. These are formed by hypertrophic folded epithelium with a core of blood vessels. The conjunctiva looks velvety in appearance.
   (c) Follicles—Follicle formation is a characteristic lesion of trachoma. The follicles are aggregates of lymphocytes in the adenoid layer (Figs. 43 and 44).

They commonly appear in the conjunctiva of the upper tarsus and fornix, but may also be present in the lower fornix and plica semilunaris, caruncle and sometimes in the bulbar conjunctiva.

In the early stage, epithelial scraping from the conjunctiva shows characteristic inclusion bodies within the cytoplasm of the cells.

2. Changes in the cornea—

Changes in the cornea occur simultaneously with the changes in the conjunctiva and not secondarily to them. They are as follows—

(a) Epithelial keratitis, i.e., superficial keratitis affecting the epithelium only. This occurs typically in the upper part of the cornea. When stained with fluorescein, minute stained areas are visible.

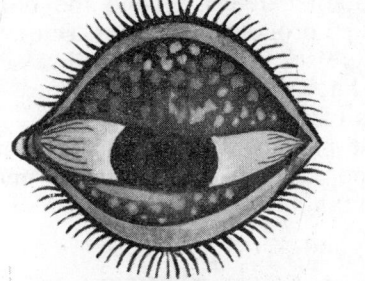 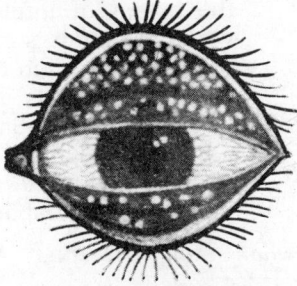

Fig. 43 Early stage of trachoma   Fig. 44. Follicles in trachoma

(b) Trachomatous pannus—This is vascularized infiltration affecting the upper part of the cornea, extending from the limbus. An inflitration of the corneal epithelium with lymphocytes occurs at 12 o'clock position, which extends into the cornea from the limbus. Along with this infiltration, blood vessels, usually parallel and with very few anastomosis, invade the epithelium from the capillary loops at the limbus (Fig. 45).

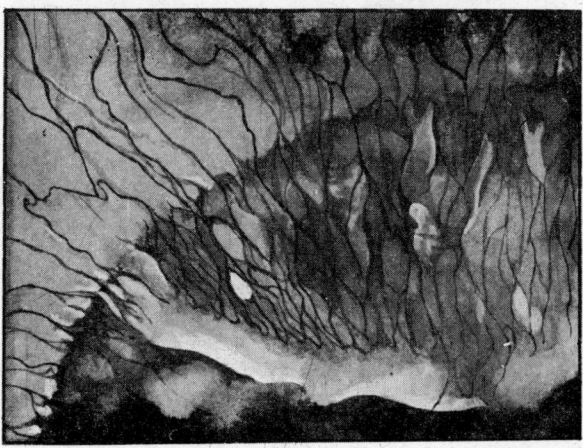

Fig. 45 Progressive pannus in trachoma (Cuénod and (Nataf)

This vascularized infiltrate, known as pannus, is, limited at first at the upper part of the cornea, but in course of time it may appear all round the limbus. The vessels are at first situated between the epithelium and the Bowman's membrane, but later on the latter becomes destroyed and the superficial layers of the substantia propria become involved. In the early stages, the extent of infiltration extends beyond the blood vessels, when it is called progressive pannus. But later on, the infiltration regresses beyond the blood vessels, when the pannus is known as regressive pannus.

(c) Corneal ulcers—Small ulcers may develop at the advancing edge of the pannus. They are shallow, not heavily infiltrated and very irritable, causing much lacrimation and photophobia.

MacCallan's stage III (Figs. 46 and 47)

It is the stage of cicatrization when healing starts. Trachoma is cured by cicatrization. The first evidence of cicatrization is in the

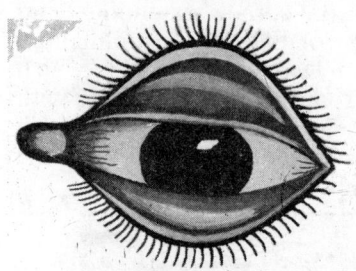   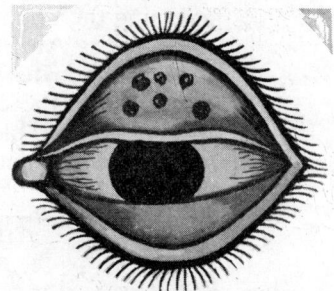

Fig. 46. Early stage of cicatrization.   Fig. 47. Advanced cicatrization.

upper lids. where white scar tissue formation can be seen underneath the epithelium. The follicles atrophy. The conjunctiva also undergoes arophic changes the blood vessels get constricted. The normal arrangement of blood vessels is permanently lost. In the cornea the pannus retrogresses, leaving behind a corneal haze and empty blood vessels. The corneal ulcers heal leaving facets, which cause great disturbance of vision.

MacCallan's stage IV

It is the stage of complications. The complications are as follows—

(a) Entropion of the upper lid.

PLATE VI

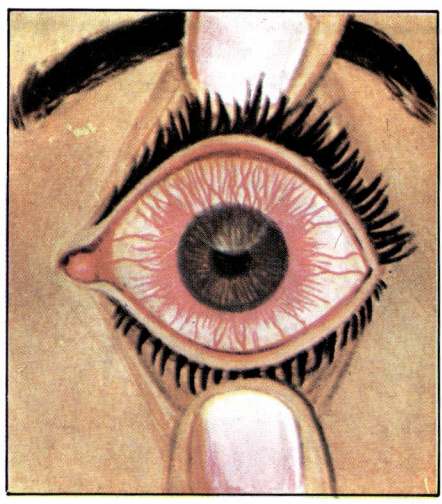

Fig. 1
Trachomatous Pannus
(Parsons)

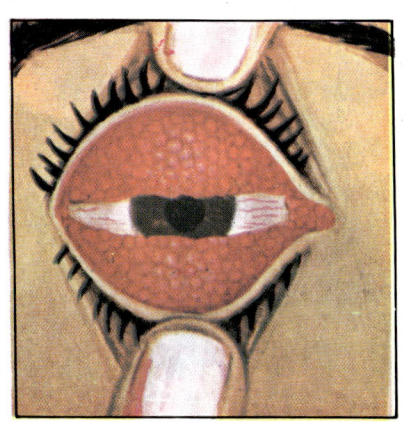

Fig. 2
Trachoma, Follicular Stage
(Parsons)

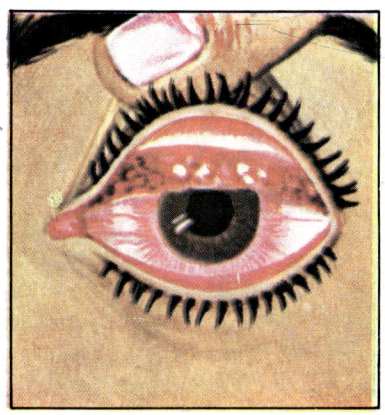

Fig. 3
Trachoma, cicatricial Stage
(Parsons)

(To face page 70)

(b) Trichiasis, i.e., misdirection of the eyelashes.

(c) Parenchymatous xerosis of the conjunctiva due to obliteration of the ducts of the lacrimal and the accessory lacrimal glands.

(d) Chalazion formation due to closure of the ducts of the Meibomian glands.

(e) Obliteration of the lower fornix or even symblepharon formation.

(f) Corneal opacities.

Also there may be pseudo-ptosis due to thickening of the upper lid.

Diagnostic criteria for trachoma

(a) Bilateral affection.

(b) Of the three groups of following clinical signs, two must be present—
  (i) Papillae, follicles and conjunctival congestion.
  (ii) Pannus.
  (iii) Signs of cicatrization and complications.

So, either there must be papillae, follicles, conjunctival congestion and pannus or pannus and signs of cicatrization and complications.

Treatment

Older method of treatment—

(a) Expression of trachoma follicles.

(b) Painting of the tarsal conjunctiva with copper sulphate stick, provided there is no corneal ulceration.

(c) In presence of corneal ulcer—painting of the conjuncitva with 1 percent solution of silver nitrate.

Recent treatment

(a) Local—
  (i) As the causative agent is a big sized virus and is susceptible to sulphonamides, sulphacetamide drop in the form of albucid 10% is instilled into the eyes four times a day for one month.
  (ii) Tetracycline ointment 1% at bed time for 1 month.
  (iii) Atropine ointment 1% once a day, if cornea is ulcerated.

(b) General—Sulphonamide tablets 1 gm 3 times a day by mouth for 10 days.

(c) Treatment of complications—

Plastic operations on lids for correction of entropion and trichiasis.

4. Conjunctivitis due to specific infection

Tuberculous Conjunctivitis

The infecting agent is tubercle bacillus, which may infect the conjunctiva from an exogenous source or from an endogenous source by blood stream.

Pathology

The lesions in the conjunctiva show giant cells, epithelioid cells and lymphocytes, with caseation and fibrosis.

Clinical signs

The conjunctival affections may be of various types—
  (a) Ulcerative type—One or more ulcers are present on the palpebral or bulbar conjunctiva.
  (b) Nodular type—Small nodules appear in the conjunctiva.
  (c) Hypertrophic or cockscomb type—There is overgrowth of granulation tissue from one of the fornices or from tarsal conjunctiva. These signs are associated with various degree of conjunctival congestion and watering. Also the pre-auricular lymph nodes are enlarged.

Diagnosis—Definite diagnosis can be done by histological examination of the scraping from the lesion and by animal inoculation.

Treatment—Usual antitubercular treatment is carried out. Locally frequent streptomycin drop in the concentration of 0.5 gm in 1 c.c. of distilled water is useful.

Syphilitic Conjunctivitis

In syphilis the conjunctiva may be affected in all its stages.
  (a) In primary chancre stage—
        Extragenital chancre in the conjunctiva is common. Associated with this lesion, there is swelling of the eye lids and enlargement of the pre-auricular and sub-maxillary lymph glands.
  (b) In secondary stage—A simple conjunctivitis may occur in association with inflammation of other mucous membranes.

(c) In tertiary stage—Gummata may develop in the conjunctiva which on breaking may produce indolent ulcers.

Diagnosis—By Wassermann,Kahn reaction or V.D.RL test.
Treatment—Usual antisyphilitic treatment.

Tularensis Conjunctivitis

The causative agent is Brucella tularens, is derived from rabbits or squirrels. Small nectrotic ulcers develop in the conjunctiva with swelling of eyelids and enlargement of regional lymphglands.

Treatment is symptomatic, as no specific treatment is known.

Conjunctivitis in Leprosy

The conjunctiva is remarkably immune to leprous infection and true leprous conjunctivitis does not exist.

In nerve type of leprosy, due to affection of the sensory nerves, the conjunctiva may be exposed to minute trauma by dust or foreign bodies. There is marked hyperaemia of the conjunctiva, leading to diffuse catarrhal conjunctivitis. In nodular or lepromatous type of leprosy, lepromata may develop in the conjunctiva.

Parinaud's Conjunctivitis

This is a condition, characterized by granuloma formation in the conjunctiva, with the enlargement of the regional glands. Several types of infection may cause this lesion, e.g., tuberculosis, syphilis and tularensis.

B. Allergic Conjunctivitis

Definition

It means inflammation of the conjunctiva due to allergic reactions.

It may occur in three forms—
1. Simple allergic conjunctivitis.
2. Phlyctenular conjunctivitis.
3. Vernal conjunctivitis or spring catarrh.

Simple allergic Conjunctivitis

Cause—The allergens may be either exogenous or endogenous, the exogenous being more common.

Exogenous allergens—Pollens, vegetable and animal dusts and drugs like penicillin, atropine, eserine and pilocarpine.

Endogenous allergens—Bacterial products from a septic focus particularly due to staphylococcu:

Symptoms

    (a) Irritation and itching of the eyes.

    (b) Photophobia and watering.

Clinical signs

    (a) Marked hyperaemia of conjunctiva.

    (b) Chemosis of conjunctiva.

    (c) Conjunctival discharge is scanty and watery but not muco-purulent.

    (d) Eosinophils in conjunctiva smear.

    (e) Oedema of the lids.

Treatment

    (a) The allergen has to be removed.

    (b) Anti-allergic and vaso-constrictor drug like Antistin-Privine drop may be used, 4 to 6 times a day.

    (c) Hydrocortisone acetate ointment 1% at bed time.

Phlyctenular Conjunctivitis

Definition—It is an allergic inflammatory reaction of the conjunctiva, to some endogenous toxin, which is bacterial in origin. Exogenous allergens like pollens or food matter are not concerned.

Etiology

    (a) Age—Usually children from 4 to 13 years of age.

    (b) Unhygienic condition.

    (c) Excessive carbohydrate diet.

    (d) Tubercular diathesis.

    (e) Exciting factor—usually tuberculo-toxin. But toxins from other organisms like staphylococcus may also be responsible for the disease.

Symptoms—

In simple phlyctenular conjunctivitis, symptoms are few. They are as follows—

    (a) Discomfort in the eye.

    (b) Irritation associated with reflex lacrimation.

On the other hand, in the presence of secondary infection or corneal involvement, photophobia becomes another prominent symptom.

Clinical signs

(a) The phlycten, which means a bleb, appears as a pinkish white nodule, varying from 1 to 3 or 4 mm. in size, usually at the limbus. (Fig. 48.)

(b) It may appear also on the bulbar conjunctiva, a little distance away from the limbus, but extremely rarely on the palpebral conjunctiva.

(c) Number of phlyctens may be one or multiple.

(d) The bulbar conjunctiva, surrounding the phlycten, becomes congested, the rest of the conjunctiva remaining clear.

(e) Usually only there is lcarimation, but no conjunctival discharge.

(f) In the presence of secondary infection, the whole of the conjunctiva becomes congested and muco-purulent discharge develops.

(g) There may be associated enlarged tonsils and cervical glands.

Pathology—On histological section, the phlycten is a compact mass of lymphocytes and polymorphs underneath the epithelium, triangular in shape, with its base towards the surface. In the presence of secondary infection, polymorphs are also present in the subepithelial tissues.

Course—Left as it is, the phlycten ulcerates and heals by granulation, but with very little scar formation. Recurrences are very common. The phlycten may spread into the cornea causing phlyctenular keratitis.

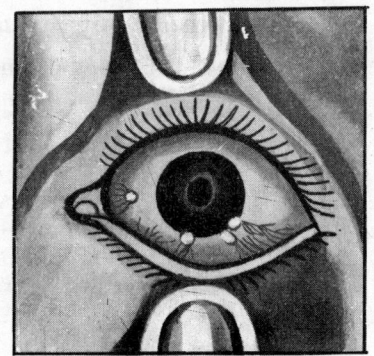

Fig. 48. Phlyctenular conjunctivitis

Diagnostic criteria

(a) A child living in bad hygienic conditions.

(b) Tiny, pinkish white, nodule, one or more at the limbus.

(c) Hyperaemia of the surrounding conjunctiva.

(d) Septic tonsils and enlarged cervical glands.

Treatment

1. Local—

(a) If no secondary infection—hydrocörtisone acetate 1 percent drops at 2 hourly intervals.

(b) In the presence of secondary infection, treatment should be like that for acute muco-purulent conunctivitis, followed by steroid therapy.

(c) If cornea is involved, atropine sulphate 1 percent ointment to be applied twice daily.

2. General—

(a) Tubercular infection should be excluded by skiagram of the chest, Mantoux test and erythrocyte sedimentation rate. If necessary, treatment should be done to combat this infection.

(b) Septic focus, in the form of septic tonsils and adenoids or carious teeth, should be removed.

(c) Vitamins and nourishing diets should be prescribed. Unless the cause is removed recurrences are bound to occur.

Vernal Conjunctivitis or Spring Catarrh

Definition—It is a hypersensitive reaction of the conjunctiva to exogenous allergens, and is mediated by Ig E as indicated by the accompanying eosinophilia

Etiology

(a) Age—6 to 20 years, usually boys.

(b) Seasonal variation—Usually prevalent during summer and subsides in winter.

(c) Exciting factor—Dust aggravated by dry heat.

Symptoms

(a) The most important symptom is marked itching.

(b) Burning sensation with photophobia and lacrimation.

Clinical signs

Two typical forms of vernal conjunctivitis are seen—palpebral type and bulbar type.

Clinical signs of the palpebral type

(a) The upper palpebral conjunctiva presents hard, flat

papillae, separated by furrows, giving a cobblestone appearance. (Fig. 49).

(b) The colour of the papillae is bluish white.

(c) Similar changes may occur in the lower palpebral conjunctiva.

(d) The fornix is not affected.

(e) Rarely the papillae may hypertrophy to produce cauli flower like excrescences.

(f) White and ropy conjunctival discharge which is alkaline in reaction, and contains eosinophils.

Pathology—Papillae consists of dense fibrous tissue, which undergoes hyaline change later on. The epithelium covering the papillae is markedly hypertrophic and sends downward prolongations in the subepithelial tissue. The fibrous tissue contains a large number of eosinophil cells.

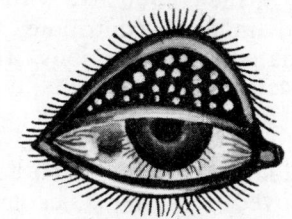

Fig. 49 Vernal conjunctivitis —palpebral type.

Clinical signs of bulbar type

It is less common. There is a gelatinous, thickened accumulation of tissue round the limbus. Symptoms are the same as in the palpebral type. The heaped up tissue may encroach the cornea. The rest of the bulbar conjunctiva is not affected.

Pathology—Same as that for palpebral type

Complications—Steroid induced glaucoma is frequently seen now a days.

Course—The disease subsides after several years.

Diagnostic criteria

(a) A child with a history of intense itching of the eyes, which is worse in summer.

(b) Flat cobble-stone like papillae in the upper tarsal conjunctiva or gelatinous, heaped up tissue around the limbus.

(c) Ropy conjunctival discharge containing eosinophils.

Treatment

(a) Cold water wash

b) Disodium Cromoglycate drop 4 times daily reduces the itching

(c) Dexamethasone drop 4 times daily for several weeks gives the best relief.

(d) In proliferative cases ß radiation is no longer practised Cryotherapy of the nodules is sometimes useful.

Degenerative Changes in the Conjunctiva

1. *Concretions*

These are minute, hard, yellowish white spots, in the palpebral conjunctiva, particularly the upper. Degenerated epithelial cells of the conjunctiva with inspissated mucous contribute to the formation of concretions. There is no calcium deposit. As they are hard and raised, they create a foreign body sensation. They are found in elderly people and can be easily removed by a sharp needle.

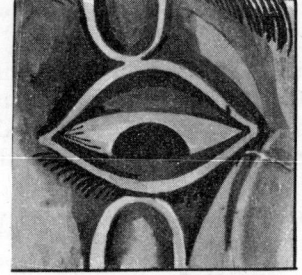

Fig. 50. Conjunctival concertions.

2. *Pinguecula*

This is a small, raised, yellowish white nodule occuring in the bulbar conjunctiva in the horizontal meridian, a little distance away from the limbus, either on the temporal or on the nasal side. (Fig. 51). It usually occurs in elderly persons exposed to wind. and dust. Histologically it consists of proliferated elastic tissue undergoing degenerative changes. Usually there is no symptom and no treatment is required.

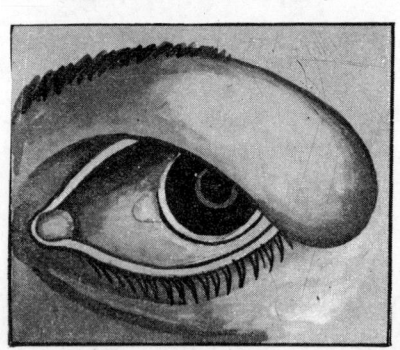

Fig. 51. Pinguecula.

3. *Pterygium*

It is a triangular fold of conjunctiva, encroaching the cornea, in the horizontal meridian, in the palpebral fissure, either from the nasal side or from the temporal side of the bulbar conjunctiva (Fig. 52), or from both the sides.

The main cause is degenerative change in the subconjunctival tissues.

Etiology—Not definitely known. It usually occurs in elderly males doing outdoor work.

Bilaterality—May be uni or bialteral, usually from the nasal side but may also occur on the temporal side.

Parts of pterygium—It consists of a head, i.e., the part which rests on the cornea, a neck and a body.

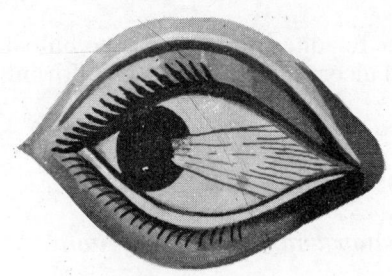

Fig. 52 Pterygium—progressive stage.

Stages of pterygium

(a) Progressive stage—The pterygium is thick, fleshy and vascular. There are also opaque spots in the cornea, just in front of the apex i.e., the head of the pterygium. It progresses in the cornea in the level of Bowman's membrane which is destroyed.

(b) Atrophic stage—The pterygium is thin, attenuated with very little vascularity. No opaque spots in the cornea in front of the head.

Symptoms—Usually no symptom unless it encroaches the pupillary area, when there is visual distrubance. Occasionally there may be diplopia, due to limitation of movement of the eyeball.

Treatment

(a) If the pterygium is stationary in the atrophic stage and is not much disfiguring, no treatment is necessary.

(b) In case of progressive pterygium, either of the following methods may be adopted for treatment—

  (i) McReynolds' transplantation operation—

    The head and neck of the pterygium is separated

from the cornea by a cataract knife. The body is then dissected and separated from sclera for a distance of about 5 mm from the limbus. The pterygium is then introduced underneath the bulbar conjunctiva at 6 o'clock position and kept in place by a mattress suture.

(ii) Excision of the pterygium—The entire pterygium is dissected and removed. The cut conjunctival margins, above and below the pterygium, are sutured.

Pseudo-pterygium

Mechanism—It is formed due to adhesion of chemosed bulbar conjunctiva to a marginal corneal ulcer. It usually occurs following chemical burns of the eye.

TABLE IV

Difference between pterygium and pseudo-pterygium

Pterygium.	Pseudo-pterygium.
1. Degenerative process.	1. Inflammatory process.
2. A probe cannot be passed underneath the neck	2. A probe can be passed.
3. Always situated in the palpebral fissure.	3. Can develop in any meridian.
4. Either progressive or stationary.	4. Always stationary.
5. Usually occurs in elderly persons.	5. Can occur in any age.

Treatment—The pseudo-pterygium may be separated from the cornea and excised.

4. *Xerosis of the conjunctiva*—

Definition—It means dry lustureless condition of the conjunctiva.

Causes of xerosis

(a) Due to local affection of the conjunctiva—when the xerosis is known as xerosis parenchymatosa. Example—

(i) Trachoma, pemphigus, membranous conjunctivitis, burns.
(ii) Following exposure as in case of ectropion or proptosis.

(b) Due to some systemic disease—when the xerosis is known as xerosis epithelialis.
Example—
Systemic disease like vitamin A deficiency.

The chief changes in xerosis occur in the epithelium of the conjunctiva which takes up the features of the epithelium of the skin and stops secreting mucous.

Treatment—Treatment is symptomatic. In vitamin A deficiency it should be treated accordingly. Locally liquid paraffin or methyl cellulose 1% may be used for the dryness.

Pigmentation of the Conjunctiva

A. *Exogenous source*

1. *Argyrosis*—This condition causes black colouration of the conjunctiva, due to prolonged use of silver preparation as eye drop or due to working with silver dust. Silver is deposited as albunate of silver around the elastic fibres of the conjunctiva.

2. *Siderosis*—There is pigmentation of the conjunctiva around an impacted body made of iron.

B. *Endogenous source*

1. Bile—Yellow discolouration of the conjunctiva as in jaundice.
2. Deposition of melanin causing black pigmentation—in Vitamin A deficiency, trachoma, Addison's disease, alkaptonuria and benign or malignant melanoma of conjunctiva.

Subconjunctival Haemorrhage

It may vary in degree. There may be minute petechial spots of haemorrhage which may be mistaken for dilated vessels or there may be extensive extravasation of blood.

Site of haemorrhage—

The exposed part of the bulbar conjunctiva is the frequent site, because this is easily liable to be injured and because blood can easily accumulate in the loose subconjunctival tissue in that area. Because of the firm attachment of the conjunctiva to the tissues in the tarsal region, subconjunctival haemorrhage in that area in extremely rare. In the early stage the haemorrhage appears bright red in colour but later .on it becomes blackish red.

Causes of haemorrhage

1. Direct trauma to the eye—The posterior limit of the haemorrhage is visible.

2. Head injury or injury to the orbit causing fracture of a wall of the orbit—

In such injuries the blood usually seeps under the conjunctiva and appears as subconjunctival haemorrhage within 12 to 24 hours after the injury. Also as the blood comes from inside the orbit, the posterior limit of the haemorrhage is not visible.

Under these circumstances the location of the blood underneath the conjunctiva varies according to the site of the injury as follows—(Duke-Elder)—

   (a) From a fracture of the roof of the orbit—To the upper lid and upper fornix along the levator muscle.
   (b) From a fracture of the floor—To the lower lid and the lower fornix.
   (c) From the apex of the orbit—Along the lateral rectus muscle.
   (d) From a fracture of the orbital plate of the sphenoid bone—To the temporal part of the bulbar conjunctiva.

3. Marked venous congestion of the neck veins as in whooping cough in children or in severe compression of the chest or neck.

4. Blood diseases—Leukaemia, purpura, haemophilia.

5. Arteriosclerosis and hypertension or local vascular anomaly like varicosity or aneurysm—in such cases there may be spontaneous rupture of a vessel.

6. Acute inflammation of the conjunctiva e.g., in acute mucopurulent conjunctivitis due to pneumococcus or Koch-Weeks bacillus, conjunctivitis of primary herpes simplex, leptospirosis ictero-haemorrhagica and viral epidemic kerato conjunctivitis.

7. Acute febrile systemic infection e.g., meningococcal septicaemia, sub-acute bacterial endocarditis, measles and yellow fever.

8. Vicarious menstruation—Bleeding may occur from ear, nose or gastrointestinal tract or from conjunctiva during menstruation

9. Idiopathic—When no cause is found.

Treatment : Besides the treatment of the cause hardly there is any treatment necessary. The blood absorbs in one to three weeks time. Hot compress may help absorption faster.. An astringent drop may be given as placebo.

Tumours of the Conjunctiva

A. *Congenital*—

(a) *Epibulbar dermoid*—The commonest congenital tumour of the conjunctiva is the epibulbar dermoid. This is flat, round or oval tumour occuring at the limbus and encroaching partly on the conjunctiva and partly on the cornea. Its rate of growth is extremely slow. It consists of fibrous tissue containing hair follicles, sebaceous and sweat glands and is covered by stratified epithelium.

(b) *Dermo-lipoma*—It is the next common congenital tumour of conjunctiva. It is slightly raised, yellowish white tumour occuring underneath the bulbar conjunctiva at the upper and outer angle and extending into the orbit. It may be associated with accessory auricles when it is known as Golden Har Syndrome.

B. *Acquired*—

The common tumours of the conjunctiva are—

1. Benign—

(a) *Papilloma*—It may arise anywhere in the conjunctiva or from the limbus. It is soft and has a raspberry-like appearance.

(b) *Angioma*—It is usually of cavernous type and may occur in any situation. It appears as a rounded or tortuously rounded tumour, with a dark bluish red surface.

Treatment of these tumours is surgical removal.

2. Malignant—

(a) *Epidermoid carcinoma*—It usually occurs at the limbus appearing at first like the head of a pterygium. As it grows, it ulcerates.

(b) *Malignant melanoma*—It may arise from a naevus. The tumour is pigmented, highly malignant and grows rapidly.

(c) *Pre-cancerous and cancerous melanosis*—A large area of pigmentation of the conjunctiva and the skin appears unilaterally. The pre-cancerous stage may remain as it is for many years, but cancerous change may supervene, when it becomes highly malignant.

Treatment of these malignant tumours is enucleation of the eyeball. In pre-cancerous melanosis, exenteration of the orbital contents has to be done.

Cysts of the Conjunctiva

1. *Implantation cysts*—These are the commonest. They occur due to implantation of conjunctival epithelial cells, following an injury or operation.
2. *Retention cysts*—They occur due to the obstruction of the ducts of the accessory lacrimal gland.
3. *Lymphatic cysts*—They arise as a result of dilatation of lymphatic spaces.

Treatment of the cysts of the conjunctiva is surgical removal.

CHAPTER V

ANATOMY AND DISEASES OF THE CORNEA

Anatomy of the cornea

The cornea is a clear transparent tissue with a smooth shining surface. Average diameter is about 12 mm. Thickness of the central part is 0.5 mm. while at the periphery it is about 0.8 mm. The central zone of a diameter of about 4 mm. is spherical but the peripheral zone is flattened.

Structure of the cornea

From before backwards cornea is made of five layers (Fig. 53)—

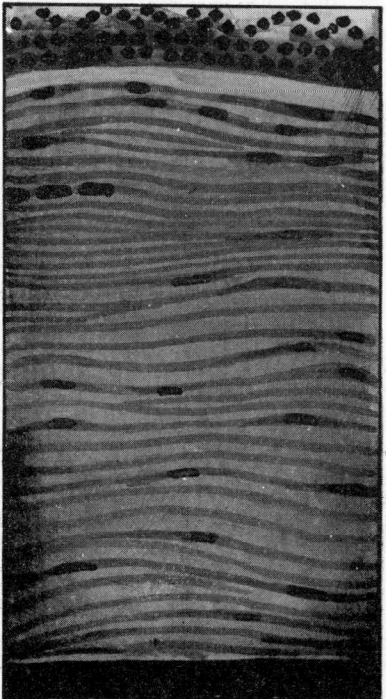

Fig. 53. Structure of the Cornea

1. Epithelium—The epithelium is stratified in nature, very regular in arrangement with uniform thickness, and consists of five layers of cells without cornification. It is continuous with the epithelium of the conjunctiva.

2. Bowman's membrane (anterior elastic lamina)—It is a homogeneous membrane on which the epithelium rests. It stops at the limbus.

3. Substantia propria—It is the corneal substance proper. It is made of corneal lamellae arranged in parallel rows and corneal corpuscles. They are held together by a transparent cement substance. This layer is continuous with the sclera.

4. Descemet's membrane (posterior elastic lamina)—It is an elastic transparent membrane. It is continuous at the angle of the anterior chamber with the pectinate ligament.

5. Endothelium—It is made of one layer of hexagonal cells resting on the Descemet's membrane. It is continuous anatomically with the uveal tract.

Nutrition of the cornea—Normally cornea has no blood vessels in it. The nutrition is derived from three sources—

(a) Perilimbal plexus of blood vessels,
(b) Aqueous humour,
(c) Oxygen from air.

Nerve supply of cornea (Purely sensory)

The ciliary nerves supply the cornea. The ultimate origin is from the 1st division of the Vth nerve through the naso-ciliary nerve. For the interest of transparency, the nerve fibrils situated in the substance of the cornea are non-meduallated. There is no kinaesthetic sensation in the cornea ; the sensory nerves carry only touch, pain and thermal sensations.

Congenital Abnormalities of Cornea

1. *Microcornea*—The normal diameter of cornea is 12-13 mm. In microcornea the diameter is very much less than normal. The eye as a whole may be small or normal in size. The refraction is usually hypermetropic.

2. *Megalocornea*—The diameter of the cornea is more than 13 mm., otherwise the eyeball is normal.

Corneal oedema

Like any other tissue in the body cornea may also be oedematous due to accumulation of fluid in its substance. For the interest of transparency of the cornea, normal fluid content of its substance is kept at a constant level and when the fluid content exceeds that level– oedema sets in.

Sources of the fluid which causes oedema—

(a) *Aqueous humour*—At first the endothelium of the

cornea must be damaged. Then the aqueous humour percolates through the damaged endothelium, and passes through the Descemet's membrane, substantia propria, and the Bowman's membrane along the nerve-canals and appears as droplets of fluid in between the basal epithelial cells.

(b) *Tears*—The epithelium of the cornea must be damaged faciliating the entrance of the tears into the corneal substance.

Clinical appearance of oedema of the cornea

The cornea appears hazy, looses its normal lusture and the surface becomes dull and uneven. Epithelial bullae may be formed. The corneal stroma may show radial or crisis-cross white lines and the condition is then known as striate keratopathy.

Symptoms of corneal oedema

(a) *Appearance of halo around the light*—This is the most characteristic symptom. The halo has red colour on the outside and blue colour on the inside.

(b) *Visual loss*—Haziness of the cornea is bound to hamper vision.

Causes of corneal oedema

(a) Break in the continuity of the epithelium or the endothelium due to mechanical trauma, ulcer or erosion ; damage to endothelium is the more potent factor for the production of corneal oedema.

(b) Increased intra-ocular pressure as in closed-angle glaucoma, absolute glaucoma, buphthalmos and epidemic dropsy glaucoma. The endothelial damage is the cause of the oedema.

(c) Inflammatory conditions of the anterior segment of the eye e.g., acute iritis of iridocyclitis. In such cases also there is damage to the endothelium.

(d) Degenerative conditions of the cornea e.g., epithelial and endothelial dystrophy of Fuchs.

(e) Neuroparalytic condition e.g., neuroparalytic keratitis following injection of alcohol in the Gasserian ganglion for trigeminal neuralgia.

(f) Oxygen deprivation of the cornea e.g., use of contact lens for several hours.

Corneal Ulcer

Classification

A. Purulent ulcer of suppurative keratitis.
  1. Ordinary pyogenic corneal ulcer.
  2. Hypopyon ulcer or serpiginous ulcer of cornea.
  3. Mycotic ulcer.
  4. Marginal ulcer.

B. Non-Purulent ulcer.
  1. Ulcer in association with trachoma.
  2. Dendritic ulcer.
  3. Lagophthalmic ulcer.
  4. Ulcer due to vitamin A deficiency.
  5. Neurotrophic ulcer as produced by injection of alcohol
in the gasserian ganglion or ciliary ganglion.

C. Allergic ulcer
  1. Phlyctenular ulcer.

D. Degenerative ulcer
  1. Atheromatous ulcer occuring in old leucoma.
  2. Mooren's ulcer.

In general the ulcers occuring in the central area of the cornea are usually due to exogenous infection whether bacterial, viral or mycotic ; those occuring in the periphery are often toxic or allergic in nature or due to endogenous infection.

Corneal Ulcer or Suppurative Keratitis

Definition—It means loss of corneal substance as a result of infection and formation of a raw, excavated area.

Normal corneal epithelium cannot be penetrated by any organism except by diphtheria bacillus and gonococcus.

So pre-conditions for an ulcer to develop are—
1. Trauma to the corneal epithelium as by a minute foreign body, misdirected eyelash or conjunctival concretion.
2. Unhealthy condition of the epithelium as evidenced in absolute glaucoma due to persistent oedema of the epithelium, in neuroparalytic condition following injection of alcohol in trigeminal ganglion to cure trigeminal neuralgia, or in keratomalacia.

These pre-conditions are then followed by infection. The infection may be exogenous, carried by a foreign body or local, from chronic dacryocystitis or conjunctivitis.

Thus after the infection has settled, there is necrosis of corneal tissue which is sloughed off, and an ulcer is .formed. A corneal ulcer may terminate in one of the three ways—

1. If the tissue resistance is sufficiently strong the ulcer. remains localized and · ultimately heals.

2. The ulcer penetrates through the corneal substance, a descemetocele is formed and then finally the cornea is perforated—perforating ulcer. (Descemetocele is due to bulging of Descemet's membrane).

3. The ulcer spreads so that whole or part of the whole thickness of the cornea sloughs off—sloughing ulcer.

Pathology of localized ulcer
It can be considered in three stages—(Fig. 54)

1. Progressive stage—
   (a) Surrounding the ulcer there is marked infiltration of corneal tissue with polymorphs.
   (b) Necrosis and sloughing off of the epithelium, the Bowman's membrane and some amount of substantia propria, corresponding to the ulcerative area take place, and ulcer crater is formed.

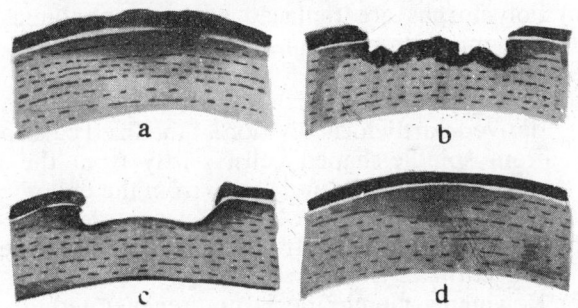

Fig. 54. Stages of localized corneal ulcer. (Parsons)
a and b—progressive stage
c—regressive stage
d—stage of cicatrization

   (c) The walls of the crater become swollen due to imbibition of fluid by corneal tissue.
Along with these changes in the cornea there are some other side effects, as follows—
      (i) Ciliary congestion.

(ii) Some degree of iritis due to absorption of toxins from ·the ulcer.

(iii) Hypopyon formation due to exudation in· the anterior chamber from the blood vessels of the iris and cillary body. This pus remains sterile so long as the Descemet's membrane remains intact.

(iv) Vascularization of cornea—It occurs particularly when the ulcer is close to the limbus and when the ulcer persists for a length of time.

(v) Due to transmission of the toxic products from the anterior segment through vitreous, there are fine opacities and cellular deposits in the vitreous. This occurs when the corneal ulcer is very virulent.

N.B. The organism which are more likely to cause hypopyon are pneumococcus, bacillus pyocyaneous, Morax-Axenfeld diplobacillus and fungi.

2. Stage of regression—

(a) A line of demarcation appears surrounding the ulcer.

(b) Necrosed tissues upto the line of demarcation slough off.

(c) Polymorphs are replaced by large mononuclear cells and infiltration diminishes.

3. Stage of cicatrization—

(a) The ulcer crater becomes filled up by fibrous tissue derived partly form division of the fixed corneal cells to from spindle-shaped cells, partly from the invading mononuclear cells and partly from the endothelial cells of the new vessels when they are present.

(b) Epithelium growing from the edge of the crater covers the cornea.

(c) Bowman's membrane is not regenerated.

(d) The newly laid fibrous tissue causes an opacity of the cornea which depending on its density is known as nebula, macula or leucoma—the last being the most dense.

Pathology of perforating corneal ulcer

The ulcerative process spreads into deeper corneal tissue and as the process reaches the Descemet's membrane, this membrane bulges forward in the form of a glistening sphere. The ulcer then erodes through the membrane and the endothelium gets perforated.

PLATE VII

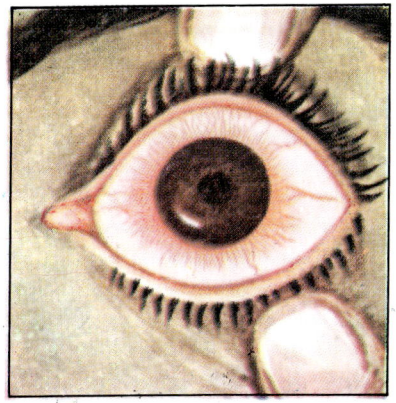

Fig. 1
Corneal Ulcer
(Parsons)

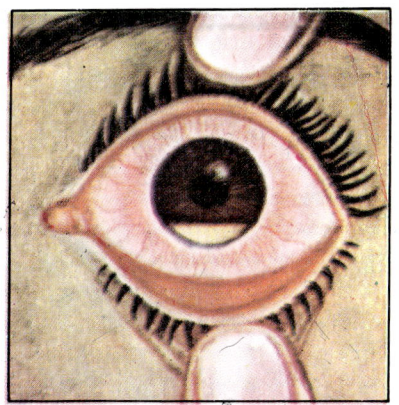

Fig. 2
Hypopyon Ulcer
(Parsons)

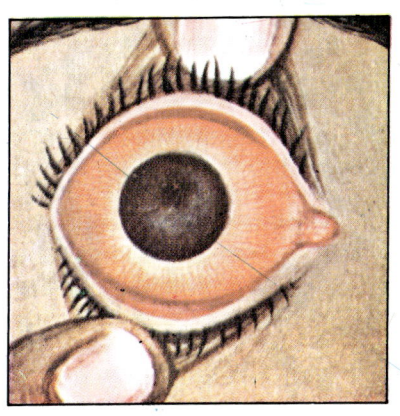

Fig. 3
Interstitial Keratitis
(Parsons)

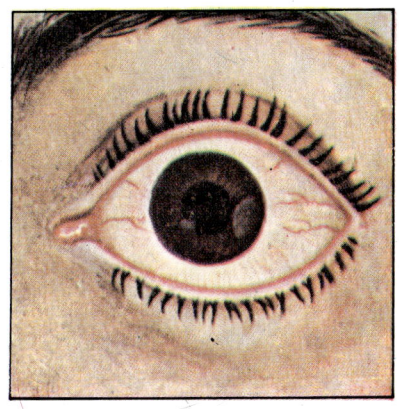

Fig. 4
Corneal Nebulae
(Parsons)

(To face page 90)

As soon as perforation of the cornea takes place, following changes occur—

(a) Drainage of aqueous humour and abolition of the anterior chamber.

(b) Iris comes forward and may prolapse through the ulcer.

(c) Usually iris gets adhered to the ulcer which now quickly heals due to the presence of vascularized iris tissue.

(d) As the ulcer heals, a leucoma is formed, but as iris remains adherent to it, it is called adherent leucoma. The anterior chamber forms as the perforation heals but remains shallow.

Adherent leucoma is the commonest end result of the perforation of a corneal ulcer. But other complications may occur as the result of perforation. They are as follows—

(a) The lens may be subluxated due to forward movement of the lens along with the iris.

(b) The lens, coming in contact with the ulcer, may develop anterior polar cataract.

(c) Expulsive haemorrhage may occur due to sudden lowering of intra-ocular pressure, following the drainage of aqueous.

(d) Panophthalmitis may develop, due to entry of the infection from the ulcer into the interior of the eyeball.

Pathlogy of Sloughing Corneal Ulcer and Formation of Anterior Staphyloma

If the infecting agent is highly virulent or the body resistance is very low, whole or some portion of the cornea may slough out. The result is the formation of a big gap in the cornea. A good amount of iris becomes exposed following drainage of the aqueous. The iris becomes inflammed and a layer of exudate covers the iris ultimately organize into a thin fibrous layer, which is known as pseudo-cornea. As it is thin, it cannot withstand the intra-ocular pressure and so it bulges forward along with the iris and the bulging is known as anterior staphyloma, which may be total if whole of the cornea sloughs off or partial if only a portion of the cornea is affected.

Other complications that may occur following sloughing of corneal ulcer—

(a) As the gap in the cornea is much bigger than a perforation, the lens, being dislocated, may be extruded.

(b) Expulsive haemorrhage may occur.

(c) Panophthalmitis may develop.

(d Later on secondary glaucoma develops due
to complete abolition of the anterior
chamber.

Clinical symptoms and signs of corneal ulcer

Symptoms

1. Pain in the eye due to exposure and irritation of the sensory
nerve endings.

2. Lacrimation, which may be profuse, due to reflex sensory
stimulation.

3. Photophobia, i.e. intolerance to light.

4. Headache and blurring of vision.

Signs

1. Marked blepharospasm, i.e., forcible closure of the eyelids
specially in children.The spasm of the eyelids is reflex in origin
due to sensory irritation. The eyelids may be oedematus.

2. Rough and raw yellowish white area on the cornea which
stains with fluorescein and does not show any window reflex.

3. Haziness of the cornea surrounding the ulcerated area, due to
infiltration of leucocytes.

4. Ciliary congestion with conjunctival hyperaemia.

5. Profuse watering but usually no muco-purulent discharge.

6. The iris is slightly muddy in colour, and the pupil is small.

7. A hypopyon may, or may not be present. The exudate
forming the hypopyon remains sterile so long as the Descemet's
membrane is intact.

8. Blood vessels may encroach the cornea from the limbus.

Diagnostic criteria of a corneal ulcer

1. Raw area on the cornea with surrounding haziness. Rawness
demonstrated by staining with fluorescein and absence of window
reflex.

2. Pain,watering,ciliary congestion and generalized conjunctival
hyperaemia.

Table V

Differential diagnosis among ulcer, keratitis and leucoma

	Corneal ulcer	Keratitis	Leucoma
1. Pain and watering.	Present	Present	Nil.
2. Ciliary congestion.	Present	Present	Nil.
3. White area in the cornea.	Stains with fluorescein and no window reflex.	No staining and window reflex present. No raw area.	No staining and window reflex present. No raw area.

Complications of corneal ulcer

1. Secondary glaucoma due to fibrinous exudation in the anterior chamber, which blocks the angle.
2. Perforation of the cornea with its sequelae.
3. Sloughing of the cornea with its sequelae.

Treatment

A. *Local*

1. Control of infection—Ideal method will be to detect the invading organism and its sensitivity to antibiotics by culturing the material scraped from the ulcer. But as it is not always possible to follow this method, crystalline penicillin 5,000 units with 0.5 gm of streptomycin sulphate dissolved in 1 c.c. of distilled water may be dropped every one hour, with a broad spectrum antibiotic ointment at bed time.

If the ulcer still tends to spread with this method of treatment, the progressive margin of the ulcer should be cauterized by thermo-cautery or with pure carbolic acid.

2. Rest to the eye—
  (i) Atropine ointment 1 percent applied twice daily gives rest to the eye by paralysing the ciliary muscle. It also causes vasodilatation and. so brings more antibodies in the aqueous humour.
  (ii) Dark glasses or shade to protect the eye from the irritating effect of strong light. But the eye must not be bandaged

3. Relief of pain—Analgesics by mouth and hot compress for the relief of pain.

4. Removal of any septic focus in the neighbourhood—The lacrimal sac must always be examined and if chronic dacryocystitis is present, the sac must be removed without delay.

B. *General*

1. To increase body resistance, injection of milk 5 c.c. intramuscularly twice a week 4 such.
2. Vitamin A and C by mouth.
  To treat a corneal ulcer the following must not be done—
  (a) Steroids must not be used so long as there is an active ulcer.
  (b) No Cocaine drops.
  (c) No bandage, as the increase of temperature due to bandage helps the organisms to grow.

Treatment of complications of corneal ulcer

    (a) For secondary glaucoma—diamox by mouth and if necessary paracentesis. Only hypopyon is not an indication for paracentesis.

    (b) For descemetocele when perforation is threatening—paracentesis and pad and bandage.

    (c) If perforation has occured with iris prolapse—pad and bandage to prevent further iris prolapse.

    (d) When the ulcer has sloughed off, with exposure of a good amount of iris, with or without the expulsion of the lens—pad and bandage with antibiotic ointment, and thereapeutic keratoplasty if donor cornea is available.

Leucoma

    Definition—Leucoma means opacity of the cornea. According to the density of the opacity, the opacity is called a nebula, a macula or a leucoma, the last being the most dense.

    The extent of the leucoma may vary. It may affect a small area of the cornea or whole of the cornea may be affected, causing a total leucoma depending upon the amount of damage of corneal tissue.

    A leucoma may have blood vessels in it or brown pigment, particulary when the iris is adherent to it.

    A long standing leucoma may develop a degenerative ulcer known as atheromatous ulcer.

Mechanisms by which a corneal opacity is formed

    (a) Healed corneal ulcer—commonest.

    (b) Healed keratitis.

    (c) Penetrating injury to the cornea.

    (d) Operative injury to the cornea.

    (e) Foreign body damaging the corneal substance.

    (f) Corneal dystrophy.

Any damage to the substantia propria leaves behind an opacity.

Changes that may occur in a corneal opacity

    (a) Clearing of the opacity—

        In infants gross opacities may almost entirely disappear. In adults sometimes clear areas or lines may appear in the central part of densely opaque leucoma. These are known as Fuch's lines of clearing and they are usually associated with newly formed blood vessels in the leucoma.

(b) Pigmentary changes—

Apart from pigmentation of the opacity in a case of adherent leucoma, a simple leucoma may show fine yellowish-brown lines in the epithelium known as the Hudson-Stahli lines. The pigment may be either haemosiderin derived from the blood vessels when the leucoma is vascularized or melanin derived from the basal layer of cells of the corneal epithelium which are potential melanoblasts.

(c) Reduction of sensitivity—Both tactile and pain sensation are diminished over the leucoma.

(d) Degenerative changes—

They occur as a rule in the old,long standing leucoma. They may be of two types—

(i) Hyaline degeneration—it is the commonest.

(ii) Calcareous degeneration of the stroma—this is accompanied by spontaneous necrosis of areas of the scar tissue which are sloughed off causing an atheromatous ulcer.

Symptoms of leucoma

(a) No symptom if the opacity is outside the pupillary area.

(b) Visual disturbance—if it is in the pupillary area.

Treatment for leucoma

1. If the leucoma is small and does not hamper vision, it does not require any treatment, except cosmetic treatment known as tattooing.

Cosmetic treatment—The white opacity in the cornea is made black, by chemicals in the following way—

(a) After local anaesthesia with xylocaine 4% drops, the epithelium over the leucoma is scraped off with a cataract knife.

(b) 2 percent gold chloride or 2 percent platinum chloride and 2 percent hydrazine hydrate solutions are applied to the raw area one after another, with swab sticks, when the opacity takes a black colour.

(c) Excess of the chemicals is washed away, atropine and antibiotic ointment are applied and the eye is kept bandaged for 48 hours.

The black colouration persists for about 2 years provided the leucoma is not vascularized. On the other hand if blood vessels are present, then the colouration disappears much more quickly.

Principle of tattooing—The hydrazine hydrate reduces the gold chloride or platinum chloride. The gold or platinum black are precipitated in the corneal tissue over which the epithelium grows. Gold produces a dark brown stain but with platinum a densely black plaque is formed. The metals are deposited in the corneal cells and between the lamellae. The epithelium is regenerated within 4 days.

2. If the leucoma is so situated that it hampers vision, then treatment becomes necessary for improvement of vision. This may be done in two ways—

(a) Keratoplasty or corneal graft—This is the ideal method, by which the opaque portion of the cornea is removed and a portion of clear cornea from a donor eye is replaced.

(b) Optical iridectomy—By this method the pupillary area is extended to the periphery by making a complete iridectomy. The site of election for optical iridectomy is downwards and inwards, provided clear cornea is available over that area ; otherwise it may be done on the temporal side, to increase the peripheral field of vision. By this method visual imporvement is not marked, as the vision is eccentric. The cosmetic treatment can follow optical iridectomy.

Adherent Leucoma

Definition—It means adhesion of a part of the iris to the leucoma.

Diagnostic criteria for adherent leucoma

(a) Presence of brown pigment in the leucoma (derived from iris pigment).

(b) Shallow anterior chamber around the iris adhesion.

(c) Pupil if visible may be seen drawn towards the adhesion.

Mechanism of formation of adherent leucoma

(a) Perforating corneal ulcer.

(b) Perforating injury to the cornea—however a tiny perforating injury exactly at the centre of the cornea, may not produce adherent leucoma, as there is no iris exactly opposite the site of the injury.

(c) Operating wound of the cornea.

Complication of adherent leucoma

Secondary glaucoma due to shallow anterior chamber.

Treatment of adherent leucoma

The treatment is the same as for leucoma but in addition, synechtomy has to be done, i.e., the adhesion of the iris to the cornea must be separated, to prevent occurrence of secondary glaucoma.

Hypopyon Ulcer of Cornea or Ulcus Serpens

It occurs commonly in the old, debilitated or the alcoholics. *Causative agent*—Pneumococcus in most of the cases. Source is the associated chronic dacryocystitis.

Clinical sings

(a) Greyish white, small, disc shaped ulcer near the centre of the cornea (Fig. 55).

(b) The ulcer spreads at one sector with a crescentic edge, then stops after a time and again spreads in another sector—thus producing a serpiginous character.

(c) Associated violent iritis and hypopyon formation.

(d) Marked ciliary congestion.

(e) Oedema of the lids.

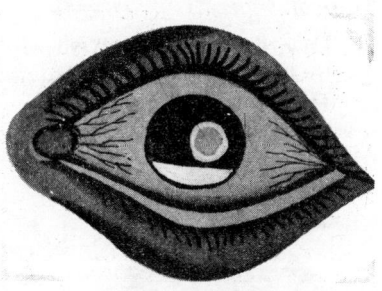

FIG. 55. Hypopyon ulcer of cornea or ulcus serpens

Symptoms

Same as for ordinary corneal ulcer but more marked.

N.B.—Any corneal ulcer may be associated with hypopyon. But a corneal ulcer with hypopyon is not equivalent to hypopyon corneal ulcer. Only when the clinical signs described above are present, the ulcer is called a hypopyon ulcer.

Course of a hypopyon ulcer—There is early tendency to perforation of the cornea and development of secondary glaucoma due to hypopyon.

Treatment : Atropine 1% drop thrice daily
Antibiotic like gentamycin drop 2 hourly
Analgesic like A.P.C. tablets twice daily.

This should be supplemented with carbolisation of ulcer and subconjuctival injection of gentamycin.

For secondary glaucoma diamox 250 mgm thrice daily.
If the lacrimal sac is blocked either syringing of sac with Penicillin solution or better dacryocystectomy is done forthwith.
Hypopyon is sterile so paracentesis is kept in abeyance.

Mycotic Ulcer
(Due to fungus infection)

Causative agents—Fungus aspergillus fumigatus,candida albicans and streptothrix actionomycosis etc.
Mode of infection—Contamination from earth or plant.
Incidence of fungi infection has increased due to indiscriminate use of antibiotic and steroid.

Clinical signs

(a) Dry, circular, yellowish white disc on the cornea, surrounded by a yellow gutter of demarcation (Fig.55a).
(b) Hypopyon formation.
(c) Ciliary congestion.
(d) Material scraped from the ulcer shows the presence of the fungus.

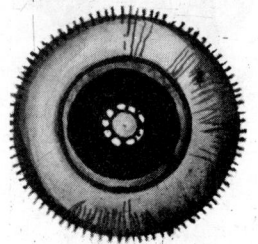

Symptoms—Same as for ordinary corneal ulcer.

After definite diagnosis has been established by microscopic examination of the scraping from the ulcer, the following treatment has to be done—

Fig. 55a. Mycotic ulcer of cornea

1. Local treatment—
    (a) Mycostatin in the form of a suspension containing 25,000 units in 1 c.c. of isotonic saline should be dropped, 1 drop every 15 minutes during the day time and every 2 hours in the night.
    (b) *Or* Amphotrecin B in the form of a suspension containing 0.1 mgm. in 1 c.c. of distilled water should be dropped, 1 drop every half an hour.
    (c) Other usual treatment for corneal ulcer like application of atropine ointment and carbolisation should be done.

(d) Recently miconazole in oily base has shown promising result when dropped hourly.

2. Keratoplasty has been reported useful in desperate case.

Marginal Corneal Ulcer

Age incidence—Usually in old people affected by gout or some debilitating disease.

It also occurs as a complication of acute muco-purulent conjunctivitis.

Causative agent Usually Koch-Weeks bacillus, but sometimes Morax-Axenfeld diplobacillus.

Cinical signs

(a) The ulcer is situated in the cornea near the limbus.
(b) The ulcer is shallow, often multiple, with infiltration in the surrounding cornea.
(c) Vascularization of the cornea is common.
(d) The ulcer may heal rapidly but recurrence is common.

In serious cases, the ulcer may spread round the limbus to form a ring ulcer, followed by complete necrosis of the cornea.

Symptoms—Same as for ordinary corneal ulcer but the pain is more severe.

Treatment—Same as for ordinary corneal ulcer.

Dendritic Ulcer of Cornea

Definition—It is an ulcer with a branched appearance caused by virus of herpes simplex.

Etiology

1. *Age*—May occur in any age.
2. *Bilaterality*—Usually unilateral.
3. *Predisposing causes*—Febrile conditions like influenza, malaria or pneumonia.
4. *Exciting cause*—Herpes simplex virus which is identical to the virus of encephalitis lethargica.

Clinical signs

(a) Tiny vesicles appear at the terminations of the corneal nerves in the corneal epithelium, which soon rupture.
(b) Those areas stain with fluorescein.

(c) Vesicles soon coalesce and produce a star-shaped or a branched figure (Fig. 56).

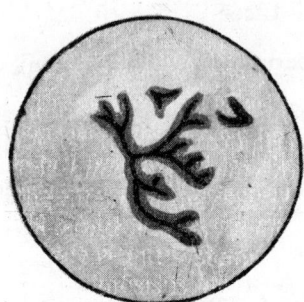

Fig. 56.   Dendritic ulcer.

(d) The attachment of the epithelium to the Bowman's membrane, close to the ulcer, becomes loose, and the epithelium can be easily removed. The phenomenon is known as epitheliolysis.
(e) Complete loss of corneal sensation as tested by a wisp of cotton wool.
(f) Ciliary congestion and lacrimation.

Symptoms—There is pain, watering and photophobia.

Course—If untreated, the condition lasts for months and invades the corneal stroma. The greater the loss of sensation, more is the time required for healing. Secondary infection may occur. Sometimes iritis develops which may be haemorrhagic.

Treatment

(a) To cauterize the ulcer and the surrounding epithelium with alcoholic solution of iodine with potassium iodide, (iodine 5 percent and potassium iodide 7 percent in alcoholic solution), with the tip of a sterile matchstick.
(b) After cautery, a drop of 4 percent cocaine hydrochloride solution is instilled, to form cocaine iodate which fixes the iodine.
(c) Application of atropine and chloromycetin ointment.
(d) The affected eye to be bandaged with pad.
(e) The treatment may have to be repeated and the eye must be kept bandaged so long the ulcer does not heal.
(f) Proflavine photoinactivation and Cryotherapy in obstinate cases.

Recent treatment

5-Iodo-2'-deoxyuridine (I.D.U.) is used as 0.1 percent solution every one hour in the day time and every 2 hours at the night time and 0.5 percent ointment at bed time for 7 days. This chemical is non-toxic to ordinary tissues. Competing with thymidine it attaches itself to DNA of the cell and thus renders the cell unsuitable for viral replication. As the drug is antimitotic so its use for more than 10 days hampers healing. Cytosine arabinoside HCl (CA), Adenine arabinoside (Ara-A) and trifluorothymidine (F_3T) are few other recent drugs.

Lagophthalmic Ulcer

Causes—This type of corneal ulcer develops, when the cornea cannot be properly covered by the eyelids, particularly during sleep. This failure to close the eyelids may be due to—
1. Serious illness producing coma vigil.
2. Paralysis of orbicularis muscle as in facial palsy.
3. Protrusion forwards of the eyeball as in proptosis.
4. Ectropion or retraction of the lids due to disease or injury.

Clinical signs and symptoms—Same as for an ordinary ulcer. The ulcer is usually located at the lower part of the cornea near the limbus, which remains exposed during sleep.

Treatment
   (a) Treatment is like that for ordinary ulcer.
   (b) Surgical operation on the eyelid like tarsorrhaphy to cover the cornea.

Neurotrophic Ulcer

It occurs as a result of defect in the sensory nerve supply of the cornea. This defect may be due to the following causes—
   (a) Injection of alcohol into the Gasserian ganglion to cure trigeminal neuralgia.
   (b) A neoplasm pressing on the Gasserian ganglion.

Clinical signs and symptoms

   (a) Oedema of corneal epithelium, which exfoliates to form an ulcer.
   (b) Ciliary congestion.
   (c) Complete loss of corneal sensation.
   (d) No pain or lacrimation, but defective vision.

Cause of the ulceration—Trophic disturbance due to loss of function of the sensory nerves.

Treatment— Tarsorrhaphy kept till the ulcer heals.

Phlyctenular Keratitis and Ulcer

Etiology
   1. Age—usually children.

2. Causative factor—Allergic reaction of the cornea to some endogenous toxin, which is bacterial in origin, usually tubercular.

Pathology—There is localized lymphocytic infiltration of the cornea which may break to form an ulcer.

Clinical signs

(a) Whitish nodule or ulcer in any part of the cornea, but usually near the limbus.
(b) Ciliary congestion and lacrimation.
(c) Marked blepharospasm

Symptoms—Pain, watering and photophobia.

Phlyctenular affection of the cornea may have the following manifestations—

1. Phlyctenular keratitis—when there is only nodular infiltration

2. Phlyctenular ulcer—when the nodule breaks.

3. Fascicular ulcer—a phlycten migrates from the limbus towards the centre of the cornea and carries a leash of blood vessels with it from the limbus (Fig. 57).

4. Phlyctenular pannus—when the cornea becomes vascularized from all the sides (Fig. 58).

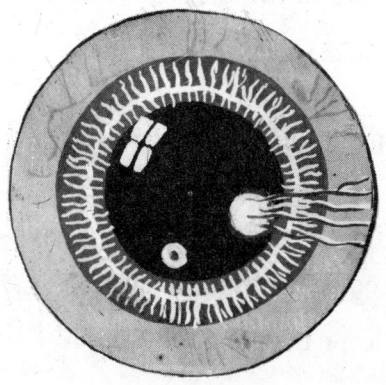

Fig. 57. Fascicular ulcer

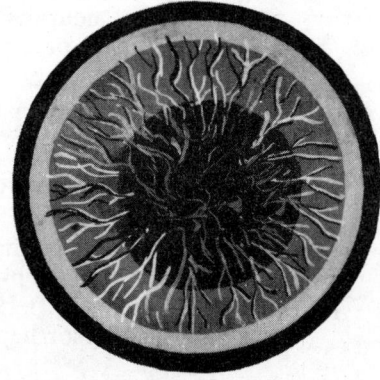

Fig. 58. Phlyctenular pannus

Complications—A phlyctenular ulcer may perforate and may have all the complications associated with perforation of an ordinary corneal ulcer. Secondary infection is common.

Treatment

1. Local—
    (a) Atropine ointment 1 percent twice daily.
    (b) Hydrocortisone acetate 1 percent solution to be dropped every 2 hours.
    (c) Broad spectrum antibiotic ointment to prevent any secondary infection
    (d) Pad or dark glasses.
2. General—same as for phlyctenular conjunctivitis.

Atheromatous Ulcer

Definition—This is an ulcer, which develops in an old leucoma, undergoing degenerative changes. The scar, with the overlying epithelium, has a low resistance due to poor nourishment and easily gets infected and an ulcer develops. the ulcer is very resistant to treatment. Ideal treatment is lamellar keratoplasty.

Mooren's Ulcer

Etiology

1. Age—Elderly persons.
2. Actual cause is not known.

Clinical signs and symptoms

(a) Superficial ulcer starting at the corneal margin, (Fig. 59).
(b) It spreads gradually over the

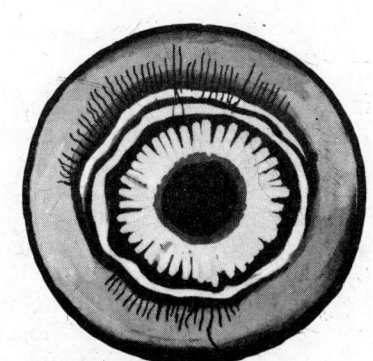

Fig. 59. Mooren's ulcer
(Duke-Elder)

whole of the cornea.

(c) At the advancing border, the ulcer undermines the epithelium and the superficial layers of the stroma forming an overhanging edge.

(d) Base of the ulcer soon becomes vasularized.

(e) Marked neuralgic pain with lacrimation and photophobia.

The ulcer never perforates the cornea.

Treatment

1. It is very unsatisfactory.

2. Ulcer may be cauterized with thermo-cautery and conjunctivoplasty may be done to cover the ulcer.

3. Beta-irradiation has also been advocated.

Keratitis

Definition—It means inflammation of the corneal tissue which may or may not form an ulcer.

Pathology—Infiltration of corneal tissue with inflammatory cells, oedema and necrosis of corneal lamellae and later on their replacement with ordinary fibrous tissue to form a leucoma.

Types of keratitis

1. Superficial—affecting the epithelium and superficial layers of stroma.

2. Deep—affecting the deeper layers of stroma.

1. Superficial Keratitis

A. Superficial punctate keratitis

It appears as punctate erosion in cornea.

Etiology

(a) Virus infection—by herpes smiplex, herpes zoster, TRIC and adeno-virus and viruses of measles, vaccinia and mumps.

(b) Following the infection of the lid with virus of molluscum contagiosum and warts.

(c) Kerato-conjunctivitis sicca—common in elderly persons.

(d) Exposure to ultra-violet rays.

Pathology

(a) Appearance of tiny infiltrates immediately underneath the corneal epithelium.

(b) Erosion of the epithelium over the infiltration and so the lesion stains with fluorescein.

Symptoms

(a) Marked discomfort.

(b) Marked lacrimation.

(c) Severe photophobia and blepharospasm.

Clinical signs

(a) Punctate erosions on cornea which stain with fluorescein. (Fig. 60).

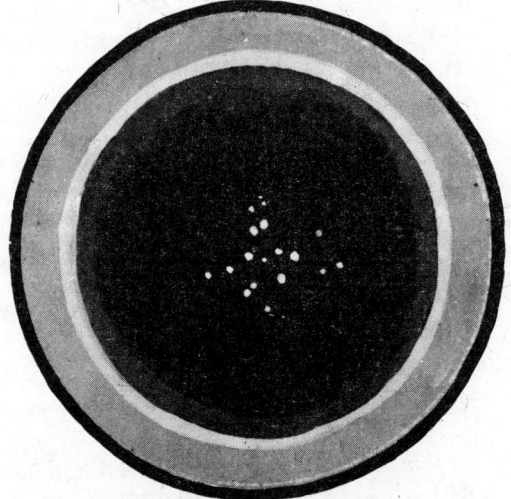

Fig. 60. Superficial punctate keratitis.

(b) Ciliary congestion.

(c) Enlargement of the pre-auricular gland, particularly when the infection is with adeno-virus.

Complications—If treated early, the lesions heal. But delay in treatment causes affection of the stroma, whereby punctate corneal opacities are left behind.

Treatment—

    (a) Atropine sulphate 1 percent ointment twice daily.
    (b) Chloromycetin eye ointment twice daily with pad and bandage.
    (c) Treatment of systemic condition in case of kerato-conjunctivitis sicca.
    (d) Local cortisone 1 percent drops if the lesions are due to ultra-violet rays.

B. Herpes Zoster Ophthalmicus

It may occur as—(a) Epidemic form or (b) Symptomatic form.

Epidemic form—

Etiology

    (a) Age—elderly persons, rarely under 40 years.
    (b) Sex—Equal in both sexes.
    (c) Causative agent—Virus identical with the virus of chicken-pox.

*Mechanism of spread of the disease—*The Gasserian ganglion is affected by the virus, causing the ganglion to be infalmed and infiltrated with lymphocytes. The virus then spreads mainly along the first division of the Vth nerve, causing affection of the supra-orbital and supratrochlear branches. The eye becomes affected if the nasociliary nerve becomes involved.

Symptoms and signs

    (a) Pre-herpetic neuralgic pain along the distribution of the 1st division of the Vth nerve, which may be severe, associated with mild fever and malaise.
    (b) This is followed within 2 to 3 days' time with appearance of vesicles on the skin of the forehead and scalp, surrounded by a zone of inflammation.
    (c) The vesicles suppurate and become cloudy and ultimately are converted into crusts, which, when fall off, leave scars behind.
    (d) The skin becomes markedly red and oedematous.

*Eye signs—*The eye becomes involved in half the number of cases on the same side. The signs are as follows—
    (a) Oedema of the lids.
    (b) Congestion of the conjunctiva.

    (c) Cornea may show—
- (i) Punctate keratitis which may ulcerate and be secondarily infected.
- (ii) Deep punctate keratitis known as keratitis profunda.
- (iii) Loss of corneal sensation.

    (d) Associated iritis which may be haemorrhagic causing hyphaema.

    (e) Low intra-ocular tension but secondary glaucoma may develop.

    (f) Nodules may appear on the sclera.

    (g) Sometimes paralysis of the 3rd, 6th or 7th nerve.

Course—The erruptive stage lasts for 3 weeks, followed by anaesthesia of the skin. But the neuralgic pain may persist for months.

Symptomatic form—

The cutaneous lesions are similar to those in the epidemic form. But, the cause of the lesions is the involvement of the Gasserian ganglion, by a malignant growth, gummatous meningitis or arsenic poisoning.

Treatment

    (a) Application of antibiotic ointment to the skin lesions to prevent secondary infection.

    (b) For relief of severe neuralgic pain, various drugs have been advocated, like injection of pitutrin or dihydro-ergotamine, but they are not effective in every case. Ordinary analgesics and sedatives may be tried.

    (c) Infection of herpes lysate, a sort of autovaccine from the fluid from the vesicles, twice a week, 6 such, is sometimes effective.

    (d) Local application of atropine ointment 1 percent, when the cornea is involved. Local cortico steroid settles the associated uveitis satisfactorily.

C. Rosacea Keratitis

It occurs usually in elderly women and is not common in this country. There are yellowish white infiltrates in the cornea, with small superficial ulcers. The cornea soon becomes vascularized.

The eye is very irritable with profuse lacrimation. Recurrences are common. Actual etiology is not known, but may be allergic in nature.

Treatment

Same as for phlyctenular keratitis.

2. Deep Keratitis

This may be of the following types—
A. Interstitial keratitis.
B. Disciform keratitis.
C. Keratitis profunda.
D. Intracorneal abscess.
E. Sclerosing keratitis.

A. Interstitial Keratitis

It is characterized by cellular infiltration of the deeper layers of the cornea followed by vascularization.

Causes

(i) Congenital or acquired syphilis.
(ii) Tuberculosis.
(iii) Leprosy.

1. *Intersitial keratitis due to congenital syphilis (is rather rare now a days.)*

It is the commonest type of interstitial keratitis.

(a) Age incidence—5 to 15 years.
(b) Eye affected—Usually both eyes are affected.
(c) Mechanism—This keratitis is an allergic manifestation as spirochoetes have never been detected in the cornea. The allergy is due to hypersensitiveness of the corneal tissue to products of disintegration of the spirochoetes, occuring somewhere in the body. The keratitis may be precipitated by trivial injuries, like a foreign body on the cornea or a discission operation for congential cataract.

Symptoms

(a) Pain in the eyes with intense photophobia and lacrimation.
(b) Marked visual loss.

Clincial signs

1. General signs—

    (a) Hutchinson's teeth and radiating scars at the angles of the mouth.

    (b) Prominent frontal eminences and depressed bridge of the nose.

    (c) Enlarged cervical glands.

2. Local signs—

    (a) Marked blepharospasm.

    (b) Ciliary congestion, aqueous flare and sometimes K.P. as the disease starts with uveitis.

    (c) Gradual appearance of more hazy patches and finally the whole of the cornea looks dull and lustureless known as 'ground-glass' cornea.

    (d) In the meantime deep vascularization of the cornea, by radial bundles of brush-like vessels, derived from the anterior ciliary arteries, takes place. The vessels appear as dull reddish patches known as 'salmon patches'.

All these changes take place within a period of 2 to 3 months.

Course—After the disease has reached its height, the cornea clears slowly from the margin towards the centre, which may remain hazy for a long time, but ultimately clears up, unless the disease is very severe. Blood vessels remain as fine reddish lines. The cornea never ulcerates.

Pathology—There is marked infiltration of the cornea with lymphocytes and oedema of both the epithelium and the endothelium. The infiltration is associated with deep vascularization but followed by lamellar necrosis. There is always pan uveitis.

Treatment

1. General—Antisyphilitic treatment with heavy doses of penicillin injection

2. Local—

    (a) Atropine ointment 1 percent twice daily.

    (b) Hydrocortisone acetate 1 percent drop every 2 hours.

II. Interstitial keratitis due to acquired syphilis

The affection is unilateral. The underlying pathology, symptoms and signs are the same as for the keratitis in congential syphilis.

III. Interstitial keratitis due to tuberculósis

The affection is usually unilateral and the lesion is limited to a sector of the cornea. The underlying pathological changes are similar to those due to syphilis.

IV. Interstitial keratitis due to leprosy

The affection may be unilateral or bilateral. There is infiltration of the deeper layers of the cornea, spreading from the periphery to the centre. The resulting opacity is dense and does not clear up easily.

B. Disciform Keratitis

This usually occurs in adults and the causative agent is herpes simplex virus. There is a greyish white disc shaped opacity in the central area of the cornea, affecting the deeper layers and marked swelling of the corneal stroma, so that the thickness of the cornea increases.

Symptoms and signs—Pain, watering, ciliary congestion and marked fall of vision. The corneal sensation may be markedly diminished.

Course—The condition lasts for months and the opacity may not disappear completely.

Pathology—The underlying pathology is marked swelling of the corneal lamellae with massive necrosis.

Treatment—It is not very satisfactory. Atropine ointment 1 percent twice daily and I.D.U. 1 percent drop every hour may be tried.

Note—The lesions produced by virus affections of the cornea are—

1. Superficial punctate keratitis.
2. Dendritic ulcer.
3. Disciform keratitis.
4. Punctate keratitis by herpes zoster virus.

C. Keratitis Profunda

It is a deep keratitis occurring in adults and usually one eye is affected. There is associated uveitis. The actual etiology is not known. The condition undergoes resolution within 3 to 4 weeks. The treatment is the same as that for interstitial keratitis. The usual signs of keratitis are present.

D. Intracorneal Abscess

It is due to purulent inflammation of the substance of the cornea. It usually occurs as a result of penetrating injury.

E. Sclerosing Keratitis

It occurs as a complication of scleritis. There is deep infiltration of the cornea, adjacent to the area of scleritis, by lymphocytes, followed by vascularization. The treatment is that for scleritis.

Degenerative Changes in the Cornea

1. *Arcus senilis*—It is seen in the aged persons. There is a greyish white circular line in the cornea, concentric with the limbus, but occurring just within the limbus, so that a clear area of cornea remains within the arcus and the limbus. The cause is lipoid degeneration of cornea, lipoid droplets being situated mainly in the substantia propria.

2. *Band-shaped degeneration*—This degenerative change is usually associated with long continued uveitis. The lesion appears as a band-shaped opacity, occurring horizontally in the interpalpebral fissure extending across the cornea. Histologically, there is deposition of lime salts and hyaline tissue, in or underneath the Bowman's membrane.

Corneal Dystrophies

1. *Endothelial dystrophy of Fuchs*—It occurs in aged persons. There are degenerative changes in the endothelium, followed by corneal opacity.

2. *Hereditary dystrophies*—They may be granular, nodular, macular or latticelike in appearance, usually affecting the central part of the cornea. All are familial and hereditary. Keratoplasty is the choice of treatment.

Keratoconus

(Conical cornea)

It is due to congenital weakness of the cornea and the cornea becomes cone shaped (Fig. 61).

It manifests itself usually in girls after puberty. There is visual impairment, as the central part of the eye becomes myopic due to bulging of the cornea. Sometimes it pulsates synchronously with the arterial pulse and this

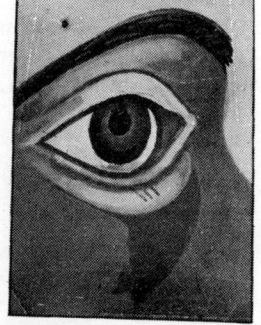

Fig. 61. Keratoconus.

may cause a subjective apparent pulsation of external objects. But the refractive error cannot be corrected by ordinary spectacle lenses. Contact lens improves vision markedly.

Megalocornea
(Keratoglobus)

The diameter of the cornea becomes bigger than normal. While the normal diameter is 12 to 13 mm., in megalocornea this becomes about 16 mm.

But the cornea remains clear and there is no rise of intraocular tension and optic disc is normal. There are differentiating points from buphthalmos (see under buphthalmos). The condition is familial and hereditary occurrring bilaterally in males.

Pigmentation of the Cornea

1. Argyrosis—Dark brown colouration due to prolonged use of silver preparation like silver nitrate, argyrol or protargol.

2. Grey-green or golden brown colour in cornea in the form of a ring, known as Kayser-Fleischer ring—It is seen in hepato-lenticular degeneration and is due to deposit of copper. The Descemet's membrane is affected.

3. Blood staining of the cornea—It is associated with severe hyphaema and rise of intra-ocular tension.

4. Deposition of melanin pigment—Usually on the posterior surface of the cornea in high myopia and diabetes.

Tumours of the Cornea

Apart from dermoid tumours of the cornea, other tumours are usually due to extensions from the limbus, such as a papilloma melanoma or epithelioma. Bowens intra-epithelial epithelioma is also included though rare.

CHAPTER VI

ANATOMY AND DISEASES OF THE SCLERA

Anatomy

The sclera constitutes the outer coat of the eye. It is opaque, about 1 mm. thick, and rigid, and white in appearance. It is made of bundles of collagenous fibrils, with connective tissue corpuscles. It is covered by Tenon's capsule and episcleral tissue. The four rectus muscles are inserted to the sclera, in front of the equator and the two oblique muscles are inserted behind the equator of the eyeball. The sclera is perforated by many vessels and nerves, the biggest vessels being four vortex veins. The inner surface of the sclera is separated from the choroid, by a potential space, called suprachoroidea.

Inflammation of the Sclera

Two types of inflammation—
1. Superficial—Episcleritis.
2. Deep—Scleritis.

1. Episcleritis

Definition—It is the inflammation of the subconjunctival episcleral tissue, along with the superficial lamellae of the sclera.

Etiology

(a) Occurs in elderly persons.
(b) Associated with rheumatism or gout.
(c) As an allergic reaction to an endogenous toxin, tubercular or streptococcal, from a septic focus.
(d) Collagen disorder.

Symptoms

(a) Pain and tenderness in the eye with ocular discomfort.
(b) No discharge, lacrimation or photophobia.

Clinical signs

(a) A hard, pinkish red nodule, of the size of a lentil,

appears underneath the conjunctiva, 2-3 mm. away from the limbus.

(b) The nodule is fixed to the deeper structures, tender to the touch, and never ulcerates.

(c) Hyperaemia of the surrounding conjunctiva (coloured plate).

Pathology—The nodule consists of an aggregation of lymphocytes in the episcleral tissue.

Complications—The lesion may extend into the deeper layers of the sclera, causing scleritis and uveitis.

TABLE VI
Differential diagnosis of episcleritis

	Episcleritis	Phlycten	Inflamed Pinguecula
1. Age	1. Elderly person.	1. Young person.	1. Elderly person.
2. Location	2. Away from the limbus.	2. Usually on the limbus.	2. Away from the limbus in the horizontal meridian.
3. Tenderness	3. Present.	3. Nil	3. Present.
4. Ulceration	4. Nil	4. Ulcerates.	4. Nil.
5. Appearance	5. Pinkish red.	5. Pinikish white.	5. Pinikish white.

Treatment

1. Local—
   (a) Hydrocortisone acetate 1 percent drop 2 hourly or sub-conjunctival injection of half c.c. of hydrocortisone once a week.
   (b) Local heat.
2. General treatement of more value than local treatment
   (a) Elimination of septic focus or tubercular focus.
   (b) Salicylates by mouth, sometimes suganril by month.

2. Scleritis

Definition—It means inflammation of the sclera.

Occurence—It is usually bilateral and women are more frequently affected than men.

Etiology—

(a) Toxic and allergic influences are the commonest

PLATE VIII

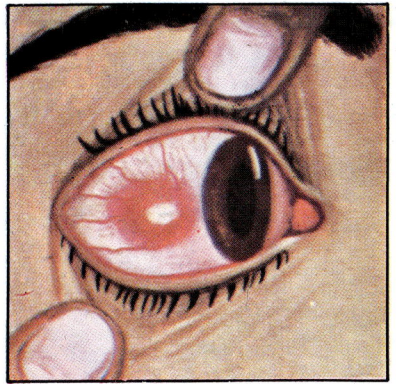

Fig. 1
Episcleritis (Parsons)

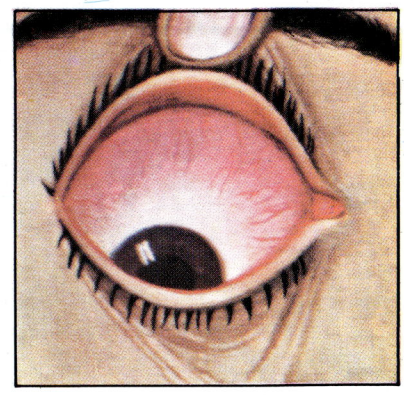

Fig. 2
Scleritis (Parsons)

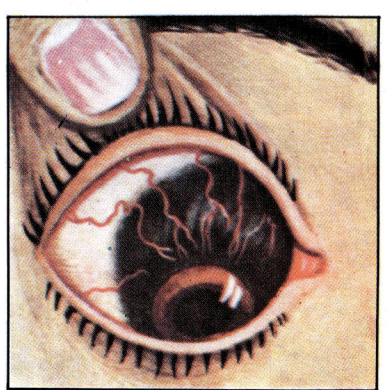

Fig. 3
Ciliary Staphyloma
(Parsons)

(To face page 114)

causes. There may be allergy to tuberculo-protein, becterial allergy and bacterial toxins from septic teeth and tonsils and allergic state in serum sickness and all of them may cause scleritis.

  (b) Endogenous infections as for example acute suppura-tive metastatic lesions, tuberculosis, syphilis, leprosy and viral infections may cause scleritis.

  (c) Secondary infections from the peri-ocular or intra-ocular tissues may affect the sclera.

  (d) Exogenous infection through the conjunctiva as a result of ulceration or injury of the latter structure may also precipitate scleritis.

  (e) Systemic and metabolic disturbances like rheumatoid arthritis or gout are frequently causes of scleritis.

Pathology—The inflammation is much more severe than episcleritis. There is marked infiltration of the scleral lamellae with lymphocytes and necrosis of the scleral fibres, with ultimate thinning of the sclera.

Symptoms

  (a) Marked pain in the eye, which may radiate to the frontal region.

  (b) Lacrimation but no discharge.

Clinical signs

  (a) Usually the anterior part of the sclera is affected in one sector.

  (b) Pinkish red area appears with hyperaemia of the surrounding conjunctiva.

  (c) The patch of scleritis is slightly elevated and markedly tender, when pressure is applied on it over the lid.

Course—Usually prolonged course.

Complications

  (a) The inflammation may spread into cornea in the form of a tongue-shaped opacity.

  (b) Associated uveitis is common in the form of iritis, iridocyclitis or anterior choroiditis.

  (c) Thinning of the sclera causes bulging of the uveal tract, known as staphyloma—usually ciliary staphyloma, which may lead to secondary glaucoma.

Treatment—Same as for episcleritis. Analgesics may have to be used frequently.

Staphyloma

Definition—It is the ectasia or bulging of the wall of the eyeball along with uveal tissue.

Types of staphyloma

1. Anterior staphyloma—as a result of sloughing of corneal ulcer.

2. Ciliary-staphyloma—due to bulging of the ciliary body due to thinning of the sclera, as a result of scleritis or injury to the sclera. This occurs in the area, extending upto 8 mm. from the limbus. It is bluish in colour and irregular in appearance.

3.Intercalary staphyloma—occurs at the limbus immediately in front of the ciliary body. Etiology is the same as for ciliary staphyloma.

4. Equatorial staphyloma—occurs at the regions of sclera which are perforated by vortex veins and also at the equatorial region of sclera.

5. Posterior staphyloma—occurs in high myopia due to bulging out of the sclera at the posterior pole of the eyeball.

CHAPTER VII

ANTERIOR CHAMBER OF THE EYE

Boundaries of the anterior chamber

(a) Anteriorly—The endothelial layer of the cornea.

(b) Posteriorly—(i) At the angle by a part of the ciliary body. (ii) The whole of the iris. (iii) The lens in the pupillary aperture.

Normal depth of the anterior chamber—about 2.5 mm. in the central part.

The important structures at the angle of the anterior chamber are the following (Fig. 62)—

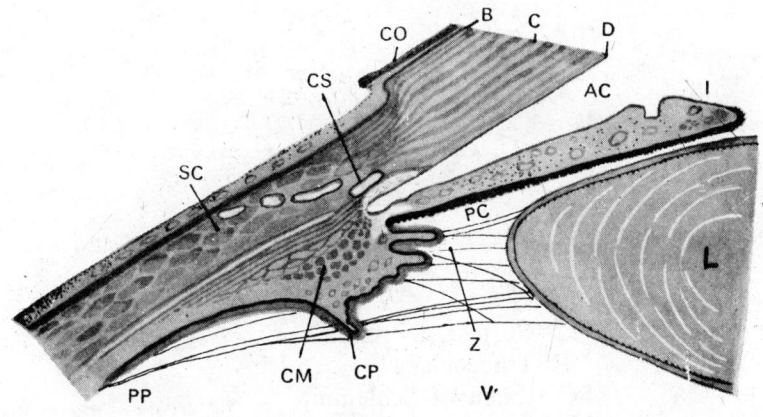

Fig. 62. Section through the anterior segment of the eye.

CO=Conjunctiva,
  B=Bowman's membrane,
  C=Cornea,
  D=Descemet's membrane
    with endothelium,
AC=anterior chamber.
  I=Iris, L=Lens,
  V=Vitreous,

PC=Posterior chamber.
  Z=Zonule
Cp=Ciliary process,
CM=Ciliary muscle,
CS=Canal of Schlemm,
SC=Sclera.
PP=Pars plana of ciliary body.

1. Trabeculae—A loose network of tissues at the extreme periphery of the anterior chamber and on the inner side of the canal of Schlemm (CS). They are continuous with the Descemet's membrane and the corneal endothelium. The spaces within the network are known as the spaces of Fontanna.

2. Canal of Schlemm—A circular sinus, normally containing aqueous humour, situated within the substance of the sclera just outside the trabeculae.

3. Aqueous veins—These are efferent channels from the canal of Schlemm, carrying in normal condition aqueous and draining into the intrascleral or episcleral venous plexus (Fig. 63).

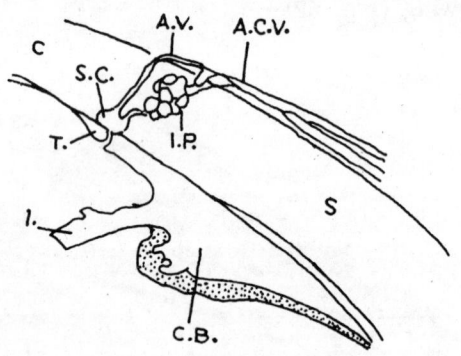

Fig. 63.   Aqueous vein.

C=Cornea, S=sclera,
T=Trabeculae,
SC=Canal of Schlemm,
AV=Aqueous vein,
IP=Intrascleral plexus of veins,
ACV=Anterior ciliary veins forming
episcleral venous plexus.
I=Iris,
C.B.=Ciliary body.

4. Scleral spur—This is a circular, condensed portion of the sclera, postero-medial to the canal of Schlemm, which gives origin to the ciliary muscle.

5. Ciliary muscle—Originating from the scleral spur, it is inserted to the choroid.

Posterior Chamber

This is a triangular space between the iris in front and the lens behind (Fig. 62).

The boundaries of the posterior chamber are—(a) Anteriorly—Iris. (b) Posteriorly—The lens and the suspensory ligament. (c) Laterally—The ciliary body.

Aqueous Humour

Normally the anterior and the posterior chamber are filled with a fluid called the aqueous humour.

Nature of the aqueous humour—It is a slightly alkaline, clear, watery fluid with a density slighty higher than water. The volume of the aqueous in the anterior chamber is about 0.25 c.c., whereas that in the posterior chamber is about 0.06 c.c.

Constituents of the aqueous humour—It consists mainly of water and also of minute traces of all the diffusible constituents of the plasma. The protein content is negligible. But the sodium and the ascorbic acid are in a higher concentration than in plasma.

Source of the aqueous humour—The chief source is from the ciliary processes of the ciliary body and a very minute quantity from the vessels of the iris.

Mechanism of formation of the aqueous—The exact mechanism is not known. But the present concept is that the aqueous is formed partly as a result of ultra-filtration through the capillary walls *i.e.,* filtration under pressure and partly as a result of secretion by the ciliary processes, the latter process being more important. The mechanism, of secretion also explains higher sodium and ascorbic acid content in the aqueous.

Functions of the aqueous humour—It maintains the nutrition of the avascular structures like the cornea and the lens and also carries away their waste products. Also the clear aqueous in the anterior chamber takes part in the refraction of the light rays. But the more important function is that it helps to maintain a constant intra-ocular pressure.

Rate of flow of aqueous humour—Depending upon the technique employed the rate of flow of the aqueous humour has been found to vary from 1 to 5 cu. mm. per minute.

Movements of the aqueous humour—There are two movements of aqueous humour—

(i) thermal circulation, and (ii) bulk-flow.

(a) *Thermal circulation*—Normally there is a difference of temperature between the cornea which is cooled by the air and the vascularized iris which is heated by the blood. This difference of temperature is about 3 to 5° C. As a result of this difference of temperature a convection current is set up in the aqueous of the anterior chamber causing a constant flow of the aqueous upwards in the region of the iris and downwards in the region of the cornea. This move- ment is known as the thermal circulation.

(b) *Bulk-flow—This type of circulation of the aqueous occurs in the following manner.*

Circulation of aqueous humour

Originated by ciliary body→posterior chamber→through pupil into the anterior chamber→through spaces of Fontanna in the trabeculae at the angle of the anterior chamber to the afferent channels of the canal of Schlemm→canal of Schlemm→efferent channels (aqueous veins)→intrascleral and episcleral plexus of veins.

Causes of deep anterior chamber

    (a) Aphakia.
    (b) Posterior subluxation of the lens.
    (c) Partially absorbed traumatic cataract. ·
    (d) Keratoconus.
    (e) Buphthalmos.

Causes of shallow anterior chamber

    (a) Closed-angle glaucoma.
    (b) Intumescence of the lens in the stage of immature or mature cataract.
    (c) Anterior dislocation of the lens.
    (d) Adherent leucoma
    (e) Iris bombé.
    (f) Delayed formation of the anterior chamber, after cataract extraction or glaucoma operation.

Normal content of the anterior chamber—A clear fluid known as aqueous humour, containing minute traces of all the diffusible constituents of plasma.

Abnormal substances in the anterior chamber

(a) Blood—Hyphaema.
(b) Exudate—Hypopyon.
(c) Lens matter—As following discission operation or after extra-capsular extraction of the lens.
(d) The entire lens—Dislocation of the lens in the anterior chamber.
(e) Nucleus of a cataractous lens due to bursting of a Morgagnian cataract.
(f) Vitreous—When there is vitreous loss during cataract operation.
(g) Air bubble—Introduced in the anterior chamber, when there is delay in formation of the chamber.
(h) Parasites.
(i) Foreign body.
(j) Tumour cells, particularly from a retinoblastoma.

Blood-aqueous barrier

It is a hypothetical barrier which exists between the blood and the aqueous and prevents free entry of substances from the blood into the aqueous and thereby maintains the difference in the composition of the two fluids. This barrier does not correspond to a single anatomical entity. As for instance in the ciliary processes the fluid has to pass through not only the capillary walls but also the two layers of the ciliary epithelium before reaching the posterior chamber, whereas on the anterior surface of the iris the barrier is only the capillary endothelium. In the posterior segment the blood aqueous barrier is formed by the retina.

Plasmoid aqueous

It means plasma-like aqueous or in other words when the composition of the aqueous resembles more or less that of plasma, particularly regarding the protein content. This condition occurs when there is breakdown of the blood-aqueous barrier and free entry of proteins into the aqueous occurs. This phenomenon takes place after paracentesis and in uveitis—both the conditions causing capillary dialatation and increased permeability of the capillary wall. If the breakdown of the barrier is complete as following a severe trauma, whole blood escapes into the anterior chamber.

CHAPTER VIII

ANATOMY AND DISEASES OF THE UVEAL TRACT

From before backwards the uveal tract is as follows :—
(a) The Iris.
(b) The ciliary body.
(c) The choroid.

Anatomically they are continuous and so disease of one part may spread to the other. The uveal tract is markedly vascular.

Anatomy of the iris—The iris is a coloured membrane hanging in front of the lens. In the periphery, it is attached to the ciliary body and centrally it ends at the pupillary margin. Anteriorly it is lined by a layer of endothelium. Underneath the endothelium is the iris stroma, consisting of spongy connective tissue, pigment containing chromatophores, vessels, nerves and two muscles—sphincter and dilator pupillae.

Posteriorly, the iris is lined by two layers of pigment epithelium. The anterior surface of the iris is uneven, and shows many crypts and fissures. The sphincter muscle is made of circular fibres close to the pupillary margin and is supplied by the 3rd nerve. The dilator muscle consists of radial fibres, extending from the ciliary body to the pupillary margin and is supplied by the cervical sympathetic. The preganglionic fibres arising from C_8, T_1, T_2, T_3 level and enter the corresponding sympathetic gangila terminating in Sup. Cervical ganglion. Then the post ganglionic fibres pass around the Internal Carotid artery→ ophthalmic division of Vth→ Nasociliary branch→long ciliary nerve →dilator Pupillae. The blood vessels are tortuous and arranged in a radial manner. The anterial supply is derived from the greater circle of the iris.

Pupil

The pupil is the circular aperture in the centre of the iris. The margin of the pupil rests on the anterior capsule of the lens. The pupillary aperture is controlled by the action of the dilator and the sphincter muscle. The normal size of the pupil is 3 to 4 mm. in diameter.

Pupillary reflexes

1. Light reflex—

    (a) Direct—the pupil contracts, as soon as light enters into the eye.

(b) Consensual—the pupil contracts, when light enters into the opposite eye.

The path of light reflex (fig. 64)

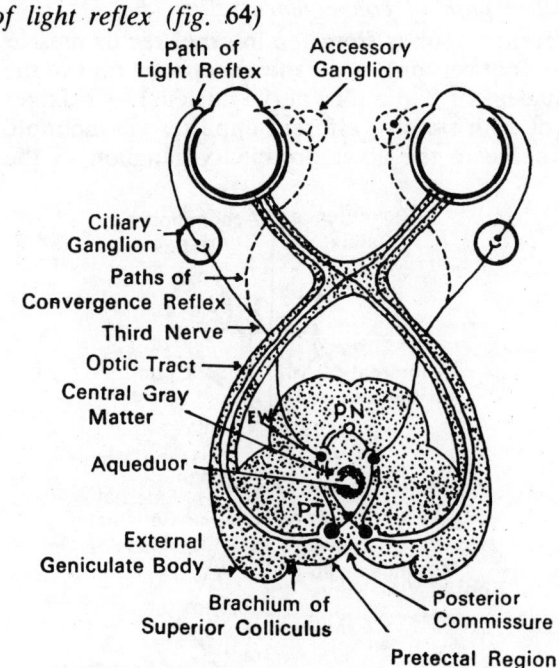

Fig 64. Pupillary pathways for light reflex
P.N.=Nucleus of Perlia
E.W.=Edinger-Westphal nucleus,
P.T.=Pretectal-nucleus

Afferent impulses from retina along the optic nerve → optic tract → pretectal nucleus in the midbrain → Edinger-Westphal nucleus of both sides → efferent impulses via the 3rd nerve → the inferior division of the 3rd nerve → the branch of 3rd nerve to the inferior oblique muscle → the short root of the ciliary ganglion → the ciliary ganglion → short ciliary nerves → the sphincter pupillae. (Parsons).

2. *Near reflex*—the pupil contracts on looking at a near object. It has two components—

(a) Convergence reflex. *i.e.*, contraction of the pupil on convergence.

(b) Accommodation reflex. *i.e.*, contraction of the pupil on accommodation.

(a) The path of convergence reflex (Fig. 65).

Afferent impulses from the internal rectus muscle along the 3rd nerve (not certain) → the mesencephalic root of the 5th nerve → the nucleus of Perlia (3rd nerve nucleus) → Edinger-Westphal nucleus of both sides → efferent impulses via the motor fibres of the 3rd nerve to the accessory ciliary ganglion → the sphincter pupillae.

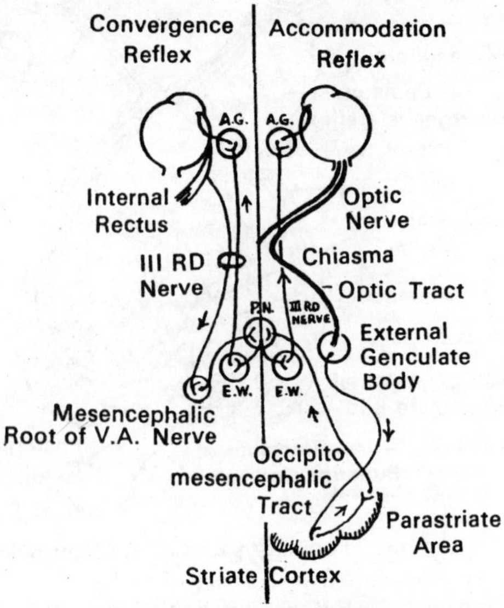

Fig. 65.   Pupillary pathways for convergence and accommodation reflexes. (Parsons)
          P.N.=Perlia's nucleus,
          E.W.=Edinger-Westphal nucleus,
          A.G.=Accessory ciliary ganglion.

(b) The path of accommodation reflex (Fig. 65).

Afferent impulses from retina along the optic nerve and tract → lateral geniculate body → along the optic radiations → striate cortex of the occipital lobe → parastriate area → along the occipito-mesencephalic tract → nucleus of Perlia → Edinger-Westphal nucleus of both sides → efferent impulses along the 3rd nerve → accessory ciliary ganglion → sphincter pupillae and ciliary muscle.

3. *Psycho-sensory reflex*—The pupil dilates due to psychic and sensory stimuli.

Functions of the pupil

1. By altering its size the pupil either allows entry of more light in darkness or prevents entry of excess of light in sunshine.
2. It prevents spherical aberration by allowing only the rays of light to enter into the eye through the central part of the lens.
3. In a similar way it prevents chromatic aberration.
4. By marked constriction the pupil may convert the eye to a pin-hole camera and thus visual improvement may be attained in spite of presence of errors of refraction.
5. By constriction, the pupil can increase the depth of focus. The depth of focus is the greatest distance through which an object point can be moved and still produce an image which falls on one retinal cone only.

Some clinical conditions of the pupil

1. Argyll-Robertson Pupil

Clinical signs—

(a) Total absence of the reaction of the pupil to light.
(b) Reactions of the pupil to convergence and accommodation are present.
(c) The pupil is constricted but may be irregular and eccentric.
(d) Patches of atrophy and depigmentation may be present in the iris.
(e) Eserine diminishes the size of the pupil but atropine dilates the pupil imperfectly.
(f) The condition is usually bilateral but may be unilateral.

Etiology and site of lesion—

Argyee Robertson pupil is a manifestation of neurosyphilis. The most probable site of lesion is in the midbrain in the nerve path connecting the pretectal nucleus with the Edinger-Westphal nucleus of both the sides (Fig. 64).

2. Inverse Argyll -Robertson Pupil

Clinical sign—The pupillary reflex to accommodation and convergence is lost but the reflex to light is retained. It is usually bilateral.

Site of lesion and etiology—

The site of lesion is in the midbrain affecting the connections of the convergence centre with the constrictor centre of the pupil *i.e.*, the connections between the nucleus of Perlia and the Edinger-Westphal nucleus (Fig. 64). This condition has been observed in diphtheria and in tumours near the corpora quadrigemina.

3. Myotonic Pupil

Clinical signs—

(a) The affected pupil is moderately dilated and the condition is usually unilateral.

(b) The reactions to light in the affected eye, both direct and consensual, are delayed, slight or absent.

(c) On convergence the constriction of the pupil may appear to be completely absent. But after prolonged near fixation, a constriction may appear and develop slowly.

(d) Reactions to atropine, homatropine, eserine and pilocarpine are normal.

(e) Knee-jerks and the ankle-jerks may or may not be absent.

(f) The condition once developed is permanent.

Etiology and site of lesion

(a) Onset is usually sudden and the age is usually the third decade.

(b) Females are more affected than the males.

(c) Site of lesion is not definitely known.

4. Hutchinson's Pupil

Clinical signs—

(a) It develops shortly after the head injury.

(b) There is widely dilated immobile pupil on the same side

as the head injury. Both the direct and the consensual reflexes to light are lost.

Etiology and site of lesion—

(a) Hutchinson's pupil is diagnostic of fractured skull with meningeal haemorrhage.

(b) Due to haemorrhage there is gross cerebral shift and herniation of the temporal lobe of the brain into the tentorial hiatus. The result is the stretching of the third nerve of the same side, whereby the pupillomotor fibres are affected first before the evidence of the third nerve palsy sets in.

Unilateral dilatation of the pupil

Causes

1. Action of mydriatic drugs—
   (a) Parasympathetic blocking agents e.g. atropine, homatropine, cyclopentolate.
   (b) Sympathetic stimulating agents e.g. cocaine, adrenaline, phenylephrine.
2. Ocular causes—

   (a) Acute congestive glaucoma.
   (b) Atrophy of the iris.
   (c) Trauma to the eyeball.
   (d) Myotonic pupil.

3. Lesion in the afferent pathway for light reflex—optic atrophy.
   4. Lesions in the efferent pathway for light reflex—
   (a) Lesions in the mid-brain affecting the 3rd nerve nucleus.
   (b) Any lesion anywhere along the course of the 3rd nerve.
5. Irritation of the cervical sympathetic pathway by neoplasm, tubercular glands, mediastinal tumour or cervical rib (Claude Bernard's syndrome).
   6. Central lesions—
   (a) Neoplasms of the cerebral cortex
   (b) Head injury (Hutchinson's pupil).

Unilateral constriction of the pupil

Causes

1. Action of miotic drugs—

(a) Parasympathetic stimulating agents e.g. eserine, pilo-carpine.

(b) Sympathetic depressants e.g. ergotamine, ergotoxine.

2. Ocular causes—

(a) Acute iritis.

(b) Injury to the eyeball.

(c) Sudden fall in tension as for example after paracentesis or after making section for cataract operation.

3. Irritative lesion of the efferent pathway—

(a) Lesion in the 3rd nerve nucleus e.g. pontine haemor-rhage.

(b) Irritative lesion anywhere along the course of the 3rd nerve.

4. Paralytic lesion of the cervical sympathetic (Horner's syndrome).

5. Central lesions—

(a) Argyll Robertson pupil.

(b) Lesion of the cropus striatum e.g. parkinsonism.

Bilateral dilatation of pupils

Causes

1 Internal administration of drugs like belladonna or hyos-cine.

2. As a·complication of diphtheria.

3. In severe anaemia and in thyrotoxicosis.

4. In n yopia.

5. Very deep general anaesthesia.

6. Bilateral optic atrophy.

7. After death.

Bilateral constriction of pupils·

Causes

1. Internal administration of drugs like opium and morphine.

2. Irritative supra-nuclear lesion, e.g., tumour of the pineal body.

3. Bilateral iritis.

4. In children and elderly persons.

5. In˙ hypermetropia.

6. During deep sleep.

Anatomy of the ciliary body

It is triangular in cross section, with its base directed anteriorly, which gives attachement to the root of the iris and the apex is continuous with the anterior choroid. The ciliary body extends upto a distance of 8 mm. from the limbus all round the wall of the eyeball. The main constituent cf the cilary body is the ciliary musole, consisting of three types of muscle fibres— meridional, radial and circualr. This muscle originates from the scleral spur and is inserted into the anterior choroid. The outer surface of the ciliary body is separated from the sclera, by a potential space known as the suprachoroidea. The anterior half of the inner surface shows folds, known as ciliary processes and the posterior half is plain. The inner surface is covered by two layers of cubical epithelium—the superficial layer being non-pigmented and the deeper one being pigmented.

Blood supply

The ciliary body is highly vascular. The blood supply is derived from the anterior and the long posterior ciliary arteries.

Nerve supply

The sensory supply is derived from the trigeminal, through the ciliary nerve. The motor nerve supply to the ciliary muscle is by the 3rd nerve.

Mechanism of accommodation

Contraction of the ciliary muscle → slight forward movement of the ciliary body → the suspensory ligament becomes loose → bulging of the anterior surface of the lens and increased converging power of the lens. Because of the vitreous, the posterior surface of the lens cannot bulge backwards. But there is no difficulty in bulging of the anterior lens surface, as some amount of the aqueous is pushed out through the canal of Schlemm.

Inflammation of the Uveal Tract
(Iritis and iridocyclitis)

As iris and ciliary body are continuous, iritis seldom occurs without some inflammation of the ciliary body and cyclitis seldom occurs without iritis. The terms iritis and cyclitis are used, depending on which structure is clinically more affected. The term iridocyclitis is used when both the components are prominent. These lesions may also be associated with anterior choroiditis.

Etiological factors for iritis and iridocyclitis

1. Exogenous infection, *e.g.*, a penetrating injury.

2. Local causes *e.g.* trauma, corneal ulcer, scleritis, herpetic infection, intra-ocular malignant tumour, sympathetic ophthalmia, orbital cellulitis etc.

3. Non-specific causes due to allergy *e.g.*,
    (a) Bacterial allergy from a septic focus.
    (b) Tubercular allergy.
    (c) Syphilitic allergy as in association with interstitial keratitis.

4. Specific causes, *e.g.*, tuberculosis, syphilis, gonorrhoea, virus infection, protozoal infection like toxoplasmosis.

5. Systemic causes, *e.g.*, Still's disease, rheumatism and gout, diabetes mellitus, sarcoidosis, ankylosing spondylitis, septicaemic condition.

6. Age and Sex—may occur in any age and equally in both the sexes.

Pathology of iritis and iridocyclitis

Both the iris and the ciliary body are highly vascular structures and so an inflammation of these structures leads to congestion of blood vessels and exudation of fibrin-rich fluid and inflammatory cells in the tissues. The nature of the inflammatory cells depends on the etiology. Polymorphs predominate in cases of exogenous infection, lymphocytes in allergic and non-specific cases, and mononuclear cells in granulomatous disease. As iris tissue is very loose, the accumulation of fluid causes oedema of the iris, the outlines of the crypts and fissures become blurred and the iris takes up a muddy colour. Due to oedema the mobility of the iris becomes hampered and so the pupil becomes sluggish. Both the sphincter and the dilator muscles of the pupil become irritated, but as the sphincter muscle is more powerful, the pupil becomes small. The radial arrangement of the blood vessels is also another cause for the small pupil. Fibrin-rich fluid and inflammatory cells also appear in the aqueous humour. In case of cyciltis, the exudation may also occur in the vitreous.

Due to the toxins liberated with the exudate, the corneal endothelium becomes oedematous and sticky and may be desquamated at places. The inflammatory cells, circulating in the aqueous by convection current, stick to the endothelial layer of the cornea as cellular deposits, known as keratic precipitates or K.P. If the exudation is profuse, a hypopyon is formed and in that case K.P. are not formed, as all the leucocytes are entangled in the fibrin-rich exudate. Oedematous and inflammed iris usually adheres to the anterior lens capsule, to form posterior synechia, which is manifested by irregular pupillary margin.

PLATE IX

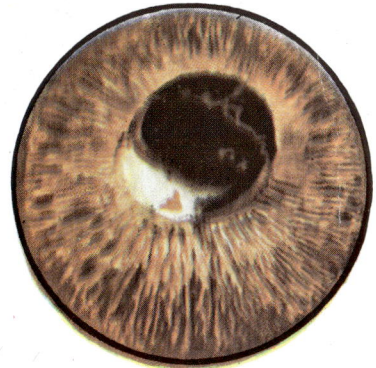

Fig. 1

Plastic iritis with
posterior synechia
(Parsons)

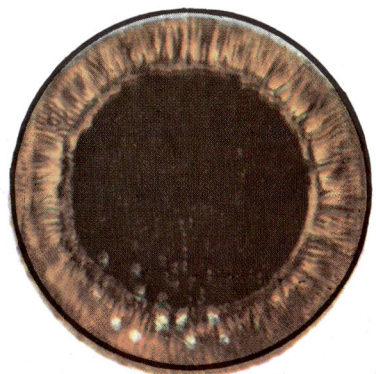

Fig. 2

Chronic Cyclitis
(Parsons)

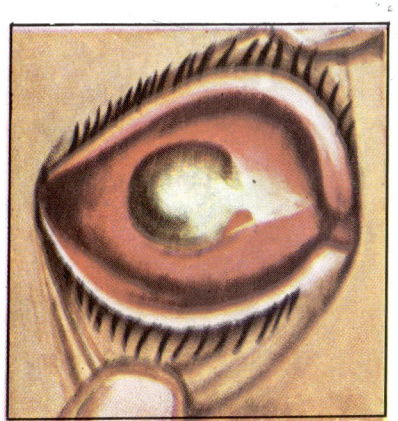

Fig. 3

Panophthalmitis
(Parsons)

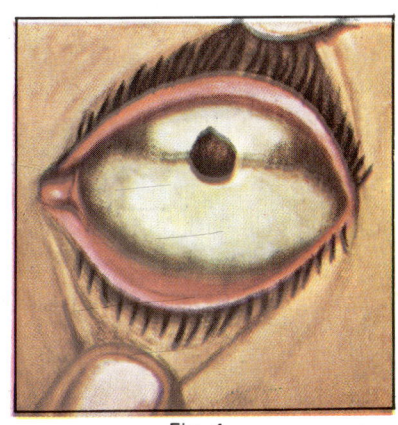

Fig. 4

Phthisis bulbi
(Parsons)

(To face page 130)

Symptoms of iritis and iridocyclitis

1. Neuralgic pain in the eye radiating along other branches of the 5th nerve. The pain is worst at night.

2. Blurring of vision due to plasmoid fluid in the anterior chamber, vitreous opacities or due to exudate in the pupillary area.

3. Lacrimation due to irritation of the sensory nerves.

4. Photophobia.

Clinical signs

1. Ciliary congestion.

2. Conjunctival hyperaemia.

3. Chemosis of the lids and the conjunctiva in severe cases.

4. Muddy colour of the iris.

5. Pupil is small, inactive and irregular due to formation of synechia—*i.e.*, adhesion between the pupillary margin and the anterior lens capsule.

6. Anterior chamber may be hazy due to plasmoid aqueous. There may be hypopyon or hyphema.

7. Keratic precipitates—when there is iridocyclitis.

8. Folds in the Descemet's membrane.

9. Opacities in the vitreous.

Diagnostic criteria

1. Severe pain in the eye.

2. Ciliary congestion.

3. Muddy colour of the iris with small, irregular, sluggish pupil.

4. Presence of K.P.

Complications

1. Secondary glaucoma due to blockage of the angle of the anterior chamber with fibrinous fluid.

2. Ring synechia leading to occlusio pupillae, due to adhesion of the entire pupillary margin to the anterior lens capsule.

3. Iris bombé—As a result of ring synechia, the aqueous humour cannot come to the anterior chamber from the posterior chamber through the pupil, so the peripheral part of the iris bulges forward and this bulging of the iris is known as iris bombe . This condition is also associated with secondary glaucoma.

4. Occlusio pupillae—Occlusion of the pupil by organization of exudate in the pupillary area.

This complication also leads to the development of iris bombe.

5. Cyclitic membrane—It is a membrane formed in the anterior vitreous, behind the lens, due to organization of inflammatory exudate.

6. Complicated cataract—The lens becomes completely opaque and appears chalky white.

7. Detachment of the retina due to contraction of the cyclitic membrane.

8. Phthisis bulbi i.e. shrinkage of the eyeball due to destruction of the ciliary body as a result of severe inflammation. Other features of phthisis bulbi are hypotony and shrunken, quadrilateral shape of the eyeball due to pressure by the four rectus muscles. Such an eye is called a quadrate eye. There is also no perception of light. Several years later on, *due to bone formation in choroid, the eye may be hard to feel.*

Special types of Uveitis

1. *Iritis and iridocyclitis due to syphilis—two types—*

(a) Plastic type—It may occur in congenital syphilis or in acquired syphilis in the secondary stage. The clinical signs are like ordinary iritis and is usually uniocular occurring more in the males.

(b) Gummatous type—It is seen in late secondary and tertiary stage and is characterized by tiny yellowish red vascularized nodules on the iris. The exudation and synechia formation are marked.

2. *Iritis and iridocyclitis due to gonorrhoea*

The infection is metastatic and may occur during an acute attack of gonorrhoea. The characteristic features are gelatinous exudate in the anterior chamber and sometimes blood in the anterior chamber. Bilateral affection and recurrences are common.

3. *Iritis and iridocyclitis due to tuberculosis*

It is a granulomatous type of iritis characterized by the formation of yellowish white nodules on the iris and mutton-fat K.P. The course is prolonged.

4. *Iritis and iridocyclitis due to leprosy*

Leprosy cases may be associated with these types of lesions. The usual signs of iritis and iridocyclitis are present, but lepra nodules may appear on the iris.

5. Sympathetic ophthalmia

It is a pan-uveitis *i.e.* iritis, cyclitis and choroiditis of plastic type of much severity, affecting the second eye when the other eye is injured. A perforating injury in the ciliary region near the limbus is the common precipitating factor. The whole of the uveal tract becomes infiltrated with lymphocytes, plasma cells and epitheliod cells. There is always iridocyclitis also in the injured eye known as the exciting eye. The K.P. in both the eyes are of mutton-fat type. The etiology of this condition is unknown.

6. Iritis and iridocyclitis associated with sarcoidosis

It is also a granulomatous type of iridocyclitis. There is formation of nodules in the iris and inflammation is severe and long continued. The K.P. are of mutton-fat variety. There are also evidences of systemic sarcoidosis.

7. Heterochromic cyclitis of Fuchs

There is low grade cyclitis affecting one eye only and associated depigmentation of the iris. There is no posterior synechia but there are fine K.P. and finally complicated cataract develops.

Treatment of iritis and iridocyclitis

1. Attempts should be made to find out the underlying cause and to treat for elimination of the cause.
2. Local treatment
   (a) Rest to the eye by instilling atropine sulphate 1 percent drop twice daily or by application of atropine ointment 1 percent twice daily. Atropine has three functions *e.g.*
      (i) it gives rest to the eye by paralyzing the ciliary muscle:
      (ii) it dilates the pupil and prevents or breaks down posterior synechia.
      (iii) it dilates the blood vessels and thus more antibodies are brought in. If atropine fails to dilate the pupil, subconjunctival injection of mydricaine 5 minims is advocated.
   (b) To control inflammation by steriod therapy—This should be done with caution. This therapy is contraindicated in the presence of a frank infection or if

granulomatous inflammation is suspected particularly tuberculosis. The treatment is done as follows :

(i) Hydrocortisone acetate 1 percent drop to be instilled every one hour or every two hours depending on the severity of the case. In addition hydrocortisone acetate 1 percent ointment may be applied at bed time.

(ii) Preparations of dexamethasone, betamethasone, or prednisolone may also be used, as 0.5 percent drops instilled every 1-2 hours.

(iii) In very severe cases, A.C.T.H. may be given 10 units intramuscularly daily for 10 days, keeping in mind general contraindications like diabetes, hypertension etc.

(c) dark glasses for photophobia.

3. *General treatment*

(a) Analgesics for relief of pain.

(b) Injection of 5 c.c. of milk twice a week intramuscularly, four such, to increase body resistance.

(c) Specific treatment for specific causes like control of diabetes, anti-tubercular or anti-syphilitic treatment etc.

Diseases of the Choroid

Anatomy of the choroid

The choroid is the vascular tunic of the eye forming the major part of the uveal tract. It is highly vascular, consisting of loose connective tissue with pigment containing chromatophores. It extends from the ciliary body upto the optic nerve head. On the outer side it is separated from the sclera by a potential space called the suprachoroidea and on its inner surface is an elastic membrane—the Bruch's membrane, on which rests the pigment epithelium of the retina. The vessels and nerves are derived from the ciliary vessels and nerves and the venous drainage is done through four vortex veins situated in four quadrants behind the equator, which drain into orbital veins.

Inflammation of the Choroid
(Choroiditis)

Usually choroiditis is acute. Types of choroiditis are as follows.

1. Localized—

    (a) Central, affecting the macular area.
    (b) Juxtapapillary, affecting an area near the optic disc.
    (c) Peripheral.
  2. Diffuse—when wide areas of the choroid are affected.
  3. Disseminated when there are scattered patches of choroiditis.

Etiology—Same as for iritis and iridocyclitis.

Clinical sings and Symptoms

  1. Defective vision.
  2. Black spots floating in front of the eye.
  3. On examination of the fundus
    (a) Greyish white patches in the choroid and retina, deep to the retinal vessels.
    (b) Marked vitreous haze.
    (c) Later on when the inflammation subsides, there is accumulation of pigment at the periphery of the patches, and portions of sclera may be visible in these areas due to atrophy of the choroid.

Treatment—Same as for iritis and iridocyclitis.

Panophthalmitis

Definition—It is a condition when there is intese purulent inflammation of all the structures of the eyeball, with particular involvement of the whole of the uveal tract.

Etiology

  1. Age and sex—May occur in any age and in either sex.
  2. Exogenous cause—Penetrating injury, operation on the eyeball or perforation of a corneal ulcer.
  3. Endogenous cause—Septic emboli lodged in choroidal or retinal vessles from a 'source of sepsis.
  4. Causative organism—Pneumococcus, Bacillus pyocyaneus, Streptococcus haemolyticus.

Symptoms

  1. Intense pain in the eyeball with headache.
  2. Fever and malaise.
  3. Complete loss of vision.
  4. Lacrimation.

Clinical sings

1. Marked oedema of the lids.
2. Chemosis of the conjunctiva with ciliary and conjunctival congestion.
3. Slight proptosis with marked limitation of movements of the eyeball.
4. Cornea is hazy.
5. The anterior chamber is full of pus.
6. In exogenous cases external signs of penetrating injury, of operation or of perforation of corneal ulcer are present.
7. Complete loss of perception and projection of light.
8. Intra-ocular tension markedly raised.
9. Cornea may give way at the limbus or the sclera may rupture and pus may come out at those places.

Pathology—There is intense purulent inflammation of the vitreous, the retina and the whole of the uveal tract. The lens becomes opaque. The cornea undergoes necrotic changes. The inflammation may spread upto the Tenon's capsule and to the extra-ocular muscles.

Treatment

1. In early stages broad spectrum antibiotics may be tried by mouth.
2. Subconjunctival injection of gentamycin may be tried.
3. Local application of heat.
4. Analgesics for relief of pain.
But usually these measures are of no avail, and ultimately the eyeball has to be eviscerated.

Endophthalmitis

Definition—It is a condition when there is acute inflammation of the structures in the posterior segment of the eyeball *i.e.* the choroid, the retina and the vitreous behind the lens. The anterior segment, apart from the presence of a few inflammatory cells in the anterior chamber and a few K.P., remians unaffected.

Etiology

1. Age and sex—Usually children of either sex.
2. Endogenous cause—Septic emboli lodged in choroidal or retinal vessels from a septic focus as in otitis media, septic tonsils or meningitis. Metastatic endophthalmitis from septic abortion are commonly seen.

The inflammation is less intense than panophthalmitis.

3. Causative agents—Pneumococcus,Meningococcus, Streptococcus haemolyticus of less virulence.

Symptoms

1. Pain in the eye but not so severe as in panophthalmitis.
2. Complete loss of vision.
3. No fever or malaise.

Clinical signs

1. Ciliary congestion.
2. K.P. may be present.
3. The cornea, the anterior chamber and the lens are clear (4th Purkinje's image is visible).
4. Whitish mass is seen through the pupil which is caused by the inflammatory exudation in the vitreous. This is known as amaurotic cat's eye reflex. This condition of whitish reflex through the pupil is known as pseudo-glioma. A similar appearance is seen in a case of glioma of the retina which is a malignant tumour. So endophthalmitis is a pseudo-glioma as it is not due to tumour formation.
5. Low intra-ocular tension and ultimately the eyeball is converted into phthisis bulbi.
6. No perception or projection of light and no reaction of the pupil. One or two posterior synechia may be present.

Treatment

The same treatment as for panophthalmitis may be tried but usually it is of no avail.

The eyeball ultimately shrinks due to the destruction of the ciliary body.

Tumours of the Uveal Tract

The commonest and the most important tumour of the uveal tract is the malignant melanoma.

Malignant melanoma originates either from the Schwann cells of the sensory nerves or from the uveal chromatophores.

The commonest site of malignant melanoma is the choroid and next is the ciliary body and the iris.

Malignant Melanoma of the Choroid

Pathology

It consists of cells containing melanin pigment with reticulin fibres in the stroma. Vascularity is high. The cells may be of spindle-shaped type which may have a fasicular arrangement or of epitheliod type or of mixed type.

Stages of the tumour

1. Intra-ocular growth—Usually symptomless unless the macular area is affected, when there is defective vision.

2. Stage of secondary glaucoma due to rise of tension.

3. Stage of extra-ocular extension—The tumour spreading into the orbital tissues.

4. Stage of generalized metastasis—Usually the metastasis is blood-borne to the central nervous system and the liver.

Treatment

As soon as detected, the eyeball must be immediately enucleated. However, light coagulation is also an effective method of treatment.

Congenital Anomalies of the Uveal Tract

1. Congenital aniridia—It means congenital absence of the iris. The condition is rare. Usually the absence of the iris is not complete, and a tiny stump of iris tissue is present at the extreme periphery. There may be associated secondary glaucoma. It is usually familial.

2. Congential coloboma of iris and choroid—Due to developmental defect there is a gap in the iris which is known as coloboma. The gap is usually situated downwards and inwards. Some part of the choroid also may show a gap and sclera becomes visible at that area.

3. Coloboma of the macula—A defect of the choroid may occur in the macular region causing marked fall of vision. This is also congenital.

CHAPTER IX

ANATOMY AND DISEASES OF THE LENS

Anatomy of the lens

The lens is a biconvex transparent structure, made of lens fibres, which are modified epithelial cells. It is enclosed in an elastic capsule. The anterior surface of the lens is less convex than the posterior and the lens is kept in position, by the suspensory ligament or zonule, which extending from the ciliary processes, is attached to the equator of the lens all round. Underneath the anterior capsule, there is a layer of cubical epithelium. The cells near the equator give rise to new lens fibres.

The lens matter consists of a superficial part—the cortex and a deeper part—the nucleus. The nucleus starts as an embryonic nucleus and as age advances, successive nuclear zones are laid down, which are known as foetal nucleus, infantile nucleus and adult nucleus. The youngest fibres are in the cortex. As age advances the older fibres are pushed towards the centre of the lens, so that the density of the nucleus increases and the nucleus becomes hard. This process is known as lental sclerosis and for this reason the lens appears grey in the elderly people.

The lens fibres meet at two suture lines—the anterior one is Y shaped and the posterior one is an inverted Y.

Function of the lens

The lens converges rays of light on to the macula, so that a clear image of the object seen is formed. In order to perform this function, the process of accommodation may have to be exerted, the mechanism for which has already been described elsewhere.

Nutrition of the lens—Upto the 8th month of foetal life by the hyaloid artery ; afterwards from the aqueous humour.

Cataract

Definition—It means opacity of the lens.

The lens, being an avascular structure, cannot develop an inflammatory disease. The commonest disease is a degenerative process leading to opacity of lens fibres, known as cataract.

Classification of cataract

A. Congenital and Developmental

This type includes
1. Blue-dot cataract.
2. Coronary cataract.
3. Capsular or polar cataract—anterior and posterior.
4. Sutural cataract.
5. Coralliform cataract.
6. Floriform cataract.
7. Central cataract.
8. Lamellar or zonular cataract.
9. Total cataract.
    (a) Soft,
    (b) Membranous.

B. Acquired Cataract

This type includes
1. Senile cataract
    (a) cortical or cuneiform,
    (b) nuclear,
    (c) posterior cortical or cupuliform.
2. Traumatic cataract
    (a) Mechanical trauma—concussion, contusion or penetrating injury of the eyeball.
    (b) Chemical trauma—due to systemic absorption of chemicals like naphthalene, lactose, galactose, or thallium.
    (c) Raditional trauma—by infra-red rays, ultra-violet rays, deep x-rays or radiations from radium.
    (d) Electric cataract—due to passage of electric current through the body.
3. Endocrine cataract—as in diabetes mellitus, hypoparathyroidism, and cretinism.
4. Cataract due to systemic diseases—as in Mongolian idiocy, myotonic dystrophy and generalized dermatitis.
5. Complicated cataract.

A. Congenital and Developmental Cataract

Congenital cataract is present at birth. Developmental cataract is that cataract, which develops during the development of the lens. These types of cataracts are developed, due to some disturbance, at a certain phase of the growth of the lens. Lens fibres, developed either previous to or later than the period of disturbance, remian normal. Therefore these types of opacities of the lens are usually stationary and they may be of various types as noted below. Underlying cause is not known but it may be due to—

    (a) maternal malnutrition,

    (b) maternal infection particularly by virus of German measles or rubella, or

    (c) deficient oxygenation due to placental haemorrhage.

    1. Blue-dot cataract—Tiny bluish white opaque spots scattered all over the lens. No visual disturbance.

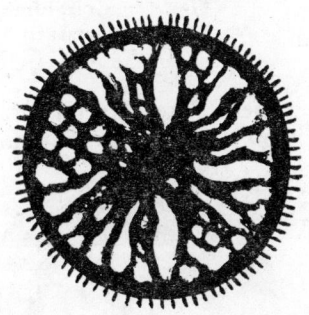

Fig. 66. Coronary cataract.

2. Coronary cataract (Fig. 66)—Club shaped opacities in the peripheral part of the cortex, arranged like a corona or crown. It develops at puberty. No visual disturbance, as the axial area of the lens remains clear.

3. (a) Anterior capsular or polar cataract—it develops as a result of delayed formation of the anterior chamber during the development of the lens. A white plaque is formed in the anterior lens capsule in the pupillary area. Sometimes this opacity may project into the atnerior chamber in the form of a pyi. mid, when it is called anterior pyramidal cataract. More commonly, the anterior capsular cataract is acquired, when it develops due to contact of the anterior lens capsule with an ulcer of the cornea, following preforation of the ulcer, and drainage of aqueous humour. Visual disturbace is not marked.

    (b) Posterior capsular cataract—Due to persistence of the posterior part of the vascular sheath of the lens. The opacity is usually tiny and visual distrubance is very little.

4. Sutural cataract—Tiny opaque dots situated in the Y sutures of the lens. No visual distrubance.

5. Coralliform cataract (Fig. 67)— Minute opacities situated in the central area of the lens in the form of a coral. No visual disturbance.

6. Floriform cataract—The opacities are annular in shape, arranged like the petals of flower and situated in the axial part of the lens. No visual disturbance.

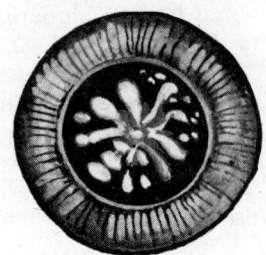

7. Central cataract—The nucleus of the lens shows opacity. The opacity may be granular when there is no visual distrubance or the whole of the nucleus may be opaque associated with visual disturbance.

Fig. 67.   Coralliform cataract

N.B. All these types of cataract may be unilateral or bilateral.

8. Lamellar or zonular cataract (Fig. 68)—It is the commonest variety of cataract in children and is usually bilateral. It may develop in the later part of intra-uterine life or in early infancy. Sometimes it is hereditary, but is usually associated with vitamin D deficiency and with evidences of rickets. The enamel of the permanent teeth, particularly the incisors and canines, is defective.

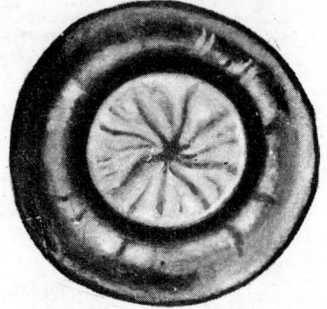

This type of cataract is characterized by the opacity of one zone of the lens fibres, while the rest of the lens, including the nucleus, remains clear.

Fig. 68. Zonular cataract

As a few lamellae of the lens fibres are affected, it is called a lamellar cataract. On dilatation of the pupil, a central, circular, disc-shaped opacity, surrounded by clear lens is seen. Sometimes linear opacities, like the spokes of a wheel may radiate towards the periphery from the opaque area and these spokes are called 'riders'. There is always visual disturbances, but the condition is stationary.

9. Total cataract—May be unilateral or bilateral and is usually congenital. The entire lens is opaque. The lens matter may remain soft or may liquify to form milky fluid contained in the capsule—the Morgagnian type or the entire lens may be converted

into a membrane due to absorption of the lens matter.

The congenital, complete cataract is due to distrubance of development, or to some intra-uterine ocular inflammation. It is common in cases of maternal rubella, occurring during the first three months of pregnancy.

How to diagnose a congenital and developmental cataract

1. Pupil must be well dilated with one percent atropine ointment.

2. The lens must be examined with a torch and a loupe or with the help of a slit-lamp, for any evidence of opacity.

Treatment of congential cataract

1. Treatment depends on the amount of visual disturbance.

2. The zonular cataract and the total cataract require treatment, as the former may cause marked visual disturbance and the total cataract always does so.

3. The other types of cataract usually do not cause much visual disturbance and they may be left alone.

4. Treatment of zonular cataract—

    (a) If the vision is 6/24, no treatment is necessary. Also if vision comes upto 6/24, after dilatation of the pupil with atropine no further treatment is necessary..

    (b) If the vision is worse than 6/24, discission operation has to be done. By this operation, the lens matter is broken with a discission needle. The proteolytic ferments, present in the aqueous, dissolve the lens matter. If there is delay in absorption of the lens matter or if secondary glaucoma develops after the operaton, a good amount of the lens matter has to be taken out through a small incision through the cornea, 2-3 mm. in front of the limbus. This operation is known as curette and evacuation. Aphakic glasses are prescribed later on. The time for doing discission operation of a zonular cataract is at puberty. A simpler and more effective treatment is "suction evacuation". After the discission a wide bone intra-muscular needle bent in the form an iris repositor fitted on a 10cc syringe is introduced into the AC through the discission puncture. The soft lens matter is gently sucked out.

5. Treatment of total cataract—The suitable time for discission operation is after the first dentition *i.e.* at the age of 6 months

to 1 year, as otherwise, the macula will not grow and nystagmus may develop.

There is no difficulty for doing the discission operation in the case of a soft or Morgangnian cataract. But in case of a membranous cataract, the membrane has to be removed, with a capsule forceps, through a keratome incision through the limbus.

B. Acquired Cataract

1. Senile cataract

General features

(i) Age—usually above 50 years, but not uncommon at a lower age in this country.

(ii) Sex—is equal in either sex.

(iii) Bilaterality—usually bilateral but develops earlier in one eye.

(iv) Heredity—Genetic influence is marked. In hereditary cases the cataract appears at earlier ages in subsequent generations.

(v) 55% of the total blindness is due to senile cataract.

Types of senile cataract

(a) Cortical or Cuneiform or Soft Cataract

Pathology

The lens fibres of the cortex are mainly affected. There is hydration due to accumulation of water droplets in between the fibres, followed by changes in the colloid system within the fibres. The proteins are first denatured and then are coagulated forming opacity. Ultimately the whole of the lens becomes opaque and assumes a pearly white appearance.

Symptoms of cortical cataract

(a) Gradual impairment of vision.

(b) Polyopia *i.e.*, one object appears multiple, as for example the person sees more than one moon. This is due to multiple refraction through the clear areas of the lens.

(c) Rainbow haloes around the light—due to accumulation of water droplets in between the lens fibres.

Clinical signs

They depend upon the stage of the cortical cataract. The stages and the signs are the following :

    (a) Incipient stage—Wedge-shaped spokes of opacity, with clear areas in between, are visible in the periphery of the lens. When examined in the dark room with dilated pupil, on throwing light into the eye with a plain mirror the opacities appear as dark lines against the red fundal glow.

    (b) Progressive stage—Further wedge-shaped opacities appear.

    (c) Immature stage—The process of opacification has advanced further. The lens appears greyish. But clear cortex is still present, and so the iris shadow is visible. The fourth Purkinje's image now has disappeared. Very little red fundal glow can be seen, because the pupillary area is almost wholly occupied by a dark shadow.

Vision is reduced to finger counting at a distance close to the eye.

Iris shadow

It is the shadow of the pupillary margin on the lens, produced when light is thrown obliquely on the pupillary margin. The significance of this sign is that, there is still a small amount of clear lens matter underneath the capsule. (Figs, 69,70).

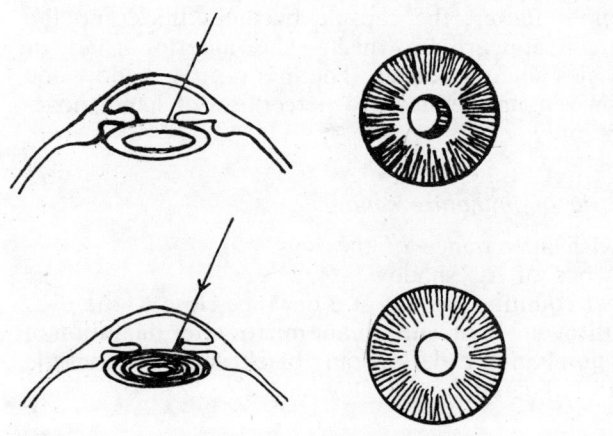

Fig. 69. Iris shadow in immature cataract

Fig. 70. No iris shadow in mature cataract

(d) Intumescent stage—The cataract is in the immature stage but the lens has swollen due to imbibition of fluid. The anterior chamber becomes shallow. This stage may persist even when the mature stage is arrived.

(e) Mature stage—The entire cortex becomes opaque white. The outlines of the opaque lens fibres are visible. The iris shadow disappears, as there is no clear cortex underneath the capsule. The vision becomes reduced to perception of hand movement only. The swelling of the lens usually subsides, but the intumescent stage may persist. On dark room examination no fundal glow is visible. The first, second and third Purkinje's images remain. The cortical type of cataract takes about one year to mature.

(f) Hypermature stage—There may be two types of hypermature cataract.

(i) Hypermature Morgagnian type—The whole of the cortical matter liquifies to form milky fluid, so that the lens is now converted into a bag of milky fluid, with the nucleus settled at the bottom of the bag. The cataract appears uniformly milky white, without any visible outlines of the lens fibres. There may be deposits of calcium on the lens capsule. There is no iris shadow. The anterior chamber may be shallow or normal. Vision is reduced to perception of hand movement.

(ii) Hypermature sclerotic type—Due to some alteration in the permeability of the lens capsule, some of the cortical matter goes out and is absorbed. The lens becomes flatter, the capsule becomes thick and the cataract appears brownish. The anterior chamber becomes slightly deeper. There is no iris shadow and vision remains reduced to perception of hand movement only.

Diagnostic criteria of immature cataract

(a) Greyish appearance of the lens.
(b) Presence of iris shadow.
(c) Finger counting present at a distance close to the eye.
(d) On throwing light with a plane mirror after dilatation of the pupil in the dark-room, black shadow is visible against the red fundal glow.

Diagnostic criteria of mature cataract

    (a) Pearly white appearance of the lens.
    (b) No iris shadow.
    (c) Absent fourth Purkinje's image.
    (d) Vision reduced to perception of hand movement.
    (e) No red fundal glow when examined in the dark-room with a plane mirror.

TABLE VII

Differential diagnosis between immature cataract and lental sclerosis

Immature Cataract	Lental Sclerosis
1. Progressive dimness of vision.	1. Dimness of vision whose progress is very slow.
2. Lens appears grey.	2. Lens appears grey.
3. Iris shadow is present.	3. Iris shadow is present.
4. Black spot against the red fundal glow when examined in the dark-room with a plane mirror.	4. No black spot against the red fundal glow when examined in the dark-room.

N.B. Lental sclerosis means hardening of the lens due to sclerosis of the lens fibres, particularly in the nucleus, as a result of ageing process.

The index of refraction of the lens is increased and so there may be dimness of vision due to development of index myopia.

TABLE VIII

Differential diagnosis between mature cataract and pseudo-glioma (organized exudate in the vitreous)

Mature cataract	Pseudo-glioma
1. White reflex in the pupillary area.	1. White reflex in the pupillary area.
2. Absence of frouth Purkinje's image.	2. Presence of the fourth Purkinje's image, as the opacity is behind the lens.

Complications of cortical cataract

    (a) In the intumescent stage—There may be an attack of acute congestive glaucoma, due to shallow anterior chamber.

(b) In the hypermature Morgagnian stage—
    (ii) The lens capsule may burst and cortical matter, coming out in the anterior chamber, may cause iritis and secondary glaucoma—a condition known as burst Morgagnian cataract with secondary glaucoma.
    (ii) If the lens remains intumescent, there may be an attack of acute congestive glaucoma.
    (iii) Lens may be subluxated or dislocated into the vitreous, due to degeneration of the suspensory ligament.
(c) In the hypermature sclerotic stage—The lens may be subluxated or dislocated in the virtreous, due to associated degenerative changes in the zonule.

Thus, the necessity for cataract operation in the mature stage is not only for improvement of vision, but also for avoiding the complications which arise in the hypermature stage.

(b) Nuclear type of Cataract or Hard Cataract

Pathology

It has already been mentioned that in lental sclerosis, the nuclear fibres undergo a process of sclerosis. When this process becomes more intensified, the nuclear cataract starts. The nucleus becomes diffusely cloudy and obstructs the light rays. The process may extend almost upto the capsule when it becomes mature, but a very thin layer of clear cortex may remain unaffected. The lens appears brown or sometimes black, due to deposition of melanin pigment, when it is known as black cataract or brunescens cataract. This type of cataract never becomes hypermature. The progress of the cataract is slow and myopic eyes are more prone to develop this type of cataract.

Sympotms
    (a) Progressive dimness of vision but no polyopia. The defect of vision is partly due to acquired myopic error of refraction and partly due to coludiness of the nucleus. In the early stages, the defect can be rectified to a great extent by concave spherical lens (minus glass).
    (b) No complaint about seeing halo around the light.

Clinical signs
    (a) The lens appears brown, dark brown or black.

(b) Iris shadow is usually present.
(c) The vision is reduced to counting fingers or perception of hand movement at a distance close to the eye, depending on how much the cataract has advanced.
(d) The fourth Purkinjil's image is absent.
(e) On dark-room examination—There is a central dark area against the red fundal glow.

(c) Posterior Cortical or Cupuliform Cataract

Pathology

The opacity develops in the posterior cortex immediately underneath the posterior capsule. At first it starts in the central area and then extends very slowly in the rest of the posterior cortex, but never extends beyond this area. The cataract is made up of minute opacities with deposition of cholesterol crystals. The progress is extre. nely slow and the cataract almost remains as it is for years. But other types of cataract, like nuclear or cortical type, may supervene. The posterior cortical cataract never matures.

Symptoms

(a) A small opacity in the lens in this type of cataract, causes marked fall of vision, because the opacity is located near the nodal point of the optical system of the eye.
(b) No polyopia or halo around the light.
(c) Defect of vision is more in the day time (day blindness) than at night. The reason for this symptom is the situation of the opacity against the pupillary area and so when the pupil constricts in strong light, light rays are prevented from entering into the eye. On dilatation of the pupil in the dark, vision improves, as more light rays can enter into the eye.

Clinical signs

(a) Blurring of the fourth Purkinje's image.
(b) On dark-room examination, there is a central dark spot against the red fundal glow.
(c) Examination by a slit-lamp shows the location of the opacity in the posterior cortex and helps to make a positive diagnosis.

Treatment of senile cataract

The cataract is removed by surgical operation called extraction of the lens which may be either intra-capsular or extra-capsular depending on the type of the cataract and other factors to be discussed later on (see under instruments and operations).

General indicaton for operation—when the vision is so much reduced that a person cannot carry out his own work efficiently, the operation is needed.

2. Traumatic Cataract

(a) *By mechanical trauma*—The injury may be penetrating, when the lens capsule is actually perforated or it may be a concussion injury, when the capsule is damaged and its semi-permeability is altered or there may be rupture of the capsule. The aqueous humour comes in contact with the lens fibres and makes the fibres opaque.

Types of traumatic cataract—

(i)   Distinct punctate opacities in the superficial cortex— They may affect only one segment and the opacity is usually stationary.

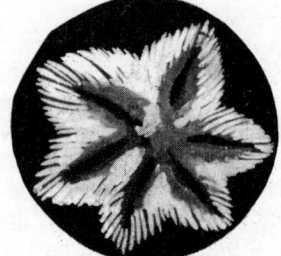

Fig. 71. Rosette-shaped cataract due to concussion injury

(ii) Rosette-shaped cataract—This develops in the posterior cortex in a star-shaped manner. The posterior capsule is very thin and so is easily damaged and the opacity develops. It may remain stationary or may progress until the entire lens becomes opaque.

(iii) Total cataract—It develops when the capsule is severely damaged. The lens fibres, coming in contact with the aqueous humour, swell and become opaque.

(iv) Vossius's ring—Sometimes a ring of brown granules of pigment with a faint opacity may form on the anterior lens capsule, just behind the pupillary margin.

(b) *By chemical trauma*—
   (i) Naphthalene cataract—Cataract may be produced in animals after feeding them with naphthalene. It develops within 2-3 weeks, and is bilateral.
   (ii) Lactose and galactose cataract—Animals, fed on only lactose or galactose, develop cataract. The cataract is bilateral, and appears very early. Similarly, bilateral cataract develops in early life, in the rare disease known as galactosaemia, when there is inborn inability to metabolize galactose.
   (iii) Thallium cataract—Animals, fed on thallium, develop cataract within 2-4 weeks, which is usually bilateral.

(c) *By radiational trauma*—
   (i) Infra-red cataract—Cataract may be induced on prolonged exposure to infra-red rays. The common example to this type of cataract is seen in glass-workers and furnace-workers. The cataract usually starts in posterior cortex of the lens.
   (ii) Ultra-violet cataract—Massive doses of ultra-violet rays can produce a cataract in experimental animals. The common cause of cataract in India is supposed to be prolonged exposure to minute doses of ultra-violet rays in sunlight.
   (iii) Irradiation cataract—Cataract develops due to exposure to X-rays or due to exposure to radiation from radium, due to direct action of these rays on the dividing cells and on the developing fibres of the lens. Usually the cataract takes a long time to develop.

(d) *Electric cataract*—This type of cataract develops following the passage of powerful electric current through the body, as when a person is struck by lightning. The cataract starts as a punctate subcapsular opacity and matures rapidly.

3. Endocrine Cataract

   (i) Diabetic cataract—It occurs in young diabetics of a severe type. The first change is the appearance of a large number of fluid vacuoles underneath the anterior and the posterior capsule. The snow-flake like opacities appear in the cortex and the entire lens becomes completely opaque very soon. It is rare now a days.

(ii) Parathyroid cataract—If the parathyroids are removed accidentally during operation on the thyroid gland, cataract develops within 2–3 months. It starts as discrete opacities in the cortex, interspersed with iridescent crystals of blue, green or red colour, and within six months the lens becomes opaque.

(iii) Cataract in cretinism—The cataract is similar in appearance to the parathyroid cataract and occurs in cretins.

4. Cataract due to Systemic Diseases

(i) In Mongolian idiocy—The cataract develops as punctate opacities in the superficial cortex.

(ii) In myotonic dystrophy—Fine dustlike opacities inter-spersed with iridescent spots appear in the superficial cortex.

(iii) Dermatogenous cataract—It develops in cases of severe dermatitis particularly in the young. The commonest skin diseases associated with cataract are neurodermatitis and scleroderma.

5. Complicated Cataract

It develops as sequence to severe intra-ocular disease like iridocyclitis, choroiditis, pigmentary degeneration of the retina or total detachment of the retina. The cataract is due to disturbance of the matabolism of the lens, caused by diffusion of toxins through the capsule. The opacity at first starts in the posterior cortex in the form of a rosette with polychromatic lustre. Then the opacity spreads in the rest of the lens, with a bread-crumb appearance. Finally the entire lens becomes opaque and takes up a chalky-white colour or white colour with a slight yellowish tinge.

Treatment

Treatment of all these types of cataract is on usual lines. If the visual defect is marked so as to cause disability, a surgical operation is the choice of treatment. If the age of the patient is below 24 years, discission operation is done and for the higher age group, extraction of the lens is the usual procedure.

6. Cataract due to Drugs

Cataract due to crotico-steroids—It has been found that posterior cortical opacities in the lens may develop following prolonged systemic administration of those drugs for more than a year. The same kind of lental opacities may also develop due to local application of those drugs for several months.

Miotic cataract—Long continued application of powerful miotics particularly belonging to the anticholinesterase group can cause lenticular opacities. The cataract appears as tiny vacuoles under the anterior capsular epithelium. If the drug is discontinued the progress of the cataract stops.

After-Cataract or Secondary Cataract

Definition—It is a membrane, formed by the remnants of the anterior and the posterior capsule, following extra-capsular extraction or discission operation.

Sometimes the membrane is very thin, but the membrane may be thick due to following reasons—
   (a) Abortive attempts by the cubical cells underneath the anterior capsule to form lens fibres.
   (b) Organization of inflammatory exudate on the membrane following post-operative iridocyclitis.
   (c) Deposition of fibrin on the membrane following post-operative haemorrhage in the anterior chamber.

The cubical cells, underneath the lens capsule, instead of developing normal lens fibers, may form large balloon-like cells, which are known as Elschnig's pearls. Sometimes the lens fibres grow between the anterior and the posterior lens capsules in the periphery, behind the iris, to form a ring known as the ring of Sommerring

Treatment of after-cataract—After dilating the pupil, a gap is made in the central area of the membrane, by a discission needle, so that light rays can enter into the eye. This operation is known as needling of the after-cataract.

Aphakia

Definition

Aphakia is the condition in which the crystalline lens is absent from its normal position.

How aphakia can be produced

1. ′ By operative measures like discission, extra-capsular or intra-capsular extraction of lens.

2. By trauma—Usually contusional injury, when the lens may be dislocated in the vitreous.

3. By couching—When the lens is forcibly dislocated into the vitreous, by a needle introduced through the limbus.

4. As a developmental anomaly—Congential absence of the lens.

Symptoms of aphakia

There is marked dimness of vision, both for the distance and for the near, due to development of acquired hypermetropia and due to complete loss of accommodation.

Clinical signs of aphakia

1. Deep anterior chamber.

2. Tremulousness of iris known as iridodonesis.

3. Jet-black pupil, provided there is no after-cataract.

4. Absence of 3rd and 4th Purkinje's images.

5. Linear scar mark at the upper half of the limbus, in cases where extraction of the lens is the cause of aphakia.

Changes occurring in an aphakic eye

1. Acquired high hypermetropia—The total dioptric power of a normal eye is about +58 to +60D, of which cornea contributes +42 to +43 D and the lens in situ contributes +15 to +18 D. Thus when the lens is removed, the dioptric power of the eye decreases and so the eye becomes hypermetropic.

2. Acquired astigmatism in cases where aphakia is due to extraction of the lens—The astigmatism is against the rule, *i.e.*, the vertical curvature of the cornea is flatter than the horizontal. This is caused by the contraction of the limbal scar.

3. Complete loss of accommodation, as there is no lens.

4. The anterior and the posterior focal lengths of the eyeball increase than normal. Thus the anterior and the posterior focal lengths of the aphakic eye become 23.3 mm. and 31 mm. as compared to 15 mm. and 24 mm. in the normal eye approximately from the cornea.

5. The retinal image of an object in an aphakic eye, even after correction with glasses, becomes bigger by 25-30 percent than that in the normal eye. So if one eye is aphakic and the other eye is normal, binocular vision is not possible even after using correct

aphakic glasses, due to the disparity of image size. So if aphakic glasses are prescribed when the other eye is normal, there is diplopia.

6.   Sometimes an aphakic eye sees objects tinged with red or blue colour, due to increased entry of infra-red or ultra-violet rays into the eye, which are normally absorbed by the lens.

Treatment of aphakia

Aphakia is treated by prescribing spectacle lenses—

   (a) The lens to be used for distant vision, provided the eye was emmetropic before operation, is +10.0 Dsp with +2.0 or +3.0 Dcyl axis 180°. The +10 dioptre spherical lens is for the correction of the acquired hypermetropia and the +2.0 or +3.0 dioptre cylinder with axis 180°, is for the correction of the acquired astigmatism.

   (b) The lens for near vision is +13.0 Dsp with +2.0 or +3.0 Dcyl axis 180°. The higher spherical lens is necessary for substituting accommodation. The astigmatic correction remains the same as for the distance.

   (c) In aphakia not due to extraction of lens, *e.g.*, due to discission operation, due to couching or due to traumatic dislocation of the lens, the astigmatic correction is not necessary. So +10.0 Dsp for distance and +13.0 Dsp for near work serve the purpose.

   (d) To restore binocular vision, when one eye is normal and the other eye is aphakic, either contact lens for the aphakic eye, which reduces the image size difference between the two eyes to about 12 percent of intraocular acrylic lens, introduced into the anterior chamber, may be used, which reduces the image size difference to 2-3 percent.

N.B.   Although the dioptric power of the lens in situ is about +18 D, a lens of dioptric power +10 D serves the purpose to' correct aphakia as this lens is placed outside the eye.

Subluxation and Dislocation of Lens

Definition

   (a) Subluxation—When a few fibres of the suspensory ligament are torn, the lens is said to be subluxated but it still remains in the pupillary area. If it is a normal lens, it remains clear even after subluxation.

   (b) Dislocation—When all the fibres of the suspensory ligament are torn, the lens is said to be dislocated. A dislocated lens may drop in the vitreous—posterior dislocation ; the lens may come into the anterior chamber—anterior dislocation or the lens may migrate into the sub-conjunctival space,through a rupture in the sclera. A dislocated lens very soon becomes opaque.

Causes of subluxation of the lens

  A. *Congenital causes*

    1. Ectopia lentis—There is bilateral subluxation of the lens, usually upwards, due to congenital weakness of the suspensory ligament. The condition is often hereditary.

    2. Marfan's syndrome—This is characterized by :
      (a) Ectopia lentis.
      (b) Arachno-dactyly of hands and feet (long fingers and toes).
      (c) Dolichocephalic skull, *i.e.*, the antero-posterior diameter of the skull is much more than the transverse diameter.
      (d) Flat foot.
      (e) Congenital anomalies in the heart.

  B. *Acquired causes*

    1. Trauma to the suspensory ligament *e.g.*, contusional injury.

    2. Degenerative changes in the suspensory ligament, *e.g.*, hypermature cataract.

    3. Inflammatory destruction of the suspensory ligament, *e.g.*, panophthalmitis.

    4. Excessive stretching of the zonule, *e.g.*, forward displacement of the lens following perforation of a corneal ulcer, in buphthalmos, and in high myopia.

Symptoms

    1. In subluxation when the lens is clear
      (a) Defective vision for the distance due to the development of myopic and astigmatic error of refraction. Myopia is due to the more convexity of the lens and the astigmatism is due to slight tilting of the lens following subluxation.
      (b) Defective near vision due to disturbance in accommodation.
      (c) Uniocular diplopia, i.e., the patient sees every object double when seen through the affected eye with the other eye closed. This occurs when the lens is shifted in such a

manner, that it only covers half of the pupillary area, so that half of the pupillary area is aphakic and the other half is phakic. In such condition, there are two different images of the same object, one through the aphakic part and the other through the phakic part of the pupil and thus there is diplopia.

2. In subluxation when the lens is already opaque, there is no symptom.

3. In dislocation

(a) If the lens is clear and is dislocated in the anterior chamber, there is marked dimness of vision due to myopia, as a result of increased convexity as well as of anterior displacement of the lens.

(b) If the lens is clear and is dislocated in the vitreous, there is marked dimness of vision due to development of aphakia.

(c) If the lens is opaque and is dislocated in the anterior chamber there is no visual symptom.

(d) If the lens is opaque and is dislocated in the vitreous, there is sudden improvement of vision to some extent, because light rays can now pass through the pupil.

Clinical signs

1. In subluxation

(a) Tremulousness of the iris and the lens, elicited on movement of the eyeball.

(b) Unequal depth of the anterior chamber at different parts.

(c) If the pupil is fully dilated, the margin of the lens becomes visible.

2. In dislocation

(a) A clear lens, dislocated in the anterior chamber, looks like a drop of oil. The anterior chamber becomes deep. An opaque lens in such a position is easily detected.

(b) In posterior dislocation in the vitreous, there are signs of aphakia and the lens is seen in the vitreous with an ophthalmoscope.

Complications of subluxation and dislocation of the lens— Development of secondary glaucoma.

Causes of this glaucoma

(a) In subluxation—due to narrowing of the angle of the anterior chamber as a result of forward displacement of the lens and the iris.

(b) In anterior dislocation in the anterior chamber—due to blockage of the angle by the lens.

(c) In posterior dislocation in the vitreous—due to low grade cyclitis as a result of irritation of the ciliary body by the lens.

Treatment

1. For subluxated clear lens
   (a) To try glasses for improvement of vision.
   (b) If part of the pupil is aphakic, aphakic glasses may be tried.

2. For subluxated opaque lens—The lens should be removed by vectis (*see* under instruments) after making an incision like cataract operation. Cryo extraction is also possible.

3. For anterior dislocation of the lens in the anterior chamber—The lens must be removed by vectis, after making an incision like cataract operation.

4. For posterior dislocation in the vitreous
   (a) It is better to treat the case as an aphakic eye, by prescribing aphakic glasses.
   (b) An attempt may be made to remove the lens with a vectis or Cryo, but there is risk of marked vitreous disturbance and vitreous loss is usually inevitable.

Congenital Anomalies of the Lens

1. Coloboma of the lens—There is a defect in the margin of the lens in the form of a notch. Usually the inferior margin is affected.

2. Lenticonus—The posterior pole of the lens becomes cone-shaped, when it is called the posterior lenticonus. Refraction becomes myopic. The condition is best detected by a slit-lamp.

CHAPTER X

ANATOMY AND DISEASES OF THE VITREOUS

Anatomy of the vitreous

It is a transparent jelly like mass, occupying the posterior part of the eyeball, behind the lens. This gel consists of the fine protein micellae saturated with fluid. The outer surface of the vitreous is condensed to some extent, which was formally known as hyaloid membrane. The vitreous forms one of the refractive media of the eye. A canal, known as the hyaloid canal, extends through the vitreous, from the optic disc to the posterior capsule of the lens, which functions as a lymph channel. The vitreous has no blood vessels and it derives its nutrition from the surrounding structures like choroid, ciliary body, and retina. The vitreous is never regenerated and the portion, which is lost as in vitreous loss during cataract operation, is always replaced by intra-ocular fluid. As there is no blood vessels in the vitreous, no inflammation of this structure is possible, and only degenerative changes occur.

Fluidity of Vitreous (Synchisis)

When the gel is converted into a sol, the vitreous becomes fluid. This change may occur due to any type of insult. The common causes of fluid vitreous are—

(a) Senility.

(b) High myopia.

(c) As a sequel to diseases of the ciliary body, choroid and retina.

Vitreous detachment or Shrinkage of the vitreous—In advanced age, the vitreous may shrink. If there is a firm attachment between the vitreous and the retina, this shrinkage causes detachment of the retina.

Muscae Volitantes

These are minute opacities in the vitreous, seen by a normal person as dark spots floating in front of the eye, particularly when he looks at a bright surface. These opacities cast shadows on the retina, which are projected in the visual field as dark spots. They are harmless and do not cause any disturbance of vision.

Opacities of the Vitreous

Causes

1. Due to changes in the vitreous itself—

(a) In association with fluid vitreous, opacities may appear.

(b) Asteriod bodies—In elderly people, snow-ball like minute white opacities appear in large numbers, in a vitreous of normal consistency, so that when the eye moves, the opacities move with the eyeball. These particles consist of soaps and salts of higher fatty acids. There is no visual disturbance.

(c) Synchisis scintillans—These are numerous flakes of golden colour, in a fluid vitreous, which move independently in the vitreous when the eye moves. They are made of cholesterol. They usually occur in a younger age group with some organic disease in the eye.

2. Due to changes in the surrounding structures—

(a) Dust-like haze or aggregated clumps, due to escape of protein material from the capillaries of the ciliary body— the condition known as plasmoid vitreous. It occurs in association with cyclitis, chorio-retinitis, choroidal tumour or contusional injury.

(b) Inflammatory exudative cells—These are usually lymphocytes, mononuclear cells or plasma cells, which come out in inflammatory conditions of the ciliary body and the retina.

(c) Blood—Usually as a result of retinal haemorrhage.

(d) Epithelial cells—They are shed from the ciliary body in the vitreous.

(e) Tumour cells—Particularly in retinoblastoma.

(f) Pigment granules—Melanotic pigment granules are common in the vitreous in senility, glaucoma, trauma and inflammation, in retinal detachment and with melanotic tumours.

(g) Membranes in the vitreous, due to organization of vitreous haemorrhage, known as retinitis proliferans.

Symptoms and signs of vitreous opacities

Symptoms—Vitreous opacities appear as black spots floating in front of the eye. If the opacities are minute, they are only annoying but there is no visual disturbance. Dense opacities may cause marked fall of vision.

Signs—The opacities are best seen by a slit-lamp. They are also visible by the ophthalmoscope with a +8 D lens. They are seen as mobile opaque matter in the vitreous.

Treatment

Slight cases of muscae volitantis needs no treatment.

(a) Treatment of the cause like uveitis or retino choroiditis.

(b) Iodides by mouth or Iodine by injection has a doubtful action.

(c) Vitrectomy in desperate cases.

Vitreous Haemorrhage

Sources of haemorrhage

(a) From retinal blood vessels.
(b) From choroidal blood vessels.
(c) From the vessels of ciliary body and iris.
(d) From vessels grown within the Vitreous.

Causes of vitreous haemorrhage

(a) Injury to the eyeball..
(b) Diabetes mellitus with retinopathy.
(c) Hypertension and arteriosclerosis.
(d) Eale's disease.
(e) Blood diseases.
(f) Malignant melanoma of choroid.

Prognosis of vitreous haemorrhage—Small haemorrhages are usually absorbed, but in recurrent haemorrhages, retinitis proliferans may be formed.

Treatment—The cause of haemorrhage should be treated. Vitrectomy when the haemorrhage is no more absorbing.

CHAPTER XI

INTRA-OCULAR PRESSURE AND GLAUCOMA

Definition of intra-ocular pressure

It is the pressure above the atmospheric pressure, maintained inside the eyeball in normal condition, created by the volume of the solid and liquid contents of the eye and the elasticity of its coats.

Normal intra-ocular pressure

It varies from 16 to 23 mm. of Hg. It is higher than that developed inside any other organ in the body, as for example the normal tissue pressure is 2 to 3 mm. of Hg., and the cerebrospinal fluid pressure is about 7 mm. of Hg., in the recumbent position.

Why this high pressure in the eye?

Compared to other organs, this high pressure inside the eye is necessary for the maintenance of the optical properties of the refracting surfaces. As for example the curvature of the cornea and the smoothness of its surface must be kept constant and also the water content of the corneal stroma has to be maintained at a constant level to keep the refractive index uniform.

Factors responsible for normal intra-ocular pressure—

The pressure inside the eyeball is created by—
    (a) Elasticity of its outer coats i.e., cornea and sclera.
    (b) The volume of its solid and liquid contents.
    (c) Elasticity of the outer coats—

The outer wall of the eye does not act as a rigid box and there is a definite although very little distensibility of cornea and sclera. This distensibility exerts an important effect upon the mechanism of intra-ocular pressure.

    (d) Volume of intra-ocular contents—
The contents of the eye which help to maintain intra-ocular pressure are—

      (i) Solid and semi-solid structures like the lens, vitreous, uveal tract and retina which by change in volume may lead to alteration in the intra-ocular pressure.

      (ii) Fluid contents like blood and aqueous humour and a variation in their volume can alter intra-ocular pressure considerably.

Measurement of intra-ocular pressure

The methods by which intra-ocular pressure can be measured are the following—

1. *Manometry*—By this method a needle is introduced either into the anterior chamber or into the vitreous which is then connected with a suitable mercury or water manometer to measure the intra-ocular pressure. This method is accurate but not suitable for clinical application.

2. *Tonometry*—

There are two types—
(a) Digital tonometry—already described under "Examination of an eye case"
(b) Instrumental tonometry—there are two types—
(i) impression tonometry i.e., to measure the depth of the impression produced upon the ocular wall by a given force.
(ii) applanation tonometry i.e., to measure the force necessary to flatten an area of the cornea.

By tonometry the tension of the outer coat of the eye is measured by assessing its impressibility as by an impression tonometer (Schiötz) or by assessing its applanability as by an applanation tonometer. As the intra-ocular pressure keeps the cornea and the sclera in a state of tension, by measuring this tension the intra-ocular pressure can be deduced. But as this deduction cannot be absolutely correct due to various factors involved, the nomenclature used for practical purposes is that the results of manometry are expressed as intra-ocular pressure and those of tonometry as intra-ocular tension.

Impression tonometry by Schiötz tonometer

Description of Schiötz tonometer (Fig. 72)

This tonometer was first devised in 1905 and later on slightly modified in 1924 by Hjalmar Schiötz. The tonometer consists of the following parts—

1. A handle (H) for holding the instrument in the vertical position on the cornea. The handle consists of two-side arms and a cuff attached to them through which passes a cylinder.

2. A cylinder the lower end of which forms a concave foot-plate (F). It rests on the cornea. The radius of curvature of the concavity of the foot-plate is 15 mm. whereas the radius of curvature of cornea is 7.8 mm. on the average. Thus when the foot-plate is placed on the cornea the central part of its concavity only touches the cornea, the periphery of the foot-plate being clear of the cornea.

3. A plunger assembly (PL)—it is a solid cylinder about 1.5 mm. in diameter which pases through a hole in the centre of the cylinder with the foot-plate and can move up and down. The lower end of the plunger has a slightly convex surface which dimples the cornea when placed over it.

4. A bent lever (L)—It has a short arm which rests on the upper end of the plunger and a long arm which acts as a pointer (P) and it moves against the scale (S).

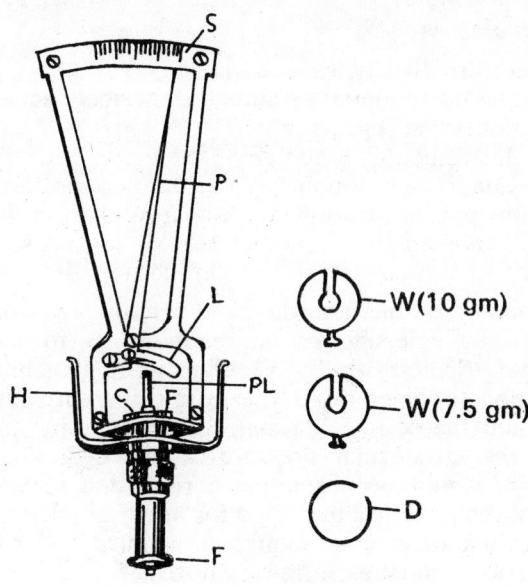

Fig. 72.　Schiötz Tonometer.

5. A scale (S) with markings—The pointer glides against this scale according to the movements of the plunger which being magnified twenty times are transmitted to the pointer through the bent lever. The intervals between the consecutive markings on the scale represent displacements of 0.05 mm. of the top of the plunger relative to the foot-plate.

6. Weights (W)—Three types of weights are used with the tonometer. The plunger itself weighs 5.5 gm. which is marked on a circular disc (C) around the upper part of the plunger. So when the tonometer is placed on the cornea, the indenting force of the plunger is 5.5 gm. Two additional loose discs (W) are

supplied with markings of 7.5 gm. and 10 gm., which when placed separately on the plunger cause the indenting force to be 7.5 gm. and 10 gm. respectively. But the actual weight of the disc having 7.5 gm. stamped on it is 2 gm. and that of the disc with 10 gm. stamped is 4.5 gm.

7. A metal sphere (D) used as dummy cornea—its radius of curvature is also 15 mm. This is used for testing the tonometer before using it for tonometry. As there is no indenting movement of the plunger, when the tonometer is placed on the metal sphere, the pointer logically should be at 0 marked on the scale because there is no downward movement of the plunger. But in actual practice, the pointer shows a scale reading—1.0 i.e., it goes 1 mark beyond the markings on the scale. This should be the correct position of the pointer when the tonometer is placed on the dummy sphere with a radius of curvature of 15 mm., so that when the tonometer is placed on the normal cornea before making an indentation on the cornea the plunger dips down in the corneal epithelium for a distance of 0.05 mm. which corresponds to 1 scale reading and then the pointer rests at 0 mark.

Conversion of scale reading to intra-ocular pressure

As soon as a tonometer is placed on the eye, the forces which come into play are shown in the Fig. 73. W the weight of the tonometer acts over an area A and indents the cornea displacing a volume Vc. The tensile forces T set up in the outer coats of the eye at everywhere tangentially to the corneal surface, with a component opposing W, so that an additional force T is added to the original intra-ocular pressure P. Thus the scale readings of the tonometer give an impression of high intra-ocular pressure (Duke-Elder). It has been calculated that an increase of volume of the eyeball of about 0.1 percent caused a sudden rise of intra-ocular pressure from 20 to 30 mm. of Hg. Clinically it is the aim to find out the

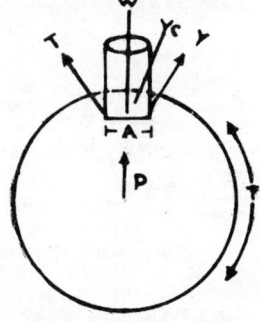

Fig. 73
Impression Tonometry

original intra-ocular pressure which is designated as Po i.e., the pressure which existed before the tonometer was placed on the eye and not the pressure shown by tonometric reading which is designated at Pt. In order to deduce Po value for Pt, obtained from tonometric readings, excised human eyes were used in which intra-ocular pressure was brought to any desired level by a manometer attached to the eye and tonometry performed. In this way it could be assessed how intra-ocular pressure would show how much scale reading of the tonometer. Various data were obtained by using various weights i.e., 5.5 gm., 7.5 gm. and 10 gm. and curves were drawn as shown in the (Fig. 74). Thus actual intra-ocular pressure of Po value is obtained by referring the scale reading to the chart.

Sterilization of the tonometer

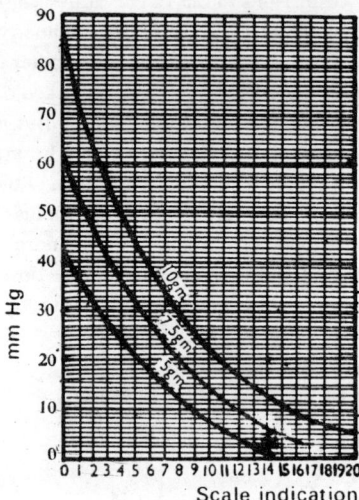

Before application the foot-plate and the lower end of the plunger have to be sterilized. This is necessary to avoid cross infection and development of corneal ulceration, if by chance the corneal epithelium gets abraded by the tonometer.

Methods of sterilization

After testing the tonometer on the dummy it is sterilized by the following methods—

1. By dipping the foot-plate in ether or absolute alcohol—after using these chemicals sufficient time must be allowed for ether or alcohol to evaporate.

2. By heating the foot-plate in the flame of a spirit lamp for 10 seconds in this process also adequate time must be allowed for cooling of the tonometer.

Fig. 74. Scale for the weighted Tonometer of Schiötz (Duke-Elder).

3. By exposure to ultra-violet radiation—this method is not generally used.

Practice of tonometry

The cornea is anaesthetized by instilling 4% xylocaine every 5 minutes three times.

The patient must lie down on a couch in a supine position without any pillow under the head.

He is then asked to look with his other eye vertically upwards towards the ceiling in order to relax accommodation. In case the vision in the other eye is poor, he is asked to raise his hand vertically upwards and then to direct his gaze towards his hand.

The surgeon separates the eye lids with the fingers of his left hand avoiding any pressure on the globe and then by holding the side arms of the handle of the tonometer in his right hand he gently rests the foot-plate of the tonometer vertically on the centre of the cornea (See under 'Examination of an eyeball').

The patient is encouraged not to move his eyes and the scale reading is recorded as soon as the pointer becomes steady. It should be aimed to take a correct reading by first application of the tonometer as repeated applications cause lowering of intra-ocular pressure.

An antibiotic ointment is then applied to the eye after tonometry.

Intra-ocular pressure is deduced by referring the scale reading to the chart.

N. B—Can tonometry be performed by placing the tonometer on the sclera, a process known as scleral tonometry ?—The answer is no ; because there is wide variation from eye to eye in the physical properties of the conjunctival and episcleral tissue overlying the sclera.

(Errors of indentation tonometry)

1. *Errors inherent in the instrument—*

As in case of any machine, instrumental errors may be present in a Schiötz tonometer. These errors are usually in the form of difference in the weight of the different parts of the instrument in different tonometers, friction arising in the working of the plunger, size, shape and curvature of the foot-plate and the plunger and the smoothness of the gliding movement of the pointer on the scale. There is a committee in U.S.A. for standardization of the tonometers to reduce the instrumental errors to minimum but still differences upto 3 mm. of Hg. are frequently found on measuring the tension of the same eye (Armaly 1960).

2. *Errors due to contraction of extra-ocular muscles—*

There is always reflex contraction of the extra-ocular muscles to some extent whenever a tonometer is placed on the eye. This process tends to increase the original intra-ocular pressure.

3. *Errors due to accommodation—*

As soon as the tonometer is brought to the eye there is a tendency to look at the tonometer and thus accommodation comes into play. The contraction of the ciliary muscle increases the facility of outflow of the aqueous due to a pull on the trabeculae at the angle of the anterior chamber and thus causes lowering of intra-ocular pressure. This process can be prevented by asking the patient to look at an object on the ceiling.

4. *Errors due to rigidity of the outer coats of the eyeball—*

As soon as a tonometer is placed on the cornea, the cornea is dimpled by the plunger causing displacement of the contents of the eyeball which distends the remainder of the globe. This process brings into play the elastic tensile forces as shown in Fig. 75. The result is that the original intra-ocular pressure is raised and more the outer coats are rigid, more is the rise of pressure. Thus the deduction of intra-ocular pressure from tonometric reading will be higher in an eye with a higher ocular rigidity than in an eye with a less rigidity although the original undisturbed intra-ocular pressure may be the same in each case.

5. *Errors due to variations with the volume of the globe—*

Tonometric readings vary with the size of the globe and curvature of the cornea. Thus errors may arise in cases of microphthalmose, buphthalmos and high myopia, because higher the radius of curvature of the cornea more is the tension as shown by the tonometer.

6. *Errors in scale reading—*

During scale reading there may be a reading error of about one scale division on either side. As for example with 5.5 gm. plunger weight if the scale reading is 5, the intra-ocular pressure is 17.3 mm. of Hg. But if the reading is 6, the pressure comes upto 14.6, whereas if the reading is 4, the pressure deduced becomes 20.6 mm. of Hg.

Thus it is obvious that tonometry is never absolutely accurate. It has been observed that in normal circumstances the limits of errors of a good Schiotz tonometer are ± 2 mm. of Hg., in the normal pressure range and ± 4 mm. in the higher ranges (Duke-Elder).

How to determine ocular rigidity

In order to determine whether the ocular rigidity is above or below average normal, differential tonometry is done i.e., tonometric readings are obtained with 5.5 gm. and 10 gm. plunger weights. The intra-ocular pressure in an eye with average normal rigidity will be the same whatever weight is used. But if the rigidity is high then 10 gm. weight will show a higher intra-ocular pressure and if the rigidity is low, the pressure with the 10 gm. weight will also lower than that determined by 5.5 gm. weight.

In such a case with abnormal ocular rigidity, a correction has to be done in the following way. The figure 75 is the nomogram by Fridenwald.

There are four slanting curves showing scale readings with 5.5, 7.5, 10 and 15 gm. weights. The ordinate shows the intra-ocular pressure in mm, Hg. The abscissa shows the volume or indentation of cornea is cu. mm. The semi-circular scale at the lower left hand corner shows the co-efficient of ocular rigidity. As shown in the figure, A represents the scale reading with 5.5 gm. and B the scale reading with 10 gm. weight during differential tonometry. The line joining A and B if

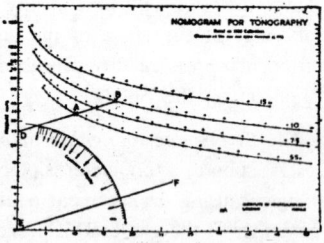

Fig. 75   Differential Schiötz Tonometry—low rigidity eye.

extended to the left, intersects the ordiante at D which shows the actual intra-ocular pressure Po. Another line EF extended from the lower left hand corner and parallel to AB corsses the semi-circular scale at F and this point shows the co-efficient of ocular ridigity. Normal average co-efficient of ocular rigidity is 0.0215.

Applanation tonometry

The underlying principle of this method is to find out the force necessary to applanate i.e., to flatten a tiny central area of the cornea of 3.06 mm. in diameter. As shown in Fig. 76, W is the force applied by the tonometer to flatten A which is a very small area of the cornea. P is the intra-ocular pressure and Vc is the displaced volume. The tensile forces T set up, lie in the plane of the plate perpendicular to the action of W and therefore there is no tendency to oppose W (Duke-Elder). So W equals to P×A. As the area A and the displaced volume Vc are very small, virtually W equals to P, and thus the pressure necessary to applanate the cornea becomes equivalent to the intra-ocular pressure.

Description of Applanation Tonometer

Applanation tonometer devised by Goldmann in 1954 is most commonly used. As shown in Fig. 77, the tonometer with the drum D and an applicator A is fitted to a slit-lamp of which C is the chin rest and H is the head rest for the patient. The observer looks at the applanted area through the eye-piece E of the slit-lamp. The applicator A consists of a cylinder at the end of which is fixed a plexiglass plate 7 mm. in diamater which is used to flatten an area of the cornea 3.06 mm. in diameter. Inside the cylinder there are two prisms with their bases in opposite direction. With the help of a coiled spring and lever system the plexiglass plate is made to press on the cornea and the force employed is controlled and recorded by a drum D calibrated directly in mm. of Hg.

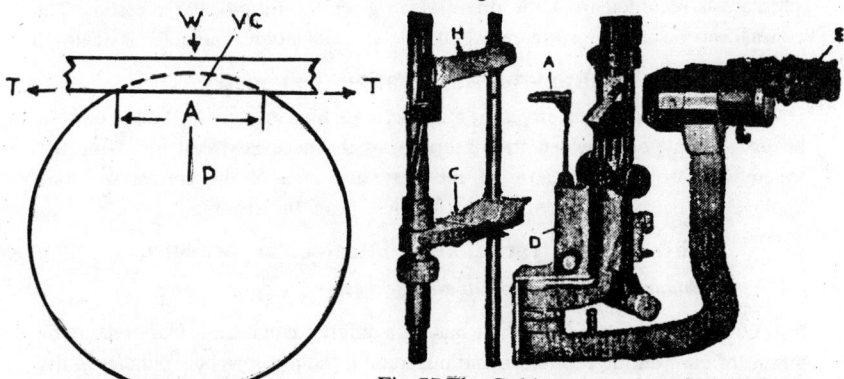

Fig. 76. Applanation Tonometer mechanism of action

Fig. 77. The Goldmann applanation tonometer mounted on the Haag Streict '900' slit-lamp (Golster).

Clinical use of Applanation Tonometer

The cornea is anaesthetized by instilling 4 percent xylocaine solution every 5 minutes three times.

The patient is seated at the slit-lamp with his chin on the chin rest and his forehead touching the head rest and he is advised to look straight ahead at a distant object in order to relax his accommodation.

The plexiglass plate of the applicator is sterilized with ether or rectified spirit. A blue filter is placed in the path of the illuminating rays of the slit-lamp.

The conjunctiva is touched with a filtered paper soaked with a definite amount of fluorescein solution.

The entire set up of the tonometer is then shifted forwards so that the plexiglass plate of the applicator touches the central part of the cornea. As soon as the plate presses on the cornea a circular green ring of tear film stained with fluorescein should be visible. But due to the presence of the two prisms with their bases in opposite direction inside the applicator, the ring is seen to break up into

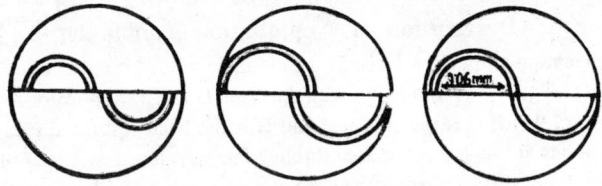

Fig. 78.   The applanation area is too small.
Fig. 79.   Area too large
Fig. 80.   Area of correct size

two semi-circles as shown in Fig. 78 to 80. The knob in the drum is then rotated to adjust pressure so that the semicircles achieve the position shown in Fig. 88. This pressure is recorded from the drum which gives the intra-ocular pressure. The normal intra-ocular pressure recorded by the applanation tonometer is 15 to 16 mm. of Hg.

Accuracy of Applanation Tonometry

This method of tonometry is far more accurate than impression tonometry by a Schiotz tonometer provided the observer has the necessary skill for doing the tonometry. Moreover because of the very tiny area of the cornea which is applanated, ocular ridigity does not interfere with the readings.

Physiological variation in intra-ocular pressure

1. *Variation with respiration and pulse beat—*

When respiration is deep, there may be a difference of intra-ocular pressure by 5 mm. of Hg., during expiration and inspiration, the pressure being higher in the former. The individual pulse beats generally produce pressure changes amounting to 1 to 2 mm. of Hg.

2. *Diurnal variations of intra-ocular pressure—*

Normally intra-ocular pressure varies in different periods in 24 hous in the following manner—(See Fig. 89).

(a) In the early morning the pressure is highest and then it falls in two phases—
  (i) a sharp fall soon after rising and then
  (ii) a slow decrease of pressure which continues until late in the evening.
(b) In the night the pressure rises again in two phases—
  (i) a slow rise for the first six hours and then
  (ii) a sharp rise increasing to maximum in the early morning bofore walking.

The maximum diurnal variation of intra-ocular pressure in normal eye is 5 mm. of Hg.

Theories regarding the cause of diurnal variation—

(a) changes in the size of the pupil,
(b) massaging effect on the eye by movements of the lids and contraction of the extra-ocular muscles and
(c) resistance in the drainage channels and increase in the episcleral venous pressure.

But exact cause for this physiological phenomenon is not yet known.

Factors responsible for maintenace of steady level of normal intra-ocular pressure

Although there are minor physiological variations of intra-ocular pressure as already descirbed, there is more or less constant steady level of intra-ocular pressure, inspite of the fact that there is a continuous drainage of the aqueous humour or in other words there is a continuous leakage from the eye. The factors which maintain this steady level are as follows—

(a) Continuous formation of the aqueous humour by secretory process of the ciliary epithelium and by ultra-filtration from the ciliary capillaries.
(b) The normal resistance offered by the drainage channels for the outflow of the fluid from the eye.
(c) The pressure in the episcleral veins in which ultimately the aqueous humour is drained.

GLAUCOMA

Definition—It is a condition where the intra-ocular pressure of the eyeball increases more than normal (normal pressure=16 to 23 mm. of Hg. by Schiotz tonometer).

Factors which cause rise of intra-ocular pressure

In general these factors are—

A. An increase in the volume of the intra-ocular contents—

    (i) Increase in quantity of the aqueous humour due to an increase in the rate of aqueous production or due to a decrease in the rate of outflow of the fluid as a result of obstruction to its drainage.

    (ii) Increase in the blood volume due to an increased arterial and capillary volume or due to a decrease in venous outflow.

    (iii) Increase in the volume of the lens and the vitreous.

B. External pressure upon the globe.

Classification of Glaucoma

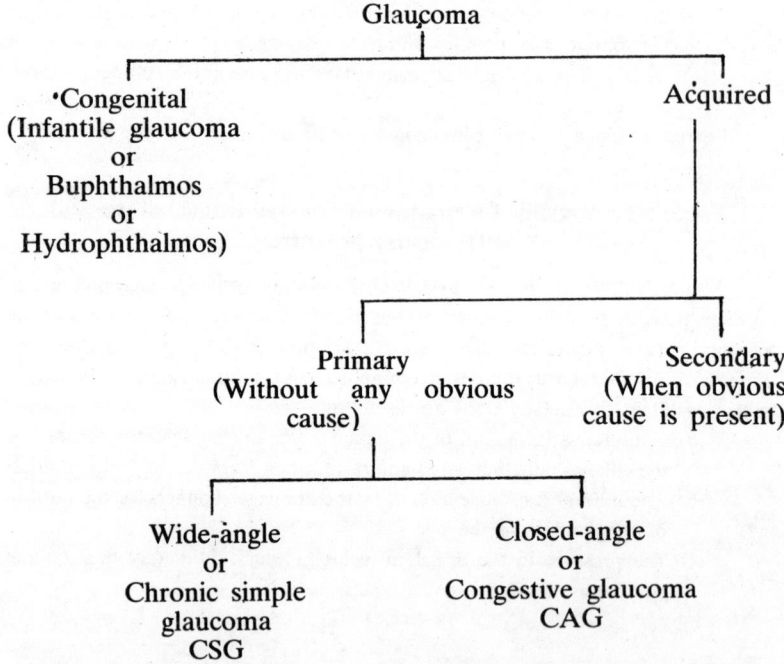

N.B. Absolute glaucoma—It is a stage of glaucoma when sense of perception and projection of light is lost. This condition may occur in the final stage of buphthalmos, wide-angle glaucoma, closed-angle glaucoma or secondary glaucoma.

Infantile Glaucoma
(Buphthalmos, Hydrophthalmos)

Etiology

1. Age—It is congenital and present from birth.
2. Sex—Boys are more affected than girls.
3. Bilaterality—Usually bilateral in 80 percent of cases.
4. Causative mechanism—Congenital abnormality at the angle of the anterior chamber, causing obstruction to the drainage of aqueous. These anomalies may be—(a) persistence of mesodermal tissue at the angle, (b) failure of mesodermal cleavage, which normally leads to opening of the angle, (c) absence of canal of Schlemm.

Symptoms

1. Photophobia. 2. Defective vision.

Clinical signs

1. The earliest clinical signs are epiphora, blepharospasm and intolerance to light. These signs may be present weeks before corneal haziness or enlargement becomes obvious to the parents. These signs are related to the irritation caused by slight oedema of the cornea due to increased intra-ocular pressure.

2. The eyeball as a whole enlarges, being elongated and oval in shape. This enlargement is due to extensibility of the sclera and the cornea in infancy.

3. Enlarged eyeball gives a false impression of proptosis. As the eyeball assumes the similarity of the eye of an ox, the term buphthalmos has been used.

4. Changes in the cornea—
   (a) Oedema of the cornea—At first most of the oedema is in the corneal epithelium, but later on it spreads to the corneal stroma. In 25 per cent of the cases the oedema is present at birth and in over 60 per cent by the sixth month. This oedema causes haziness of the cornea.
   (b) Enlargement of the cornea—Under the influence of the raised intra-ocular pressure there is progressive enlargement of the infant cornea. If there is no rise of pressure until after the age of 3 years, the eyes usually, resist distention. Most infant corneas measure under 10.5 mm. in the horizontal meridian. A measurement over 12 mm. is diagnostic of enlargement of the cornea. Prognosis becomes poor if the corneal diameter exceeds 14 mm.

(c) Tears in the Descemet's membrane—The major part of the enlargement of the eye of an infant occurs at the corneo-scleral junction. As the Descemet's membrane is less elastic than the corneal stroma, the membrane ruptures. These splits in the Descemet's membrane appear as single or multiple ridges and are situated at first at the peripheral part of the cornea. These ruptures also increase the haziness of the cornea.

5. The aqueous veins are absent and so they are not visible. The drainage of aqueous is partially carried out through the anterior ciliary veins.

6. The sclera becomes thin due to stretching and appears blue due to the underlying uveal tissue showing through it.

7. The anterior chamber is deep.

8. The lens becomes flat due to stretching of the suspensory ligament and may be subluxated.

9. The iris becomes tremulous due to flattening of the lens and may show atrophic patches.

10. The fundus, when examined by an ophthalmoscope, shows cupping of the disc.

11. There is rise of intra-ocular pressure, which is neither marked nor acute.

12. There is myopic error of refraction due to expansion of the eyeball, but the myopia is not upto that extent which is expected. This effect is due to flattening and slight posterior displacement of the lens.

13. There may be other associated congenital malformations like neuro-fibromatosis (von Recklinghausen's disease) or facial angioma (Sturge-Weber syndrome).

N.B. It may be required to examine the child under general anaesthesia and this is particularly necessary for the measurement of intra-ocular pressure and the corneal diameter. The most suitable method is induction by nitrous oxide and oxygen and not with ether; because by this method there is no marked fall of intra-ocular pressure.

Diagnostic criteria of buphthalmos

1. Enlarged eyeball with raised intra-ocular tension in a child.
2. Oedema or linear opacities of cornea.
3. Cupping of the optic disc.

TABLE IX

Differential diagnosis between buphthalmos and megalocornea

Buphthalmos	Megalocornea
1. Familial occurrence rare.	1. Familial occurrence common.
2. Males to females=5 : 3	2. Almost entirely in males.
3. Unilateral in 35% of cases.	3. Bilateral.
4. Corneal opacities and ruptures in Descemet's membrane.	4. No corneal opacities.
5. Visual impairment is marked.	5. No visual impairment.
6. Intra-ocular tension raised	6. No rise of tension.
7. Gross abnormalities at the angle of the anterior chamber.	7. No malformation at the angle.
8. Cupping of the disc present.	8. No cupping of the disc.

Course and prognosis of a case of buphthalmos

(a) Equilibrium may be established and further loss of vision may be checked.

(b) In other cases, rapid fall of vision may occur, particularly after puberty and ultimately absolute glaucoma develops, if not treated in time.

Treatment—Not very satisfactory.

1. Miotics are of no value.
2. Operative treatment—

   (a) Ordinary fistulizing operations, like trephining or iridencleisis have been replaced by trabeculectomy.

   (b) Goniotomy—i.e., to cut through the mesodermal tissue at the angle of the anterior chamber, with the point of a specially constructed knife, introduced through the limbus. If successful, the angle opens and tension becomes controlled.

Primary wide-angle Glaucoma
(Chronic simple glaucoma)

Definition

It is a type of primary glaucoma, where there is no obvious cause for the rise of intra-ocular tension and the angle of the anterior chamber remains wide.

Etiology

1. Age—Middle aged and elderly people are usually affected. Incidence increases rapidly after the age of 40.

N.B. The term-juvenile glaucoma is a misnomer. This condition is either due to a wide-angle glaucoma of early onset or due to an infantile glaucoma of late onset.

2. Sex—Mostly equal in both sexes but there is slight preponderance of the males.

3. Bilaterality—Usually bilateral.

4. Nature of the patient and associated factors—
   (a) This type of glaucoma is more common with high degree of myopia.
   (b) Capillary fragility is normal.
   (c) Although the patients are subjects of vascular sclerosis, systemic high blood pressure is not an etiological factor.
   (d) Disturbance of sympathetic nervous system is not the underlying cause.

5. Causative mechanism—The actual cause for the glaucoma is not known. But it is certain that the increased intra-ocular pressure is due to interference with the aqueous outflow, caused by some changes in the trabeculae, the Schlemm's canal or in the exit channels from the Schlemm's canal. There is also associated vascular sclerosis, which may hamper the absorption of the aqueous humour.

Pathology

   (a) Due to increased intra-ocular pressure, there is atrophy of retinal nerve fibre bundles as well as atrophy of the ganglion cells.
   (b) The lamina cribrosa is depressed backwards and this condition is called cupping of the optic disc.
   (c) There is cavernous atrophy of the optic nerve, *i.e.*, cavity formation in the nerve without gliosis.
   (d) There is sclerosis of the trabeculae at the angle, with deposition of pigment.
   (e) In later stages, whole of the uveal tract becomes atrophic. The angle of the anterior chamber remains clear, without any peripheral synechia.

Symptoms

1. The onset is very insidious and symptoms may be practically nil in the early stages.

2. Mild headache and eyeache may occur but the pain and the headache are never severe.

3. Presbyopic glasses may require frequent change due to accommodative weakness, as a result of pressure upon the ciliary muscle and its nerve supply.

4. An intelligent and observant patient may notice defect in his field of vision at a little more advanced stage.

5. Gradual dimness of central vision is noted at a later stage.

6. Also in the later stages there may be night-blindness, due to peripheral field defect and loss of function of the peripheral parts of the retina.

Clinical signs

1. The eye remains quiet with a clear cornea, normal anterior chamber and normally acting pupil. At a very late stage, the cornea may be slightly hazy and the pupil reaction may become sluggish. Continued high tension may cause a visible dilatation of the anterior ciliary arteries particularly the perforating branches.

2. Rise of intra-ocular tension—It is indicated by both digital tonometry and by Schiotz tonometer. But the state of the intra-ocular tension requires careful study and repeated observation, particularly in the early stages. For this purpose, the patient should be admitted in a hospital and a tension curve has to be drawn by recording intra-ocular tension at frequent intervals. The diurnal variation of tension takes up the following pattern in chronic simple glaucoma.

　　(a) In the early stage, the normal diurnal variation is exaggerated. Normal variation is shown in the curve below.

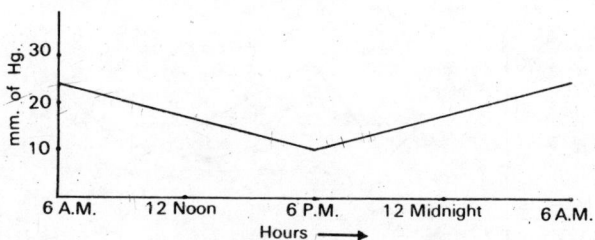

Fig. 81. Normal diurnal variation
on intra-ocular pressure.

　　(b) There may be morning rise of tension in 20 percent of cases as shown in the curve below.

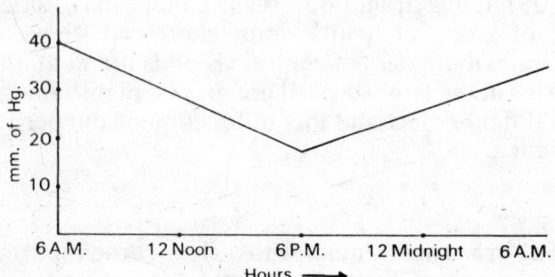

(c) There may be afternoon rise of tension in 25 percent of cases as shown in the curve below.

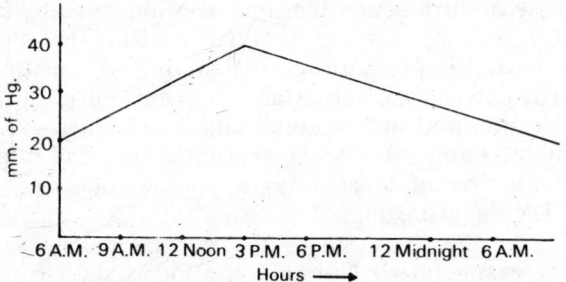

(d) There may be biphasic variation or double rise in 55 percent of cases as shown in the curve below.

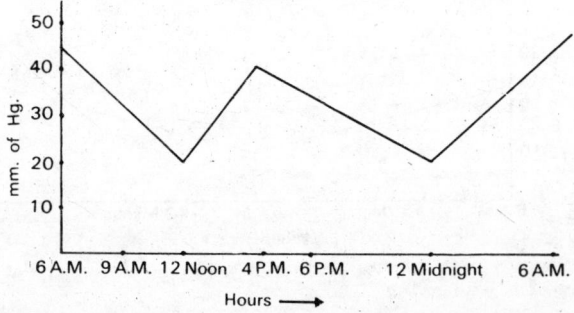

Between the phasic rises, the tension comes to normal. So if the patient is examined during the phase when the tension is normal, the diagnosis may be missed and for this reason a 24-hour tension curve is necessary.

(e) In the established stage of glaucoma later on, the normal level of intra-ocular tension is never attained.

The difference between the peak pressure and the base pressure diminishes and permanent elevation of tension persists.

The intra-ocular tension in chronic simple glaucoma is never very high. Usually it varies between 30 to 40 mm. of Hg. In the early stages, although the tension may remain within the normal range, a variation of tension of over 5 mm. of Hg should excite suspicion about glaucoma.

3. Cupping of the optic disc—The cupping of the optic disc is detected when examined by direct or indirect method of ophthalmoscopy. This is an early sign. The cupping means excavation of the disc (Fig. 82).

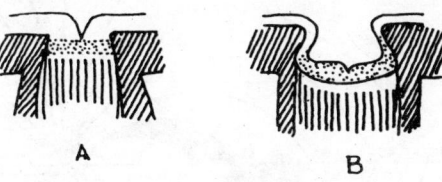

A B

Fig. 82

A—Normal optic nerve head B—Excavated optic nerve head or cupping.

The disc appears pale, the excavation reaches upto the margin of the disc, and the sides of the excavation are steep. The retinal vessels have the appearance of being broken off at the margin of the disc (Fig. 83).

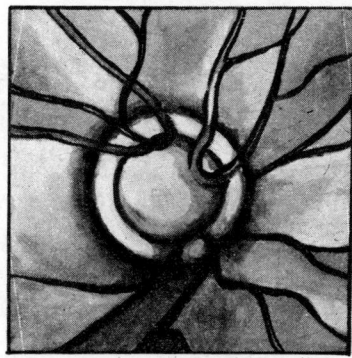

Fig. 83. Glaucomatous cupping of the optic as seen by an ophthalmoscope (Parsons).

The pulsation of the retinal arteries may be seen at the margin of the disc—a very pathognomonic sign of glaucoma.

The underlying mechanism for cupping of the disc.

(a) Mechanical factor—increased intra-ocular pressure forces the lamina cribrosa backwards.

(b) Vascular factor—This is more important. The associated vascular sclerosis, affecting the arterial supply of the optic nerve near the disc, produces ischaemic atrophy of the optic nerve, without corresponding increase of supporting glial tissue. As a result, cavernous spaces are formed within the optic nerve, the support of lamina cribrosa is lost and consequently the lamina bulges backwards.

4. Defects in the field of vision—

The changes in the field of vision run parallel with the changes in the optic disc. The normal course of nerve fibres in the retina is shown in Fig. 84.

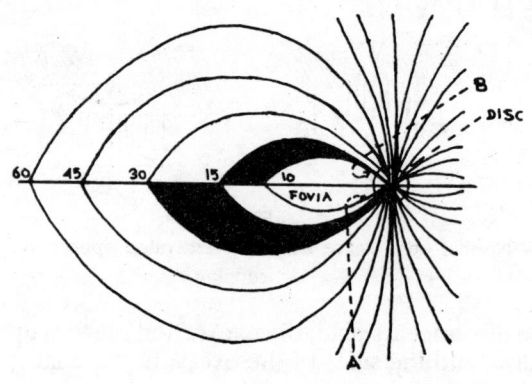

Fig. 84. Normal course of nerve fibres in retina (Parsons).
The shaded areas indicate the nerve bundles which when affected produce the filled defects as shown in Fig. 88.

It is already known that in chronic simple glaucoma, there is damage of nerve fibre bundles and so the field defects are clinically manifested according to the nerve fibre bundles affected.

(a) Earliest field defect is the baring of the blind spot (Fig. 85).

When the central field is plotted on a 2 metre Bjerrum's screen with a white object 1 mm. in diameter, normally the line limiting the visual field (known as isopter) is a 30° circle. But in glaucoma, the line curves inwards to exclude the blind spot. The actual mechanism for this early field defect is not definitely known.

(b) In a somewhat later stage, small wing-shaped scotomata appear above and below the blind spot, which join
the blind spot very soon to form a sickle-shaped
scotoma, with its concavity towards the fixation point.
This type of field defect is known as Seidel's sign. (Fig.
86).

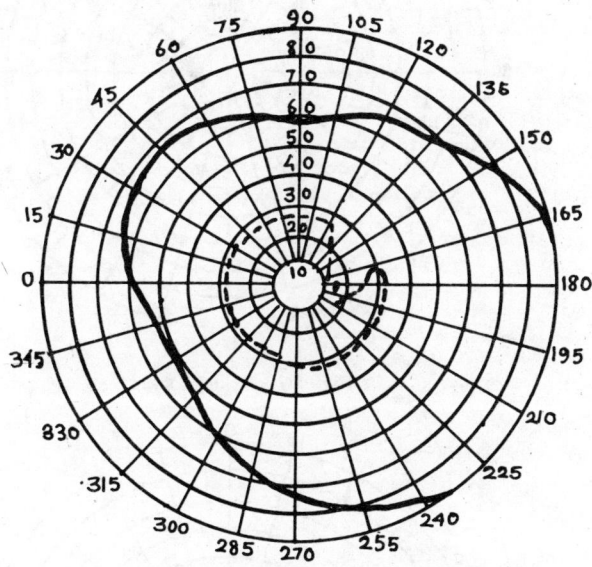

Fig. 85.   Baring of the blind spot.

(c) At a later stage, the sickle-shaped field defect extends
in an arc either above or below the fixation point to
reach the horizontal line. This type of field defect is
known as arcuate scotoma or Bjerrum's scotoma (Fig.
87). Two arcuate scotomata, on joining each other,
form an annular scotoma.

(d) The two arcuate scotomata may run in different arces,
one above and the other below the fixation point. On
reaching the horizontal meridian at the periphery, the
two scotomata meet to form a sharp right angle defect,

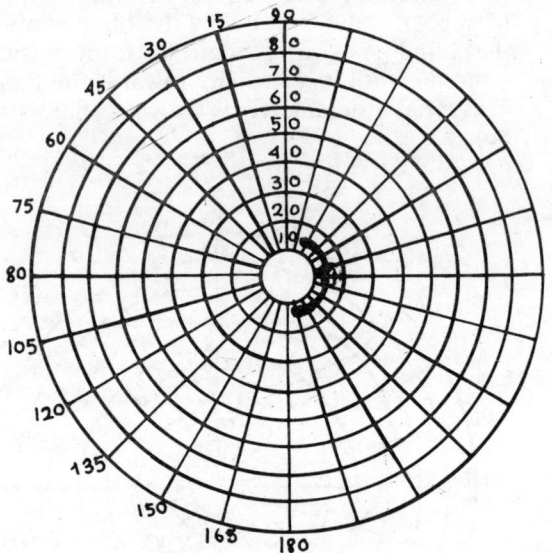

Fig. 86.   Seidel's sign.

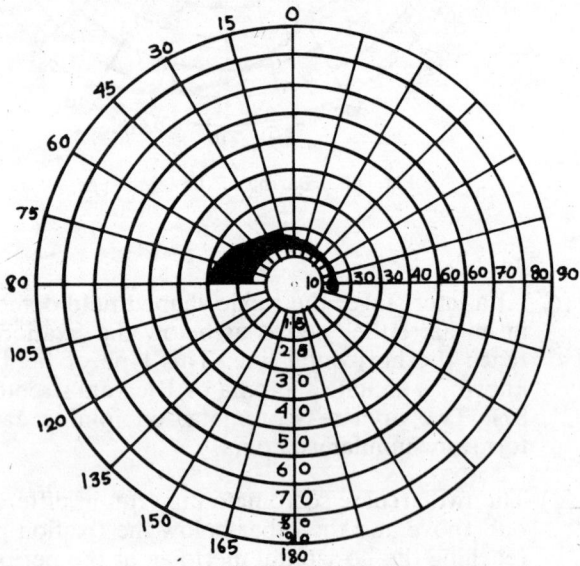

Fig. 87.   Bjerrum's Scotoma.

one side of the angle corresponding to the horizontal meridian., This defect is known as Roenne's nasal step (Fig. 88.).

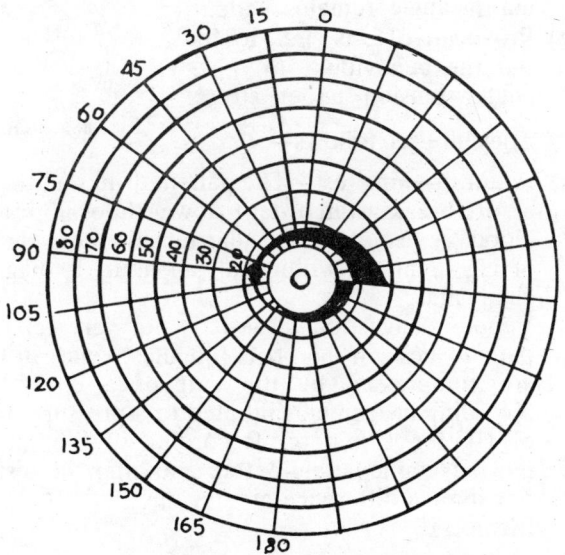

Fig. 88. Roenne's Nasal Step.

All these defects are elicited by scotometry on a Bjerrum's screen.

(e) Defects also appear in the peripheral field sometimes at an early stage or sometimes at a late stage. The peripheral field defect is usually either in the upper or in the lower nasal field. These defects are usually sector defects. This is how there is contraction of the nasal field in glaucoma. This defect is elicited by perimetry.

(f) In advanced stage of glaucoma, the peripheral field defect gradually extends all round the periphery, until only a central tubular field remains.

(g) Finally in the absolute stage, the central field is also abolished and the eye becomes blind.

Other diagnostic tests for chronic simple glaucoma

(a) Gonioscopy.—A gonioscope is a special instrument, which when placed on the cornea, reveals the angle of

the anterior chamber with the
help of a plane mirror incorporated in the insturment (Fig.
88 a).In chronic simple glaucoma the angle remains wide.

(b) Provocative tests, *i.e.,* to find
out the behaviour of intra-
ocular tension under stress.

They are as follows—

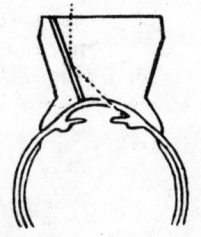

Fig. 88a. Gonioscope

(i) Water drinking test—The patient drinks a litre of water
before breakfast in order to lower the osmotic tension of
blood. A rise of intra-ocular tension more than 6 mm.
of Hg (Schiotz) within half an hour, is diagnostic of
glaucoma.

(ii) Venous congestion test—It is not very reliable. The
patient lies on his back, jugular veins in the neck
are compressed by the cuff of a blood pressure
recording instrument, inflated to a pressure of 50 mm.
of Hg for 1 minute. Recording of the intra-ocular
tension, immediately before and after the test, should
not show a difference greater than 9 or 10 mm. of Hg
(Schiotz).

Diagnostic criteria of chronic simple glaucoma

1. Elderly person complaining of gradual dimness of vision.
2. Raised intra-ocular tension.
3. Field defects.
4. Cupping of the optic disc.
5. External appearance of the eye—normal.

Differential diagnosis— This is done on the basis of gradual
dimness of vision in an elderly person—

1. Immature cataract.
   (a) Intra-ocular tension normal.
   (b) Black spot in the lens seen against the red fundal glow
       on dark room examination.
   (c) No cupping of the disc.
2. Optic atrophy
   (a) The optic disc is pale but no glaucomatous cupping.
   (b) Concentric contraction of the field.
   (c) Intra-ocular tension normal.

Treatment of chronic simple glaucoma

As soon as diagnosis is made treatment should be started.

1. Treatment by miotic—Pilocarpine nitrate 2 per cent drop is the best treatment is such cases. The medicine is dropped 2-3 times a day. Eserine sulph 0.5 to 1 per cent solution may be combined with pilocarpine.

Pilocarpine dilates blood vessels and in this way helps absorption of aqueous humour and lowers the intra-ocular tension. It also increases the tone of the ciliary muscle and as a result there is a pull on the trabeculae and so the trabecular meshwork is opened up which helps more outflow of the aqueous. In chronic simple glaucoma, constriction of the pupil does not help to lower the tension as the angle remains wide.

2. Recently Timolol maleate a β_1 and β_2 adrenergic antagonist in the trade name of Timoptic is used as 0.25% & 0.5% twice a day along with pilocarpine. Though its mode of action is not definitely known it acts primarily by reducing aqueous production.

3. Treatment by carbonic anhydrase inhibitor or diamox— Treatment by diamox is a temporary measure to tide over a crisis. 250 mgm. tablets are given by mouth twice or thrice daily. Because of its side effects, this drug cannot be continued for a long time.

If the intra-ocular tension remains controlled by miotic and so long as there is no further change in visual field defect and no change in the cupping of the disc, miotic should be continued. However, the patient must remain under observation and check up should be done every two months.

4. Operative treatment—If miotic fails to control the tension and the field defect progresses, operative measures have to be taken. The common operations are—

(a) TRABECULECTOMY OPERATION :—

This has become very popular now a days and it acts by subscleral filtration helped by some drainage through the opened Canal of Schlemm.

The limbal based conjunctival flap is reflected down at 12 O'clock position. A trap door of 2/3rd thickness of sclera is fashioned so that it is a 5 mm square and hinged at the limbus. A deeper trap door measuring 4 mm square is fashioned to expose the ciliary body, its attachment to the scleral spur and the root of the iris. This deep scleral flap is excised which contains in its anterior part the trabecular tissue and the canal of Schlemm. A peripheral iridectomy is performed. Superficial Scleral flap is sutured with two 8/0 virgin silk. Conjunctival flap is closed by continous silk suture.

(b) Iridencleisis operation—An incision is made through the sclera, underneath the conjunctiva, just beyond the limbus at 12 o'clock position and a piece of iris is drawn out and is kept in the scleral wound. The tag of iris works like a wick and drains the aqueous into the sub-conjunctival space (for further details *see* under operations).

(c) Elliot's Sclero-Corneal trephine. This once popular sub-conjunctival drainage operation is almost obsolete now a days.

Low-tension Glaucoma Or Pseudo-glaucoma

This is a condition which is not glaucoma in the true sense. It occurs bilaterally in elderly persons. There are cupping of the disc and visual field changes similar to those in chronic simple glaucoma. The angle of the anterior chamber is also wide. But the intra-ocular pressure remains either normal or subnormal. This pressure does not elevate during diurnal variations and also it can not be raised by provocative tests. The cupping and the field changes are due to vascular insufficiency of the optic nerve-head and the optic nerve. Thus this condition should be best considered as ischaemic neuropathy of the optic nerve.

Primary closed-angle Glaucoma

(Acute congestive glaucoma)

This is a condition in which the intra-ocular pressure is raised as a result of obstruction to the outflow of the aqueous due to extreme narrowness on closure of the angle of the anterior chamber consequent upon the close proximity of the iris to the cornea in the absence of any other disease of the eye.

Etiology

1. Age—Common at 45 to 50 years of age.
2. Sex—Women are more affected than men.
3. Type of individual—Highly strung, nervous individual, with unstable vasomotor system.
4. Type of the eye affected.
   (a) Usually the hypermetropic eye, *i.e.,* a small eye.
   (b) Eye with a shallow anterior chamber, with the lens-iris diaphragm situated forwards.

(c) Eye with a narrow angle. The narrowness of the angle may be due to—
    (i) smallness of the eye,
    (ii) bigger size of the ciliary body,
    (iii) relative bigger size of the lens.

5. Eye affected—Usually one eye is affected first and then the other eye.

6. Hereditary influence—Narrowness of the angle is often influenced by heredity.

7. Seasonal incidence—The peak incidence in this country is said to be in the rainy season. This occurrence is due to pupillary dilatation as a result of diminished light.

Grading of the angle width

(after Becker-Shaeffer)

The angle of the anterior chamber can only be examined with the help of a gonioscope. To compare the width of different angles it is convenient to have the following grading system—

Angle grade	Numerical grade	Implied clinical interpretation
Wide open angle (Fig. 89)	3 to 4	Closure impossible
Narrow angle, moderate (Fig. 90)	2	Closure possible
Narrow angle, extreme (Fig. 91)	1	Closure probable
Narrow angle, complete or partial closure (Fig. 92)	0	Closure present or imminent

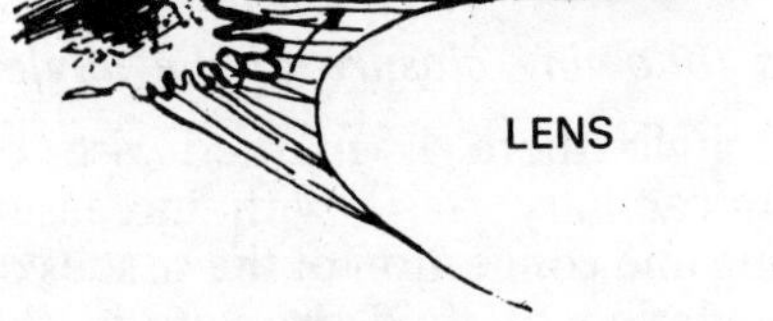

WIDE-OPEN ANGLE-GRADE 3-4

Fig. 89. Grading of angle width (Becker-Shaeffer).

Fig. 89.

Mechanism of closure of a narrow angle—It varies and is commonly due to the following factors—

(a) Dilatation of the pupil—The iris, on dilatation of the pupil, collects at the angle and so closes the already narrow angle. Thus it is dangerous to put atropine in the eye of an elderly person with a shallow anterior chamber.

    (b) A swelling or anterior displacement of the ciliary body due to congestion and oedema of the ciliary body following vasodilatation.

    (c) Relative pupillary block—If the lens is relatively large and the anterior chamber is shallow, a greater surface of the iris comes in contact with the anterior surface of the lens than is usual. There is tendency for the sphincter muscle to exert a posteriorly directed force on the lens surface. Thus resistance is created in the path of flow of aqueous from the posterior chamber through the pupil to the anterior chamber. As a result of this reistance the pressure in the posterior chamber rises and so there is physiological iris bombe and there is ballooning of the peripheral iris forwards and thus the already narrow angle becomes closed.

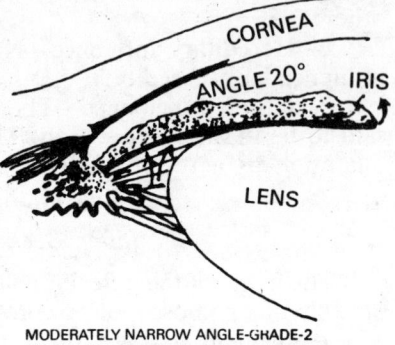

MODERATELY NARROW ANGLE-GRADE-2

Fig. 90. Grading of angle width (Becker-Shaeffer).

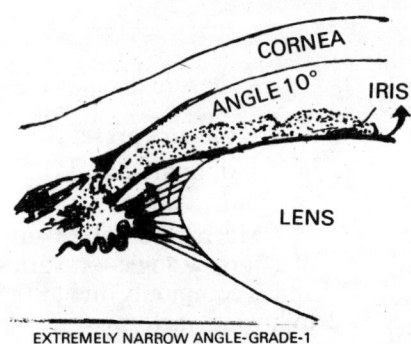

EXTREMELY NARROW ANGLE-GRADE-1

Fig. 91. Grading of angle width (Becker-Shaeffer).

Sequence of pathological events following closure of the angle

Following closure of the angle there is marked rise of intra-ocular pressure leading to capillary stasis with increased permeability resulting into oedema and congestion of the tissues of the eye, so that there is accumulation of fluid droplets in the corneal epithelium and congestion of the anterior ciliary veins of the conjunctiva. This is congestive glaucoma.

Pathological changes in the optic nerve and the retina.

Optic nerve—Immediately following the acute attack there is neither papilloedema *i.e.*, oedema of the optic disc nor cupping. Seventy two hours after the attack there is mild papilloedema and hydropic degeneration of the nerve fibre anterior to the lamina cribrosa. After six days if the tension remains unrelieved, the papilloedema increases and disintegration of nerve fibre becomes evident. Later on the papilloedema subsides and if the glaucoma persists after a period of two weeks, cupping of the disc with cavernous spaces in the optic nerve as seen in chronic simple glaucoma become apparent.

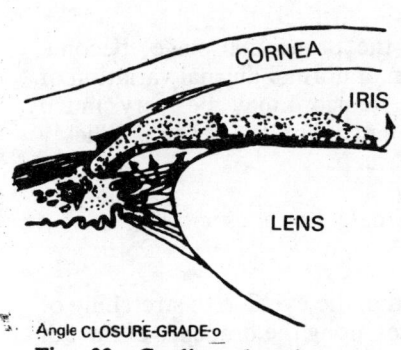

Angle CLOSURE-GRADE-o

Fig. 92. Grading of angle width (Becker-Shaeffer).

Retina—If tension remains unrelieved for three days, retinal changes appear in the form of spotty disappearance of the ganglion cells of the retina near the macula (Duke-Elder).

Clinical course of the disease has been divided into five stages

    A. Prodromal stage.
    B. Phase of constant instability.
    C. Acute congestive attack.
    D. Chronic congestive stage.
    E. Stage of absolute glaucoma.

A. Prodromal stage—

Symptoms

    1. Occasional attacks of blurring of vision with haloes around the light.
    2. Mild headache.
These symptoms are transient.

Clinical signs

    1. Sudden rise of intra-ocular tension for a short period, which may reach 40 or 60 mm. of Hg.
    2. The eye remains white and there is no congestion.

3. The cornea becomes slightly oedematous.

The rise of tension in this stage is transient and the attacks may be intermittent. Such transient ' attacks in this stage are precipitated by overwork, anxiety, fatigue or due to dilatation of the pupil in darkness as caused by a visit to a cinema or the use of mydriatic during refraction.

B. Phase of constant instability—

The attacks, as described in the prodromal stage, become more regular. There is exaggeration of normal diurnal variation of intra-ocular tension, so that the tension may be very much increased, particularly in the evening. But the tension quickly comes to normal on rest, or on sleep.

C. Acute congestive attack—

It is precipitated, when the angle becomes closed.

Symptoms

1. Sudden onset of intense pain in the eye due to stretching of the sensory nerves. The pain radiates along the branches of the 5th nerve.

2. Severe headache.

3. Marked dimness of vision and vision may be reduced to perception and projection of light only. This defect of vision is partly due to oedema of. cornea but is mainly due to pressure on the optic nerve fibres in retina.

4. Photophobia and lacrimation.

Clinical signs

1. Oedema of the lids.

2. Marked congestion of the conjunctiva—both ciliary and conjunctival congestion.

3. There may be chemosis of the conjunctiva.

4. Cornea becomes steamy and insensitive.

5. Anterior chamber is very shallow.

6. Pupil is moderately dilated, vertically oval and reaction to light and accommodation is abolished.

7. Iris is discoloured.

8. Intra-ocular tension becomes markedly raised and eyeball is very tender.

9. Examination of the fundus by an ophthalmoscope is not possible due to corneal oedema. But a drop of glycerine temporarily clears the cornea and then on examination of the fundus, the disc appears congested but there is no cupping.

10. Vision is reduced to perception and projection of light.

Along with these clinical signs there are associated systemic disturbances such as—

1. Vomiting with prostration.

2. Rise of body temperature with pulse becoming irregular.

Due to these systemic distrubances, an acute congestive glaucoma may be misdiagnosed as a case of acute abdomen.

Termination of an acute congestive attack.

1. If the tension is not controlled, either by medication or by operation, the eye becomes blind due to pressure atrophy of the nerve fibres of the retina.

2. But spontaneous improvement may occur, when the pain subsides, the tension becomes lowered and vision improves to some extent.

3. Recurrences of acute attacks are however common. With each recurrent attack following changes occur—

(a) Further lowering of visual acuity.

(b) Concentric contraction of the field of vision.

(c) Permanent adhesion of the congested root of the iris, to the inner surface of the cornea, forming peripheral anterior synechia. This synechia formation at first starts at the upper part of the angle and then spreads around the periphery. When three quarters of the circumference of the iris becomes attached to the cornea, the stage of chronic congestive glaucoma is reached.

D. Chronic congestive stage—

Clinical signs

1. The eye remains congested and irritable.

2. The tension remains permanently elevated.

3. Field defects appear, which are similar to those in chronic simple glaucoma.

4. Cupping of the disc becomes visible.

5. Vision remains depressed.

If no treatment is done, gradually the eye passes on to the final stage of absolute glaucoma.

E. Stage of absolute glaucoma—

Clinical signs

1. The eye is completely blind, as there is no perception of light. Such an eye is usually painful.

2. The anterior ciliary veins are dilated, with a slight ciliary flush around the cornea. In long standing cases constant engorg-

ment of the veins leads to formation of an irregular venous anastomosis around the limbus which is knows as "the Medusa head"

3. Cornea is hazy and insensitive. There may be epithelial bullae or filaments on the cornea formed by partially shed epithelium.

4. The anterior chamber is very shallow.

5. The iris is atrophic.

6. The pupil is dilated and there is no reaction to light. The pupil appears greyish or greenish.

7. The optic disc is deeply cupped if it could be seen.

8. The tension is very high—the eye may be stony hard. Sooner or later other changes take place—

1. The cornea becomes ulcerated due to lowering of the resistance of the epithelium as a result of persistent oedema and superficial vascularization of cornea takes place—glaucomatous pannus.

2. The corneal ulcer may perforate leading to panophthalmitis and later on to phthisis bulbi.

3. As a result of continued high intra-ocular pressure, the sclera may give way either in the ciliary region or in the equatorial region giving rise to ciliary and equatorial staphyloma.

4. In the long run, the eye may shrink as a result of pressure atrophy of the ciliary body.

Provocative tests for closed-angle glaucoma

These tests are of value in the early stages of narrow-angle glaucoma, *i.e.*, in the prodromal stage and in the stage of constant instability. Acute congestive stage as well as the chronic congestive stage does not require provocative tests for diagnosis.
The provocative tests are as follows—

(a) Dark-room test—The patient is placed in a completely dark room for half an hour, so that his pupil dilates. If the difference between the intra-ocular tensions measured before and after the test, goes above 8 mm. of Hg the test is positive. The dark-room test is reinforced by making the patient lie prone.

(b) Mydriatic test—The pupil of the suspected eye is dilated with homatropine hydrobrom 1 percent drop. If the tension rises more than 8 mm. of Hg due to the mydriatic, the test is positive. After this test miosis is mandatory.

Diagnostic criteria of closed-angle glaucoma in the early stages

(a) Attacks of sudden, transient, blurring of vision with rainbow halo around the light in an elderly person.

(b) Narrow angle of the anterior chamber revealed on gonioscopy.

(c) Positive provocative tests.

N.B. Circumstances in which a patient sees rainbow halo around a light are as follows—

(a) In the early stages of closed-angle glaucoma, when corneal oedema is the cause.

(b) In the early stages of cataract, when accumulation of water in between the lens fibres is the cause of halo.

(c) In the acute muco-purulent conjunctivitis, when a layer of mucous on the surface of the cornea breaks the white light into its component parts.

Differentiation between glaucomatous halo and lenticular halo

The patient is asked to look at a light around which he sees rainbow halo. A stenopaeic slit, which is nothing but a vertical slit in a disc or in a square plate, is moved in front of the eye from one side to the other. In glaucoma, the halo remains as it is, but the intensity of illumination of the halo diminishes due to the slit. In the case of a cataract, the halo breaks and rotates like a fan as shown in the figure. This test is known as Emsley-Fincham test. (Fig. 93).

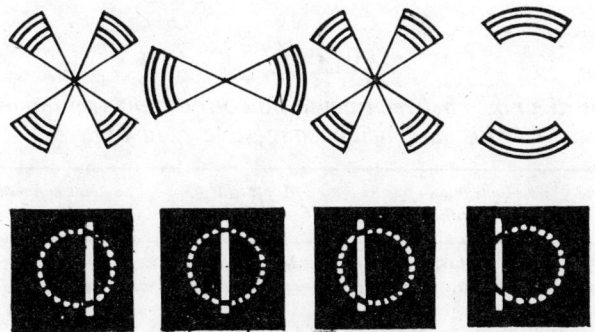

Fɪɢ. 93 Breaking up of the lenticular halo into a fan-Emsley-Fincham test (Parsons).

Different types of halos

A halo becomes best visible when a person looks at a bright source of light in an otherwise dark room. Two rings are seen around the light, of which the outer one is reddish yellow and the inner one is bluish violet. The angular diameter of the ring varies according to the origin of the halo. When the light is at a distance of 10 ft., the diameter of the halo due to conjunctival mucous is 14°, that due to oedema of corneal epithelium is 7°−12°, that due to changes in the lens is 6°−7° and that due to oedema of the corneal endothelium is about 4°.

Treatment of closed-angle glaucoma

1. In the prodromal stage and in the stage of constant instability—the patients seldom seek medical advice in these early stages.

The treatment to be followed in these stages are—
   (a) Instillation of miotic drops like pilocarpine nitrate, 2 percent or eserine sulph 0.5 to 1 percent 3 times daily. The miotics by contracting the pupil help the angle to remain open.
   (b) If miotics fail to stop the prodromal attacks, a surgical operation in the form of a peripheral button-hole iridectomy at 12 o'clock position is done. This operation helps the aqueous humour to pass directly to the anterior chamber from the posterior chamber and thereby the physiological iris bombe is prevented and the angle remains open. The iridectomy is done through a limbal incision.

TABLE X

Differential diagnosis between acute muco-purulent conjunctivitis, acute iritis and acute congestive glaucoma

Symptoms and signs	Acute muco- purulent conjunctivitis	Acute iritis	Acute congestive glaucoma
1. Pain	1. Mild discomfort	1. Moderate pain.	1. Severe pain radiating along the branches of the Vth nerve.
2. Tenderness.	2. Nil.	2. Marked.	2. Marked.
3. Vision.	3. Normal but may be slightly blurred. There may be halo around the light.	3. Impaired to some extent.	3. Marked impairment.
4. Onset of the disease.	4. Gradual.	4. Gradual.	4. Sudden.
5. Secretion.	5. Muco-purulent discharge.	5. Only lacrimation.	5. Only lacrimation.

6. Congestion.	6. Conjunctival type.	6. Mainly ciliary type.	6. Ciliary type and conjunctival hyperaemia.
7. Cornea.	7. Normal with normal sensation.	7. Normal with normal sensation.	7. Steamy and insensitive.
8. Anterior chamber.	8. Normal and clear.	8. Normal or may be hazy due to exudation, but not shallow.	8. Very shallow.
9. Pupil.	9. Normal in size and shape, and reactions are normal.	9. Irregular and small due to posterior synechia. Reactions are sluggish.	9. Dilated, vertically oval, and not reacting to light.
10. Tension.	10. Normal.	10. Normal, unless there is secondary glaucoma.	10. Markedly raised.
11. Systemic disturbance.	11. None.	11. Very little, like headache.	11. Many, such as vomiting, prostration and fever.

2. In the acute congestive stage—

A. Medical treatment—

(a) Treatment intended to lower the intra-ocular pressure—

(i) Pilocarpine 2 percent drop every 15 minutes for 1 hourly. It should also be instilled in the other eye, 3 times a day, as a prophylactic measure to prevent an acute attack.

(ii) Diamox 250 mgm. tablets by month 3 times a day—Potassium bicarbonate should be taken by mouth 1 to 3 gm. daily, during the treatment with diamox, to prevent the side effect of diamox. Diamox lowers the intra-ocular pressure by reducing the formation of aqueous humour.

(iii) Intravenous injection of 20 percent mannitol.

(b) Treatment for relief of pain—An injection of pethidine 100 mgm. should be given intramuscularly for the relief of pain.

(c) Treatment for relief of congestion—
Hydrocortisone acetate 1 percent drop every 1 hour.

B. Surgical treatment—

(a) If the tension is not controlled within 12 hours by medical treatment, a surgical operation has to be done.

However in majority of cases with above medical treatment the congestion and tension subside when the condition is reasonably quiet the condition of the angle is ascertained by gonioscopy. If there are no peripheral anterior synechiae, a peripheral button-hole iridectomy at 12 o'clock position is sufficient to keep tension under control.

But if peripheral anterior synechiae have already formed, a fitration operation has to be done.

(b) As a prophylactic measure, a peripheral button-hole iridectomy should be done in the other eye.

3. In chronic congestive stage—

There are already peripheral anterior synechiae in this stage, so, only peripheral button-hole iridectomy is of no avail. A fistulizing operation either in the form of Trabeulectomy or in the form of iridencleisis, should be done to control the tension. Miotics are useless in this stage.

4. In the stage of absolute glaucoma—

(a) The eye may be enucleated if the pain is troublesome.

(b) If enucleation is not desirable, the following procedures may be adopted—

(i) For relief of pain—Retrobulbar injection of 1 c.c. of 2 percent xylocaine followed by a retrobulbar injection of 1 c.c. of 80 percent alcohol to destroy the ciliary ganglion.

(ii) To lower the intra-ocular tension—Application of cryo or diathermy points to the sclera over the ciliary body along half the circumference of the eyeball.

Secondary Glaucoma

Definition—It means glaucoma secondary to some pre-existing disease. So, cause of the rise of intraocular pressure is known.

Causes of secondary glaucoma

1. Glaucoma due to inflammation—

(a) Acute iridocyclitis—The rise of tension is due to engorgement of uveal vessels, increased osmotic tension due to plasmoid aqueous and blockage of the angle of the anterior chamber by inflammatory exudate.

(b) Acute scleritis—The rise of tension is due to associated uveitis.

(c) Corneal ulcer with hypopyon—The glaucoma is due to blockage of the angle with the exudate.

(d) Panophthalmitis—The whole of the vitreous becomes converted into purulent matter and so the rise of tension is due to increased bulk of the ocular contents.

(e) Orbital cellulitis—The glaucoma is due to obstruction to the venous drainage from the eye, caused by inflammatory infiltration of orbital tissues.

2. Post-inflammatory causes—

(a) Ring synechia or occlusio pupillae with iris bombe — The glaucoma is due to obstruction to the drainage of aqueous humour from the posterior to the anterior chamber.

(b) Occlusio pupillae with iris bombe —The cause of glaucoma is the same as above.

Peripheral anterior synechia following acute iritis or iridocyclitis—The inflammed and swollen root of the iris adheres to the posterior surface of the cornea. The rise of tension is due to blockage of the angle.

(d) Adherent leucoma following perforation of corneal ulcer—The rise of tension is due to shallow anterior chamber and persistent drag on the iris.

3. Lens induced glaucoma—

(a) Intumescent cataract—The rise of tension is due to shallow anterior chamber.

(b) Burst Morgagnian cataract—The lens matter in the anterior chamber causes iritis which is the cause of glaucoma.

(c) Subluxation of the lens in the anterior chamber—The glaucoma is due to blockage of the angle.

(d) Dislocation of the lens in the vitreous—The lens in the vitreous causes low grade cyclitis which is the cause of the rise of tension.

(e) Flocculent lens matter in the anterior chamber either following discission operation or following the rupture of the lens capsule as a result of concussion or penetrating injury—The glaucoma is due to blockage of the angle by the lens matter.

4. Glaucoma following intra-ocular haemorrhage—

(a) Massive haemorrhage in the anterior chamber—The glaucoma is due to increased osmotic tension of the aqueous due to the presence of proteins of the blood and due to blockage of the angle by the cellular elements of the blood.

(b) Massive haemorrhage in vitreous—The lens-iris diaphragm may be pushed forwards making the angle very narrow and thereby causing glaucoma.

5. Haemorrhagic glaucoma—This type of glaucoma follows thrombosis of the cental vein of the retina. The glaucoma is due to formation of new vessels at the drainage angle.

6. Glaucoma due to intra-ocular tumour—The glaucoma may be due to increase in volume of ocular contents, venous engorgement, or infiltration of the angle of the anterior chamber by tumour cells.

7. Post-operative causes—
   (a) Aphakic glaucoma following extraction of the lens.
   (b) Glaucoma due to cyst formation in the anterior chamber, following extraction of the lens—If by chance conjunctival epithelium is left introduced in the anterior chamber due to faulty reposition of the conjunctival flap after cataract operation, there is formation of a thin-walled cyst in the anterior chamber. This cyst invariably leads to secondary glaucoma and the treatment is very difficult. The condition is however rare.

Treatment of secondary glaucoma

It depends on individual conditions. The cause of the glaucoma must be treated. Paracentesis may be done to lower the intra-ocular pressure temporarily. In cases of intra-ocular tumour, the eye should, be removed.

Special types of Glaucoma with clinical importance

1. Aphakic glaucoma

It occurs as a delayed complication following cataract operation, usually several weeks to several months after the operation. It is in fact a secondary glaucoma and the causes are as follows—
   (a) Delayed formation of the anterior chamber after cataract operation and adhesion of the iris to the cornea at the periphery.
   (b) Iris or lens capsule, incarcerated in the incisional wound during healing, thereby blocking the angle.
   (c) Vitreous protruding through the pupil into the anterior chamber, thereby blocking the pupil and obstructing the circulation of the aqueous humour.
   (d) A mass of vitreous into the anterior chamber which blocks the angle.

Clinical signs·

   (a) Gradual dimness of vision.

   (b) Raised tension.

   (c) Cornea may be slightly hazy.

   (d) Eye is quiet.

   (e) Cupping of the disc.

   (f) Field defects.

Treatment

   (a) To prevent such an incidence, post-operative care should be taken to help the formation of the anterior chamber.

   (b) Proper care during operation so as not to disturb the vitreous or not to leave tags of the lens capsule or the iris in the wound.

   (c) Miotics may be tried but not very useful.

   (d) Operative measures cyclodialysis operation is seldom practised now a days. Scheie's operation or Trabeculectomy with Vitrectomy are more useful.

   (e) Cyclo cryopexy or cyclo diathermy.

2. Malignant glaucoma

It is usually the sequela of primary closed-angle glaucoma, when the tension remains high, even after a filtration operation. The cause of persistent rise of tension is the forward displacement of the lens, so the angle remains permanently closed.

Treatment—Posterior sclerotomy in the equatorial region to release the beads of vitreous, or sucking out of vitreous with a wide bore needle.

3. Steroid glaucoma

It is an open-angle glaucoma induced as a result of prolonged local or systemic use of steroids. The cause of glaucoma is not known.

4. Glaucomato-cyclitic crisis

There are recurrent attacks of raised intra-ocular pressure with signs of mild cyclitis. The ·clinical features are as follows—

   (a) Very high rise of tension, but the eye remains quiet and pain is slight.

   (b) Temporary blurring of vision and halo may be seen around the light.

   (c) Pupil slightly dilated.

   (d) Keratic precipitates present.

   (e) No cupping of the optic disc.

(f) Attacks may recur, but the prognosis is good.
The cause of rise of tension is cyclitis.

Treatment

(a) Hydrocortisone acetate 1 percent drop, every two hours, is the most effective treatment.
(b) Diamox 1 tablet by mouth twice daily.
(c) Miotics, mydriatics and surgical intervention are contraindicated.

Ocular hypotension

Definition—It is a condition in which the intra-ocular pressure remains below average normal. In its extreme condition, when in association with persistent low pressure there is structural and functional changes as in a case of phthisis bulbi, the condition is known as ophthalmomalacia.

There are two types of ocular hypotension—
1. Essential hypotension.
2. Secondary hypotension.
   (a) Secondary to some disease of the eye.
   (b) Secondary to systemic causes.

1. Essential hypotension—
This is a condition in which there is bilateral and persistent low tension without any obvious local or systemic disease. This is a normal condition in some people, as there is no functional or structural change in the eye. Heredity may have some influence and the condition does not require any treatment.

2. Secondary hypotension—
   (a) Secondary to a local condition in the eye as for example long continued iridocyclitis, trauma to the eye in the form of either perforating or concussion injury or operative trauma as following cataract operation and cyclodialysis operation, high myopia with vitreous degeneration, detachment of the retina or detachment of the choroid.
   (b) Secondary to some systemic diseases as for example diabetic coma, uraemic coma, marked dehydration as in cholera and malnutrition.

Ocular hypertension

It is the persistent presence of higher ocular tension than the generally accepted normal, in the absence of optic disc anomaly or visual field defect and with a normal aqueous outflow facility. It may be considered as "Glaucoma Suspect" and repeated examination of tonometry and perimetry are required.

CHAPTER XII

ANATOMY AND DISEASES OF THE RETINA

Anatomy of the retina

The retina is a delicate and thin membrane, extending from the optic disc behind to the ciliary body in front being situated between the choroid on the outer side and the hyaloid membrane of the vitreous on the inner side. The thickness of the retina is about 0.5 mm. near the optic disc, 0.2 mm. at the equator of the eyeball and 0.1 mm. most anteriorly. Normally the retina is transparent, but immediately after death it becomes white. The anterior termination of the retina, where it is continuous with the epithelium of the ciliary body, is known as ora serrata.

On the inner surface of the retina, at the posterior pole of the eyeball, is the macula lutea or the yellow spot, an area about 1-2 mm. in diameter and in its centre is a small depression known as fovea centralis.

Minute anatomy of the retina

On microscopical examination, the retina is found to consist of the following layers (Fig. 94)

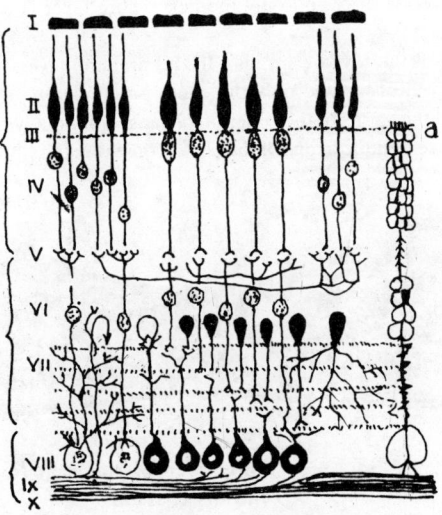

Fig. 94. Different layers of retina.

From the outer side—1. Layer of pigment epithelium—a single layer of hexagonal cells containing melanin pigment and resting on the membrane of Bruch.

II. Layer of rods and cones—the end organs for visual sensation.

III. External limiting membrane.

IV. Outer nuclear layer—consisting of nuclei of the rods and cones.

V. Outer plexiform layer—consisting of arborizations of the axons of the rod and cone nuclei and the dendrites of the bipolar cells.

VI. Inner nuclear layer consisting of—

(a) Bipolar cells, which are rod-bipolars connecting with the rods and cone-bipolars connecting with the cones.

(b) Association elements, which are of two types—horizontal cells and amacrine cells. They inter-connect different cells with one another.

VII. Inner plexiform layer—consisting of the arborizations of the axons of the bipolar cells with the dendrites of the ganglion cells.

VIII. Layer of ganglion cells—consisting of large ganglion cells.

IX. Nerve fibre layer—consisting of the axons of ganglion cells.

These fibres are non-medullated and are continued as optic nerve fibres.

X. Internal limiting membrane.

All these neural elements are bound together, by a supporting neuroglial tissue known as fibres of Muller (Fig. 94 a, b). The interlacement of these fibres on the outer side forms the outer limiting membrane and that on the inner side forms the internal limiting membrane. The outer layers of the retina stop abruptly at the margin of the optic disc, and only the nerve fibre layer is continued as the optic nerve.

Structure of the fovea centralis—In this area, all layers of the retina are very thin. There are no rods and only the cones predominate. There is also no nerve fibre layer and the axons of the cones are arranged obliquely to reach the margin of the fovea. These oblique axons of the cones constitute the fibre layer of Henle (Fig. 95)

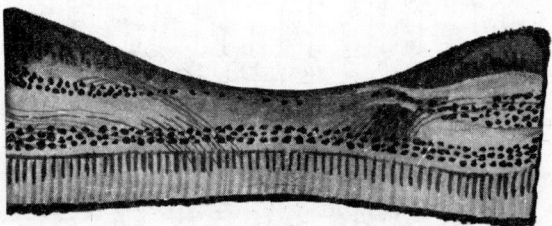

Fig. 95. Fibre layer of Henle at fovea
centralis (Parsons).

Blood supply of the retina

1. The pigment epithelium, the layer of rods and cones and the outer nuclear layer have no direct blood supply. But the nutrition of these layers is maintained by

PLATE X

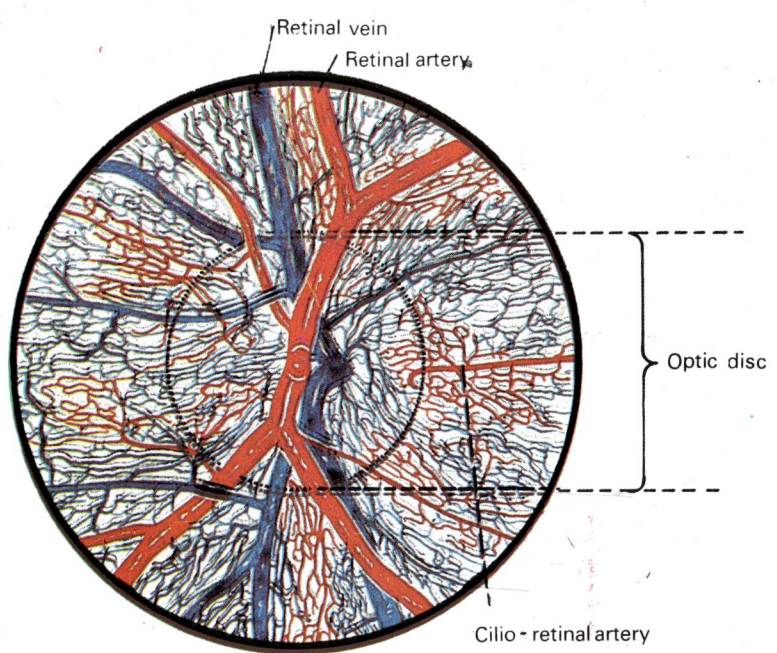

Retinal vein

Retinal artery

Optic disc

Cilio - retinal artery

(To face page 202)

in size, or macropsia—when objects appear larger in size.

(b) If the peripheral part of the retina is involved, there is only blurring of vision due to vitreous haze.

Clinical signs

(a) The affected part of the retina appears hazy.

(b) There may be one or two spots of minute haemorrhages in the area.

(c) The vitreous over the lesion becomes hazy.

(d) Later on when inflammation subsides, there is chorioretinal atrophy, the sclera becomes visible and accumulation of retinal pigment takes place at the margin of the lesion.

Treatment—The same as that for choroiditis.

2. *Periphlebitis of retinal veins (Eale's disease)*—

Etiology

(a) Usually occurs in young adults.

(b) Males are more commonly affected.

(c) Usually both eyes are affected in succession.

Causative agent—It is not definitely known, but it may be allergic or toxic in origin from a tuberculous or septic focus.

Clinical signs

(a) There is phlebitis of the peripheral retinal veins, which appear thickened, tortuous and congested.

(b) There is sheathing of the affected veins.

(c) Retinal haemorrhages appear near the affected veins. If the haemorrhage is massive, it enters into the vitreous.

(d) Good central vision is maintained, provided there is no vitreous haemorrhage.

Symptoms—Usually none, but there is sudden defective vision, if there is haemorrhage in the vitreous.

Course—The haemorrhages clear up but recurrences are common. If the haemorrhage organizes in the vitreous, retinitis proliferans is formed, which is fibrous tissue of mesodermal origin.

Treatment—It is not very satisfactory. But the following treatments are usually done—

(a) Anti-tubercular treatment has been tried.

diffusions from the choriocapillaries. Similarly the fovea centralis has no blood vessel but nutrition is derived from the choriocapillaries.

2. The rest of the layers of the retina are supplied by the central artery of the retina, which is a branch of the ophthalmic artery. The central artery is an end artery.

Venous drainage

(a) The outer layers are drained by the vortex veins of the choroid through the choriocapillaries.

(b) The inner layers are drained by the central vein of the retina, which ends in the cavernous sinus.

Functions of the retina—

(a) The central part, i.e., macula lutea consists mainly of cones and is responsible for the greatest visual acuity in daylight and for colour vision.

(b) The peripheral part of the retina, which consists mainly of rods, is responsible for night vision. The ability to see in the darkness is due to the presence of a pigment, known as visual purple, in the rods.

Affections of the retina

A. Congenital and developmental defects

1. *Coloboma of choroid and retina—*
It is an area where the choroid and the retina fail to develop. It is situated either downwards and inwards at the site of the foetal fissure or at the macula.

2. *Opaque nerve fibres—*
Normally the medullation of the optic nerve fibres stops at the lamina cribrosa. But sometimes, a patch of nerve fibres in the retina near the disc, becomes myelinated. These fibres appear as a white patch with feathery margin.

B. Inflammatory and exudative affections of the retina

1. *Retinitis—*
Pure retinitis is rare. It is usually associated with the inflammation of the choroid, when it is called chorioretinitis or with inflammation of the optic nerve head, when it is called neuro-retinitis.

*Etiology—*Same as that for choroiditis and optic neuritis (*see* choroiditis and optic neuritis).

Symptoms

(a) If the macular region is involved, there is blurring of the vision with micropsia, when objects appear smaller

(b) Aspirin by mouth and long continued steroid is sometimes useful.

(c) Diathermy coagulation of the affected veins has also been tried. But more effective is photo coagulation.

(d) Vitrectomy may help to clear off old haemorrhage and retinitis proliferans.

3. *Central Serous Retinopathy* (C.S.R.) is caused by exudation from parafoveal or choroidal capillaries. This is attributed to angiospasm which is either allergic or toxic in nature.

It occurs mostly in young males and looks like a circular dark swelling about the size of a disc over the macula with a surrounding ring-shapped reflex like "Budha halo".

The oedema may be pre or subepithelial so that the affected macula is raised above the level of retina. Fluorescein 'angiography reveals leakage of dye through a defect in Bruch's membrane.

The patient complains of sudden dimness with a black patch in front of his vision. Vision ranges from $6/_{12} - 6/_{60}$ with micropsia and metamorphopsia and improves considerably with + 1.0 Dsph addition.

The condition is usually transient and resolves in most of the cases leaving a few brown exudative dots or even a scar on or around macula. Though the overall prognosis is good in few cases with macular scar the relative central scotoma may be replaced with a small central scotoma.

Treatment with antitubercular drugs, vasodilators and retrobulbar injections of steroids have been out dated. A course of Calcium, Vitamin C and anti-allergic drugs are more fruitful. Anthelmintics and anti–amoebic treatment may also be done emperically. Photo-coagulation is an accepted treatment now.

4. *Massive exudative retinitis (Coat's disease)*—

It is a rare condition, usually occurring in one eye in young boys. There is haemorrhage with exudation between the outer layers of the retina due to unknown reason. One theory is that the disease is due to vascular anomaly. The eye fundus shows large, raised, yellowish white areas. The eye is usually lost due to secondary glaucoma and retinal detachment.

C. Vascular affections

1. *Hyperaemia of retina.*

It may be arterial or venous or both. Arterial hyperaemia is due to inflammatory lesions. Venous hyperaemia is due to obstruction to the venous return, which may be local as in the case of thrombosis of the central retinal vein or one of its branches, or general as in the case of congenital heart disease and congestive cardiac failure. Both types of hyperaemia occur also when there is excess of blood cells as in polycythaemia vera and leukaemia.

2. *Anaemia of the retina.*

It may be due to local eye condition or as an expression of general condition.

Local condition

(a) Occlusion of the central artery of retina.
(b) Spasm of retinal arteries.
(c) Quinine poisoning causing narrowing of retinal arteries.

The arteries become extremely narrow, the disc becomes pale, the retina becomes pale white and there is loss of vision.

General condition—Usually following profuse haemorrhage. The appearance of the fundus is more or less the same as in local condition.

3. *Oedema of the retina*

An oedematous area in the retina appears pale white and cloudy. It may be localized or diffuse.

Causes of oedema of retina

(a) Inflammatory condition as retinitis.
(b) Occlusion of the central artery of the retina or one of its branches.
(c) Concussion injury to the eyeball producing commotio retinae.
(d) Papilloedema associated with pressure of the surrounding retina.

In the macular area, due to the presence of Henle's fibre layer, oedema tends to throw the retina into radiating folds and the whole area appears like a star. This is known as macular star and is usually seen associated with papilloedema and various retinopathies.

4. *Retinal haemorrhages—*
They may be of the following types—

(a) *Intra-retinal haemorrhage*—When the haemorrhages from the retinal vessels *i.e.,* arteries or veins are small, they are situated within the retinal tissue and are known as intra-retinal haemorrhages. According to the location, *i.e.*, the layer of the retina in which haemorrhage has taken place, the haemorrhages assume different shapes as follows—

   (i) flame-shaped haemorrhage—when the haemorrhage is in the nerve fibre layer.

   (ii) rounded or irregular haemorrhage—when the haemorrhage is in deeper layers.

   (b) *Pre-retinal or subhyaloid haemorrhage*—If bleeding takes place from a large vessel the blood bursts through the internal limiting membrane and lies between the retina and the vitreous. Such a haemorrhage usually occurs in the macular area and very soon due to gravity the upper margin of the haemorrhage becomes horizontal as shown in Fig. 96.

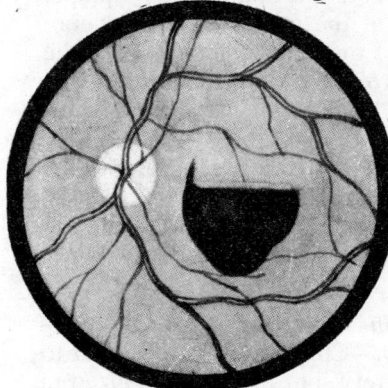

Fig. 96. Subhyaloid haemorrhage (Parsons).

Fate of retinal haemorrhages—They are usually absorbed ; the time required for absorption varies with the amount of haemorrhage.

Causes of retinal haemorrhage—

   (a) Trauma.

   (b) Venous obstruction.

   (c) Local inflammatory condition.

   (d) Toxic states as infective fevers.

   (e) Vascular retinopathies due to nephritis, diabetes, hypertension, and toxaemia of pregnancy.

   (f) Blood diseases like anaemia, purpura and leukaemia.

Symptoms

If blood enters into vitreous there is marked visual disturbance.

5. Occlusion of the central artery of the retina or one of its branches—Causes

   (a) Thrombosis of the artery due to arteriosclerotic or atheromatous change.

   (b) Embolism of the artery—the embolus usually coming from the heart, in case of heart disease.

   (c) Severe spasm of the artery as following intake of quinine.

The fundus picture in occlusion of the central artery of the retina is as follows—

   (a) The branches of the artery become extremely narrow.

   (b) The blood column in the retinal veins breaks up and takes up beaded appearance.

   (c) Within a few hours, the entire retina appears opaque and milky white, except at the fovea centralis, where because of the thinness of the retina, at that area, the red reflex from the choroid is visible. This red area appears as a cherry-red spot which is known as cherry-red macula.

   (d) Within the next few weeks, the white appearance of the retina clears up, the tissue becomes transparent again, but becomes completely functionless due to degeneration of the cells of the retina. The optic disc becomes pale.

Symptom of arterial obstruction—complete loss of vision.

Obstruction of an arterial branch—Clincial signs are similar to those for obstruction of the main artery, but they are localized in the area surrounding the affected branch. A permanent defect in the visual field develops corresponding to the lesion.

Treatment :

If the occlusion is due to spasm then there is a visual recovery if treated with vasodilators. Loss of vision is irrecoverable when it is due to embolism. Vasodilator either by mouth or through retrobulbar injection are useless. Amyl nitrite inhalation, pressure on the globe, paracentesis all hardly prove effective.

6.   **Obstruction of the central retinal vein or one of its branches**

The usual cause of obstruction is thrombosis of the vein.

Causes of venous thrombosis

   (a) Arteriosclerotic and atheromatous change in the central artery which compresses the vein at the arteriovenous crossing.

   (b) Endo or periphlebitis of veins.

   (c) Diabetes mellitus.

   (d) Increased viscosity of blood as in polycythaemia vera.

Symptoms

    (a) If the central vein itself becomes affected, the symptom is sudden loss of vision which becomes reduced to perception and projection of light only.

    (b) If a branch of the vein is obstructed, a sector shaped field defect takes place corresponding to the area of the retina affected.

Clinical signs

    (a) When the trunk of the central vein is affected—

        (i) Retinal veins are markedly distended.

        (ii) Numerous extensive haemorrhages occur throughout the retina.

        (iii) The optic disc becomes oedematous.

        (iv) Later. on, new anastomotic collateral vessels develop on the disc.

Course of thrombosis of the central vein—The haemorrhages take several months to disappear. The visual improvement depends on the retinal damage done by the haemorrhages. In 20 percent of the cases, secondary glaucoma, known as thrombotic glaucoma, may develop after a period of 2-3 months.

    (b) When a tributary of the central vein is affected, the fundus picture is the same, but is confined to the area of drainage by the tributary. There is no risk of glaucoma.

Treatment:

    It is not as hopeless as central artery occlusion. Anticoagulant therapy is the treatment of choice, after controlling the associated B.P. & diabetes.

    Persantin and aspirin have proved to be effective in many cases.

    The thrombotic glaucoma may respond to cyclocryopex or retrobulbar absolute alcohol injection.

D. Retinopathies

    Ocular Fundus is the only region in the body where the blood vessels can be visualised for any change in different systemic disorders.

1. *Retinopathy of benign hypertension*—

    In benign hypertension, if the person is young, the retinal arteries become narrow due to hypertonus of the vessels. But in elderly persons, where there are already arteriosclerotic changes, the narrowing is not so marked.

If the hypertension is long continued, there are changes in the arterial wall, which make the vessels pale due to increased reflection of light from the wall. These changes are due to arteriosclerotic changes. In more advanced stage, the arteries appear as copper wires and later on as silver wires, with sheathing. The veins become compressed at the arterio-venous crossings.

But before these extreme arteriosclerotic changes occur, flame-shaped haemorrhages and hard, white and tiny exudates appear in the retina. This stage is known as the stage of arteriosclerotic retinopathy.

2. *Retinopathy of malignant hypertension or hypertensive retinopathy*—

If the malignant hypertension occurs in a young adult the retinal changes are as follows—

    (a) Marked narrowing of the arteries.
    (b) Flame-shaped haemorrhages.
    (c) Wooly exudates.
    (d) Papilloedema to some extent.

If the malignant hypertension is superimposed on a case of long continued benign hypertension, the retinal changes are similar to those already described under arteriosclerotic retino-pathy and in addition there are wooly exudates and papilloedema.

3. *Retinopathy associated with renal disease—chronic glome-rulo-nephritis—*

The retinal changes are similar to those in hypertensive retinopathy. But the wooly exudates and generalized oedema of the retina are more marked.

4. *Retinopathy of toxaemia of pregnancy—*

The retinal changes are similar to those in hypertensive retino-pathy. But there may be transudation in the subretinal space which causes detachment of the retina.

5. *Diabetic retinopathy—*

It usually occurs 8 to 10 years after the onset of diabetes mellitus, controlled or uncontrolled.

The signs in the early stage

    (a) Micro-aneurysm formation in the retinal capillaries which appear as tiny circular red dots.

PLATE XI

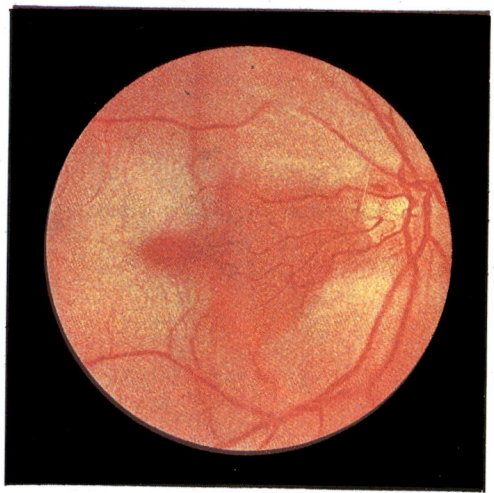

Fig. 1

Central retinal artery occlusion with a cherry
red spot and sparing of a temporal
cilio-retinal vessel.

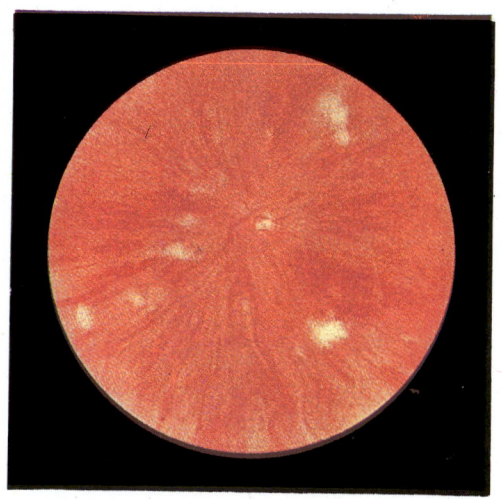

Fig. 2
Central retinal vein thrombosis
(Parsons)

(To face page 210)

PLATE XII

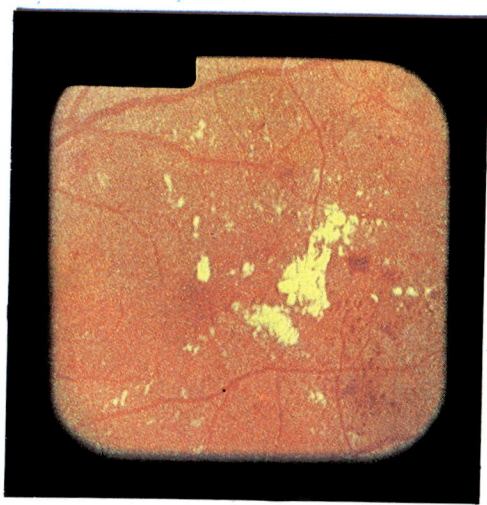

Fig. 1

Diabetes—background retinopathy

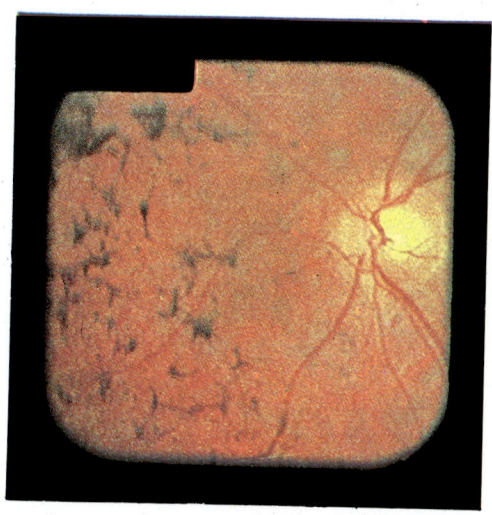

Fig. 2

Retinitis pigmentosa with bone corpuscle
formation, attenuated retinal arterioles
and a yellowish disc (Parsons)

(To face page 210)

(b) Yellow, waxy exudate in the retina usually described as hard exudate.

The signs in the later stage
(a) The micro-aneurysms rupture producing circular 'dot' to 'blot' haemorrhages in the deeper layers of the retina.
(b) The exudates increase but there is no ọedema of the retina or of the optic disc.
(c) A branch of the retinal vein may be thrombosed producing massive retinal and vitreous haemorrhage.
(d) As a result of vitreous haemorrhage, retinitis proliferans and vitreous neovascularisation may develop.

Fluorescein angiography gives a more detailed picture of diabetic retinopathy.

Diabetic retinopathy may, sometimes be associated with retinal oedema and cotton wool exudate resulting from hypertension of glomerulosclerosis in the kidney. This is called Kimmel Steil Wilson Syndrome.

Treatment :

Background Diabetic retinopathy is best treated with Pan Photo Coagulation, Cryo retinopathy of the peripheral retina is an alternative if there is no light coagulator.

For proliferative diabetic retinopathy vitrectomy may be necessary followed by photo coagulation.

Laser coagulation is a variety of photo coagulation.

E.   Detachment of Retina

Retina develops from the two layers of the embryonic optic vesicle. The outer layer forms the pigment epithelium and the inner layer forms the retina proper. Normally they lie in apposition and the space between them in a potential space. When fluid collects in this potential space there is separation of the neural elements (embryonic inner layer) from the pigment epithelium (embroyonic outer layer). So the terminology of the detachment of retina should be in true sense 'Separation of Retina.'

Clinically it may be divided into two types—
(a) Simple ;
(b) Secondary.

Simple Retinal detachment of Rhegmatogenous retinal detachment :
This is mostly due to a break in the retina in the form of a hole

or tear. There is percolation of fluid to the subretinal space through the break. If the virtreous gel is healthy and solid such a detachment rarely occurs; if it is fluid or detached and if there is vitreoretinal adhesion a detachment readily develops.

Causes of hole and tear

    (a) Degenerative changes in the retina in old age, high myopia and aphakia;

    (b) Trauma to the eyeball. Many a times the trauma is a very trivial one causing a detachment. These are essentially in eyes which are predisposed from myopic or senile degeneration. Trauma can also cause a massive dialysis.

    (c) Jerky eye movement can tear off the vitreo retinal adhesion resulted from chorio retinitis.

Retinal holes vary in shape and size. It may be single or multiple. Holes are mostly associated with lattice degeneration of retina. Broadly they may be classified as follows :

    (a) Dialysis or disinsertion at ora serrata. It looks like a semilunar area of bright red choroid bounded centrally by the greyish margin of the detached retina.

    (b) Horse shoe shaped tear or arrow shaped tear with a lid like tongue or operculum may be seen in the equatorial region more frequently in the upper two quadrants.

    (c) Round holes may be single or multiple and are seen in the peripheral retina near ora serrata. Round holes are also seen around the macular regions.

Clinical features :

    Premonitary symptoms like flashes of light, muscae volitantis and distortion of objects are common. This is followed by profound dimness of vision. The field of vision corresponding to the area detached becomes defective. In the early stage it may be difficult to detect a shallow detachment with direct ophthalmoscopy. However indirect method of opthalmoscopy gives a wider view of the retina and more helpful for the detection of holes in the periphery. Retina assumes a white, grey colour which shows bright sheen at the summits and appear greenish grey in the depressions. During slight movements of the eye the detached retina show oscillations. The reitnal vessels appear darker than usual and may be almost black showing no central light streak. In an extensive case great balloon like folds may be seen obscuring all view of the disc. Associated lattice degeneration and pigment disturbance may be seen. There may even be spots of haemorrhage and exudate. In total detachment retina looks like a funnel. Treatment of simple detachment is by operation with the following principle.

(a) Apposition of retina with the choroid by draining the subretinal fluid.

(b) Aseptic inflammation by diathermy, cryopexy orphoto coagulation over the retinal break. Thus obliterating the hole or holes.

The prognosis in simple detachment is good and in 80% of the cases anatomical reapposition is obtained. Functional recovery is good if the case is operated early before the macula is lifted up.

Symptoms

The field of vision corresponding to the area detached becomes defective. Thus if there is detachment of the upper temporal retina of the right eye, the lower nasal field for the right eye becomes defective.

Clinical signs

By ophthalmoscope, the detached retina is seen to be raised, bluish in appearance and thrown into folds. A hole or a tear in the retina may be visible.

Treatment of detachment of the retina—Sealing the retinal hole or tear by application of diathermy points on the sclera around the break in the retina, followed by drainage of the subretinal fluid by puncturing the sclera opposite the hole.

This treatment is applicable when the detachment is due to a hole or a tear in the retina.

F. Degenerative changes in the Retina

1. Senile macular degeneration

It occurs in the aged persons. One or both the eyes may be affected. Fundus picture shows fine pigmentary changes, fine exudates and tiny haemorrhages all restricted in the macular area.

Symptoms

The central vision is lost but the patient never becomes completely blind. The loss of vision is due to degeneration of the cells of the outer nuclear layer and degeneration of the rods and cones.

There is no satisfactory treatment, however telescopic lens or magnifying lenses are of some help.

2. Disciform degeneration of macula

It also occurs in the aged. One or both the eyes may be affected. Fundus picture shows a round, white, and slightly elevated patch about the size of the optic disc in the macular area.

Pathology

There is sclerosis of the chorio-capillaries in the macular area, followed by haemorrhage from the capillaries. The blood breaks through the membrane of Bruch and collects underneath the pigment epithelium. Finally the haemorrhage is converted into fibrous tissue.

There is no satisfactory treatment. Low visual aids are of some help.

3. Primary pigmentary degeneration of the retina. Retinitis pigmentosa—

It is a chronic progressive degeneration of all the layers of the retina with proliferation of the retinal pigment, occurring usually in the young and there is hereditary tendency.

Pathology

At the begining, there is degeneration of the rods and cones along with the pigment epithelium and migration of the pigment into the retina particularly around the blood vessels of the retina. Later on, the ganglion cells and their axons also degenerate and they are replaced by neuroglial tissue. The blood vessels become attenuated and the disc assumes a waxy yellow colour due to consecutive atrophy.

Fundus picture

    (a) Black pigment spots like bone corpuscles, along the blood vessels, mainly in the equatorial region.

    (b) Yellow waxy appearance of the optic disc.

    (c) Retinal arteries markedly narrow.

Field defect—An annular or ring scotoma is usually detected in the early stage—ultimately the field contracts around the fixation point leaving a tube vision.

Symptoms

    (a) Night blindness.

    (b) Later on dimness of vision.

Prognosis

In advanced life, the central vision becomes very poor, there may be nuclear cataract as well.

G. Neoplasm of the Retina
RETINOBLASTOMA

The commonest tumour originating from the retina is a highly malignant tumour, known as retinoblastoma, which was formerly called glioma of the retina.

Etiology

(a) Age incidence—Most probably it is congenital and becomes manifest within first. 5 years of age.

(b) Sex—No difference between male and female.

(c) Bilaterality—Usually unilateral but in 20 percent of cases it is bilateral. The growth in the second eye is independent of the growth in the first eye.

(d) Heredity—Most of the cases are sporadic, but a hereditary factor is well-recognized.

Origin of the tumour—From the outer or the inner nuclear layer of the retina. Usually the tumour grows inwards into the vitreous. But sometimes it may grow in the subretinal space, causing detachment of the retina or sometimes in the plane of the retina.

Pathology

The tumour consists of small, round, densely packed cells with basophilic large nuclei. They may be arranged in a single layer round a central space, when this arrangement is called a true 'rosette or there may be several layers of cells around a blood vessels, when this arrangement is called a 'pseudo-rosette'. The cells, furthest from the blood vessel, undergo necrotic changes. There may be areas of calcification.

Symptoms

Usually there is no pain and as it occurs in the very young, they usually cannot detect any defect of vision.

The clinical picture may be considered in four stages—

1. The stage of intra-ocular growth—

The *signs* are—

(a) Externally the eye is quiet.

(b) Whitish reflex in the pupillary area and this condition is known as amaurotic cat's eye reflex.

(c) With the opthalmoscope, a yellowish white growth is seen protruding into the vitreous, the surface of the growth showing new vessels or even spots of haemorrhage.

2. The stage of glaucoma—
The *Signs* are—
(a) There is rise of intra-ocular pressure.
(b) The size of the growth increases.
(c) The size of the eyeball may be bigger.
3. The stage of extra-ocular extension—
The *signs* are—The growth perforates through the sclera and enters into the orbit. The eyeball becomes proptosed. The extraocular portion of the tumour grows rapidly and assumes a fungating appearance.
4. The stage of metastasis—
The metastasis usually occurs in the following ways—
(a) Intracranially along the optic nerve.
(b) From the extra-ocular growth along the lymphatics to the regional lymph glands and to the cranial bones.
(c) By blood stream to the distant bones, like humerous, sternum or ribs. This occurs when by chance the tumour erodes into a blood vessel.

Prognosis
Prognosis is very poor. Death occurs due to intracranial extension.

TABLE XI

Differential diagnosis between pseudo-glioma and retinoblastoma.

	Pseudo-glioma	*Retinoblastoma*
1. Nature of the disease	1. Inflammatory in origin and it is the terminal phase of endophthamitis.	1. It is a neoplasm.
2. Inflammatary signs.	2. (a) Cilliary flush. (b) Posterior synechia. (c) K. P.	2. Nil.
3. Tension.	3. Usually low or normal.	3. High.
4. Progress.	4. Non-progressive	4. Progressive.

Treatment
(a) If one eye is affected, the eye must be enucleated as

soon as diagnosis is made, followed by deep X-ray for therapy of the orbit .

(b) In bilateral cases, that eye, with a more advanced tumour, must be tried.

(c) When there is a fungating growth, exenteration of the orbit has to be done *i.e.*, removal of all the orbit including the periosteum, followed by deep X-ray therapy.

Fluorsecein Angiography

Fluorescein Angiography has sparked a major ophthalmic revolution by providing a unique dynamic document of pathological changes in the eye. Sodium Fluorescein following its injection in the antecubetal vein reaches the ocular circulation within 8-11 seconds and courses the arteries, capillaries and veins over a retinal circulation time of 2−3 seconds where it may be viewed and sequentially photographed by a conventional fundus camera by sending light through a excitor filter (480 nm) for activation and screening the emittedfluoresced light through a barrier filter (520 nm) thereby producing valuable informations of flow and perfusion. Nature's grace has extended the barriers to the eye at two very important sites the normal a retinal vasculature and pigment ep-ithelium and disurption of these as in various pathological indentit-ies immediately unmasks characteristic patterns in the angiogram ex-tending diagnostic clarifications and at the same time pin pointing the defect for therapeutic considerations with photocoagulation.

Ultrasonography

When sound waves with frequencies between 5000 H_z + 20,000 H_z are directed towards the eye, some reflected at interfaces separating media of differeing dersities, these reflected waves are converted into electrical potential and displayed on a oscilloscope.

(1) A scan-Traces a series of spikes on the oscilloscope. The hight of each spikes depends on the tissues cellular composition. The distance between the spikes gives a measure of distance between intra-ocular structures. This is useful recording the axial light of an eye before inserting an intra-ocular lens during cataract surgery.

(2) B. Scan-This is obtained by moving the transducer across the eye to give a two dimensional picture of ocular structure. This is useful to detect retinal detachment when there is vitreous opacities or lental opacities or to locate an intra-ocular foreign body which in radiotranslucent.

An ultrasonic transducer omits narrow beam of waves similar to sound energy but of a high frequency. The degree of reflection of Such waves is differennt from different intra-ocular tissue.Such reflections can be monitered on a cathode ray tube.

CHAPTER XIII

ANATOMY AND DISEASES OF THE OPTIC NERVE

Anatomy of the optic nerve—The optic nerve extends from the lamina cribrosa upto the optic chiasma. The entire optic nerve is covered by the meningeal sheaths *i.e.,* the dura, the arachnoid and the pia. The meningeal spaces of the nerve are continuous with those of the brain. The nerve can be divided into four parts—1. Intra-ocular part—1 mm. 2. Intra-orbital part—25 mm. 3. Intra-osseous part—4-10 mm. 4. Intracranial part—10 mm. (Duke-Elder).

1. **The intra-ocular part**—It is the part of the nerve, within the lamina cribrosa of the optic disc, which is situated slightly on the inner side of the posterior pole of the eyeball.

Optic disc—At about 3 mm. on the inner side of the fovea centralis, at the posterior pole of the eyeball, is the optic disc. The optic disc is slightly pinkish white, oval or round area and represents the optic nervehead or the beginning of the optic nerve. The optic disc is normally flat and is in the same place as the retina, but there is normally a depression in its central part which is known as physiological cup.

Structure of the optic disc—It consists of a transverse network of connective tissue, containing much elastic fibres—the lamina cribrosa. The fibres of the nerve fibre layer of retina pass through the meshes of the lamina cribrosa to be continuous with the optic nerve.

2. **The intra-orbital part**—It extends from the lamina cribrosa to the optic canal. This part of the nerve presents a 'S' shaped curve, which allows free movement of the eyeball. This part of the nerve lies within the extra-ocular muscle cone. At a short distance from the eyeball the central artery of the retina enters the optic nerve and the central vein of the retina leaves the nerve.

3. **The intra-osseous part**—It lies within the optic canal. This part of the nerve is accompanied by the ophthalmic artery, which lies on the lateral side of the nerve.

PLATE XIII

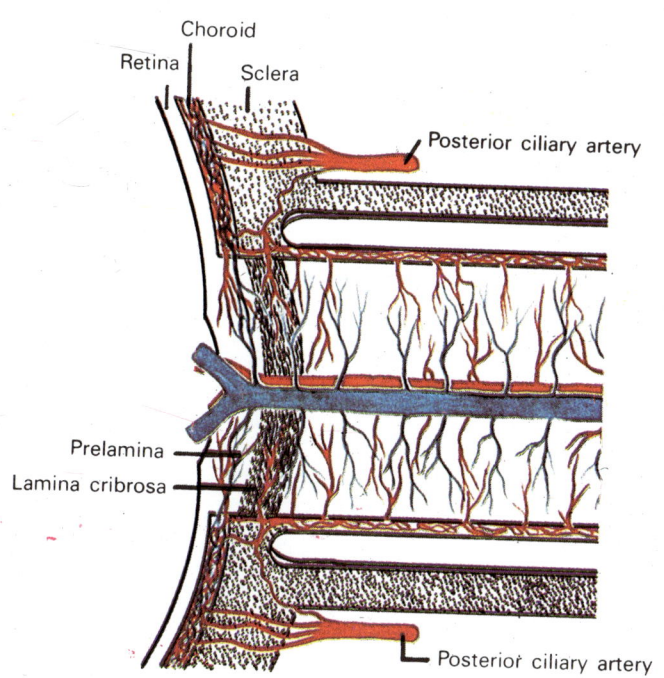

(To face page 218)

4. The intracranial part—This part of the nerve is short and flat. It extends from the cranial end of the optic canal to the lateral ·end of the optic chiasma.

The optic nerve consists of the axons of the ganglion cells of the retina. It is not strictly a nerve, but a tract of nerve fibres of the central nervous system. There is a myelin sheath for the fibres of this nerve, but there is no neurolemmal sheath. For this reason there is no regeneration of the optic nerve fibres after injury or destructive disease.

Blood supply of the optic nerve—The intracranial and the intra-canalicular part of the optic nerve are supplied by the branches of the anterior cerebral and the ophthalmic artery. The intra-orbital and the intra-ocular portions are supplied by the branches from the ophthalmic artery, the short posterior ciliary arteries and the central artery of the retina.

Congenital anomalies of the Optic Disc
1. Coloboma of the disc—The disc appears bigger in size and much excavated.
2. Congenital coloboma of the choroid and retina may involve the disc.

Inflammation of the Optic Nerve
(Optic Neuritis)
This disease can be divided into two groups—
1·. Papillitis—when the optic nerve head is inflamed.
2. Retrobulbar neuritis—when the nerve behind the eyeball is affected.

1. Papillitis
Etiology
It is not always clear. Some septic condition like tonsillitis and sinusitis or general febrile illness may precipitate the lesion. Usually one eye is affected. It may occur in any age or sex.

Symptoms
Rapid and marked fall of vision which may be reduced to perception and projection of light only. But there is no pain in the eye.

Clinical signs
  (i) Pupil reaction to light becomes very sluggish and the reaction
      is not sustained.
 (ii) The Optic disc becomes hyperaemic, the margins become
      blurred and later on the disc swells.
(iii) The retinal veins are markedly congested.
 (iv) Flame-shaped retinal haemorrhages appear round the disc.
  (v) There is no external sign.

Prognosis
  If treated early, the inflammation subsides, appearance of the
disc becomes normal and vision is regained. But if the disease is
allowed to continue for sometime, the optic nerve undergoes
atrophy.

Treatment
        (a) Treatment of the cause, such as treatment of the septic
            focus.
        (b) Injections of heavy doses of vitamin B_1, B_1, and B_{12}
            daily for at least 20 days.
        (c) Steroids and broad spectrum antibiotics by mouth.

2.   Retrobulbar Neuritis

  It may be acute or chronic.

A.   Acute Retrobulbar Neuritis

Etiology
  Septic focus, acute infectious diseases, diabetes, disseminated
sclerosis and local inflammatory conditions like orbital cellulitis
are the usual causes. Usually one eye is affected and it may occur
in any age or in any sex.

Symptoms
        (a) Rapid fall of central vision.
        (b) Slight pain in and around the orbit.
        (c) Pain on moving the eye upwards, because of the
            attachment of the sheath of the superior rectus muscle to
            the sheath of the optic nerve near the optic foramen.

Clinical signs
        (a) Externally the eye is normal.
        (b) The pupil reaction to light is very sluggish and the
            contraction is not sustained.
        (c) The fundus picture including the optic disc is normal.

Prognosis
  Recovery is usually complete. But a central scotoma may

remain. Recurrent attacks may lead to optic atrophy.

Treatment
Same as for papillitis.

B. Chronic Retrobulbar Neuritis
(Toxic Amblyopia)

This is a bilateral condition, caused by exogenous poisons, affecting primarily the ganglion cells of the retina. As there is atrophy of the macular fibres of the optic nerve, the condition was formerly known as chronic retrobulbar neuritis. But as the lesion is primarily in the retina, the toxic amblyopia is considered now-a-days as toxic retinoneuropathy.

Etiology
The toxic amblyopias are due to the following poisonous agents—

(a) Tobacco.
(b) Ethyl alcohol or a combination of both alcohol and tobacco.
(c) Methyl alcohol.
(d) Arsenic.
(e) Lead.
(f) Quinine.

(a) *Tobacco amblyopia*—
(i) It usually accurs in elderly persons consuming tobacco who have also general ill health and suffer from vitamin B_{12} deficiency.
(ii) The causative agent most probably is not nicotine, but one of its decomposition products such as collidine or lutidine.
(iii) *Symptoms*—Gradual dimness of vision and inability to distinguish colours.
(iv) *Clinical signs*—On scotometry, a central or centrocoecal scotoma, both for white and coloured objects. On ophthalmoscopic examination, there is no sign except a slight pallor of the optic disc.

Treatment
(i) Complete withdrawal of tobacco.
(ii) Administration of vitamin B_1 and B_{12}.
(iii) Improvement of general health.

(b) *Ethyl alcohol amblyopia*—Symptoms and signs are the same as for tobacco amblyopia. The only difference is that the person consumes alcohol instead of tobacco. Treatment also is similar to that for tobacco amblyopia.

(c) *Methyl alcohol amblyopia*—It is caused by drinking wood alcohol or methylated spirit. It may occur in an acute or chronic form.

Acute form

There is nausea, headache, giddiness and coma. If the patient survives, there is rapid fall of vision, which may end in total blindness. The optic disc becomes completely white.

Chronic form

There is progressive loss of vision with optic atrophy.

Treatment

    (i) To withhold methyl alcohol.

   (ii) Injection of heavy doses of vitamin B_1, B_6, B_{12}.

(d), (e) *Arsenic and lead poisoning* also lead to gradual dimness of vision and optic atrophy. The treatment is to remove the chemicals from the system.

(f) *Quinine amblyopia*—Even small doses of quinine may lead to blindness. There is sudden fall of vision, following administration of quinine. The pupils are dilated and do not react to light. The eye fundus shows oedema of the retina with cherry-red macula, very narrow arteries and a very pale disc.

Treatment—Withdrawal of quinine and vasodilator drugs.

Papilloedema (Choked disc)

Definition—It is the non-inflammatory oedema of the optic disc.

Causes of papilloedema

1. Increase intracranial tension due to a space-occupying intracranial lesion, as for example, brain tumour, brain abscess, and subdural haematoma. Brain tumour is the commonest cause, particularly the cerebellar tumours. The exception is the pituitary tumour, because so long it lies within the sella turcica, there is no papilloedema.

2. Venous stasis as in association with carotico-cavernous aneurysm, orbital tumour, thrombosis of the central vein of the retina or thrombosis of the superior sagittal sinus inside the cranium.

3. Local causes, e. g., hypertensive retinopathy and hypotony of the eyeball following glaucoma operation.

Pathology

There is oedema of the optic nerve head which affects the nerve fibres at the optic disc, which become swollen and varicose and ultimately degenerate.

Symptoms

(a) In the early stages there is no symptom, except sudden black out of vision from time to time due to spasm of retinal arteries.

(b) In the later stages there is fall of vision.

Clinical signs

The fundus picture is as follows—

(a) Blurring of the disc margin with filling of the physiological cup.

(b) Gradually the disc swells and becomes raised anteriorly.

(c) The retinal veins become markedly congested.

(d) Flame-shaped haemorrhages and soft white exudates appear around the disc.

(e) A macular star may be formed.

(f) On scotometry, there is enlargement of the blindspot.

If the papilloedema is allowed to continue for sometime, the nerve fibres undergo atrophy. So the clinical signs in a late stage are the following—

(a) Loss of vision becomes marked.

(b) The disc becomes pale with blurred margins. The swelling of the disc subsides.

(c) On testing the field of vision, there is concentric contraction of the field.

(d) Ultimately complete blindness ensues due to postpapilloedemic optic atrophy.

Treatment

The cause must be detected and the treatment should be aimed at removal of the cause. Meanwhile a shunt operation will be helpful to relieve the intracranial pressure.

Optic Atrophy

Any damage of the optic nerve fibres, either due to disease or injury, at any point between their origin in the ganglion cells of the retina and their termination in the lateral geniculate body, is followed by optic atrophy.

According to the ophthalmoscopic appearance of the optic nerve-head, the optic atrophy has been classified into three groups—

1. Consecutive atrophy—The optic atrophy is the sequela to certain diseases of the retina as for example retinitis pigmentosa, occlusion of the central retinal artery and glaucoma.

2. Primary optic atrophy—the chief features are as follows—
   (a) The disc is very pale. The margins of the disc are clear cut. The physiological cup is present.
   (b) The blood vessels are of normal calibre and there is no sheathing of the retinal vessels.
   (c) There is contraction of the visual field.

Causes of primary optic atrophy
   (a) Trauma to the optic nerve or chiasma or compression of these structures by a tumour.
   (b) Demyelinating disease like disseminated sclerosis.
   (c) Toxic conditions producing toxic amblyopias.
   (d) Malnutrition—particularly vitamin B_1 deficiency.
   (e) Syphilis—particularly tabes dorsalis.

3. Secondary optic atrophy—the chief features are as follows—
   (a) The disc is very pale, but the margins are blurred and the physiological cup is filled up.
   (b) The retinal arteries are narrow and there is sheathing of the arteries and veins near the disc margin.
   (c) Field—contraction of the field of vision.

Causes of secondary optic atrophy
   (a) Following papillitis.
   (b) Following papilloedema.

Symptoms of optic atrophy—There is fall of vision, which depending on the cause may be gradual or rapid.

Treatment of optic atrophy—Treatment is according to the cause.

Tumours of the Optic Nerve

The primary tumours of the optic nerve are rare and they are of two types—
1. Glioma of the optic nerve.
2. Meningioma of the optic nerve.

1. Glioma of the Optic Nerve

It usually occurs in the young children The growth originates from the neuroglial tissue of the optic nerve. There is axial proptosis of the eyeball, without any limitation of its movements.

The vision graudally falls due to optic atrophy. X-ray of the optic foramina reveal enlargement on the affected side.

2. Meningioma of the Optic Nerve

It occurs in the elderly persons. The tumour is in fact an endothelioma, as it originates from the endothelial cells of the meningeal sheaths of the optic nerve. There is also proptosis, but it is not axial. The eyeball may be pushed to any direction, depending on the situation of the growth. There is limitation of the movements of the eyeball due to involvement of the extra-ocular muscles. There is fall of vision and later on optic atrophy.

Both these tumours are locally malignant but usually there is no distant metastasis.

Treatment
Surgical removal of the tumour through orbitotomy.

CHAPTER XIV

VISUAL PATHWAY AND ITS LESIONS

The visual pathway consists of—
(a) Two optic nerves
(b) An optic chiasma.
(c) Two optic tracts.
(d) Two lateral geniculate bodies.
(e) Two optic radiations
(f) Visual cortex on each side.

A. The Optic Nerves

The general description of the nerves has already been given in the chapter on diseases of the optic nerve.

Arrangement of the nerve fibres in the optic nerve—Immediately behind the eyeball, the middle of the temporal half of the nerve contains papillomacular nerve fibres, derived from the macula The fibres from the upper and lower temporal parts of the retina are placed in the upper and lower parts of the temporal half of the nerve. The fibres from the nasal part of the retina are placed in the nasal half of the nerve. But more posteriorly, the papillo-macular bundle is situated in the central part of the nerve, and the rest of the fibres occupies corresponding positions.

B. The Optic Chiasma

It is a flat, oblong band, 8×12 mm. in size, and lies in the majority of cases above the pituitary fossa. The optic nerves are joined to the antero-lateral angles of the chiasma. From the postero-lateral angles of the chiasma, the optic tracts originate.

The optic nerve fibres continue into those of the optic chiasma. But in the chiasma semi-decussation of nerve fibres takes place. The fibres from the nasal half of each retina cross over to join the optic tract of the opposite side, whereas the fibres from the temporal half of each retina continue uncrossed to the optic tract of the same side (Fig. 97).

Further details of the decussation in the chiasma—The fibres from the infero-nasal quadrant of the retina, cross in the anterior part of the chiasma. The fibres, from the supero-nasal quadrant of the retina, cross in the posterior part of the chiasma.

Macular fibres—The fibres from the nasal half of the macula, cross in the posterior part of the chiasma to the opposite optic tract, whereas the fibres, from the temporal half of the macula, continue uncrossed to the optic tract of the same side (Fig. 97).

C. The Optic Tracts

Two optic tracts, one on each side, are cylindrical bands, running outwards and backwards from the postero-lateral angle of the chiasma. They wind round the crus cerebri to end in the lateral geniculate bodies. Each tract consists of uncrossed fibres from the

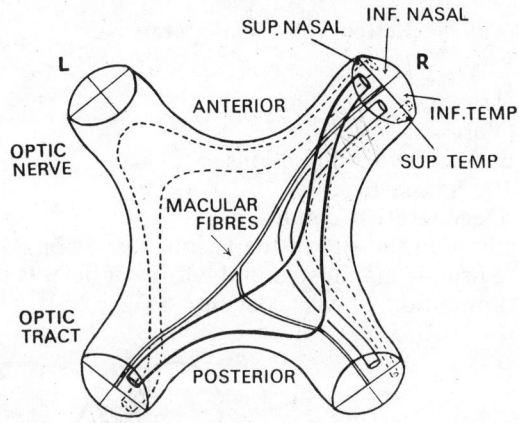

Fig. 97. Arrangement of optic nerve fibres in chiasma (May and Worth).

temporal half of the retina, including macula of the same side and crossed fibres from the nasal half of the retina and macula of the opposite side. The arrangement of the nerve fibres in the tracts are not regular.

D. The Lateral Geniculate Bodies

They are ovoid bodies situated at the posterior end of the optic tract. The fibres of the optic tract end in the geniculate bodies and new fibres for the optic radiations originate from them.

E. The Optic Radiations

The relay fibres for visual pathway, from the lateral geniculate body, constitute the optic radiations. They pass through the posterior portion of the internal capsule and end in the calcarine cortex surrounding the calcarine fissure in the occipital lobe. This area is also known as the visual cortex. In the radiation, the nerve fibres are arranged in order, so that upper half of the radiation represents the upper quadrant of the temporal half of the ipsilateral retina and the upper quadrant of the nasal half of the contralateral retina. Similarly the lower half of the radiation represents lower quadrants of the corresponding retinae.

F. The Visual Cortex

It is spread above and below the calcarine fissure extending into the floor of the fissure and reaches upto the occipital pole of the occipital lobe.

Lesions of visual pathways

Causes

    (a) Trauma.
    (b) Vascular lesions.
    (c) Inflammatory affections.
    (d) Neoplasms.
    (e) Degenerative conditions.

Depending on the site of the lesion, the lesions of the visual pathway are usually manifested in the form of defects in the visual field and diminution of visual acuity. (Fig. 98).

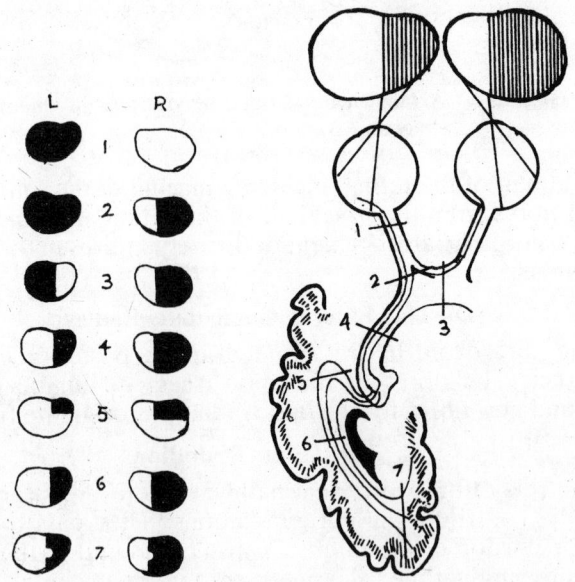

Fig 98. Field defects due to lesions of visual pathway at different levels (Parsons).

1.Lesions of the optic nerve

(a) Affection of the papillomacular bundle produces central scotoma.

(b) Affection of temporal or nasal fibres of the nerve causes corresponding field defects, *e.g.,* temporal lesion causes defect in the nasal field and vice versa.

(c) Total lesion of the optic nerve causes total blindness due to optic atrophy.

2. Lesions of the optic chiasma

Usual field defect following a lesion through the middle of the chiasma is bitemporal hemianopia, *i.e.,* loss of temporal field of vision in each eye, due to the affection of the crossed fibres from the nasal half of each retina.

Binasal hemianopia, *i.e.,* loss of nasal field in each eye, is extremely rare. It is produced by lesions on either side of the chiasma, so that the uncrossed fibres from the temporal half of each retina are affected. In both the conditions, there is partial optic atrophy.

3. Lesions of the optic tract

The usual field defect is homonymous hemianopia, *i.e.* loss of nasal field of the same side and temporal field of the opposite side. The field defects are incongruous, *i.e.,* the defects in two sides are not exctly equal and also the macula, *i.e.,* the fixation area is not spared. The incongruous defect is due to irregular arrangement of nerve fibres in the tracts.

Due to proximity of the crus cerebri and oculomotor nerves to the tracts, ocular palsies aand hemiplegia may be associated with tract lesions. There is also partial optic atrophy.

Right homonymous hemianopia causes difficulty in reading.

4. Lesions of the lateral geniculate body

The field defect caused by this lesion is also homonymous hemianopia.

5. Lesions of optic radiation

A lesion across the entire radiation produces homonymous hemianopic field defect. But the field defects in the eyes are congruous, *i.e.,* the extent of the defect is the same in each eye. There is also sparing of the fixation area. The congruous nature of the field defect is due to the regular arrangement of the nerve fibres in the radiation. There is no optic atrophy and pupil reactions are normal. The cause for sparing of the fixation area is not known.

A lesion in the upper or lower part of the radiation produces quadrantic hemianopia in which corresponding quadrants of each field are lost.

6. *Leisons of the visual cortex*

If the lesion is extensive as due to thrombosis of the calcarine artery, the field defect is homonymous hemianopia with sparing of the fixation area. But if only the area above or below the calcarine fissure are affected, quadrantic hemianopia is produced.

CHAPTER XV

OCULAR MOTILITY AND SQUINT

(Strabismus)

Anatomy of the extra-ocular muscles

There are six extra-ocular muscles in each eye, of which four are rectus or straight muscles and two are oblique muscles.

The rectus muscles are—
    (a) Superior rectus.
    (b) Inferior rectus.
    (c) Medial rectus.
    (d) Lateral rectus.

The oblique musecles are—
    (a) Superior oblique.
    (b) Inferior oblique.

The four rectus musecles originate from the common annular tendon of Zinn situated around the optic foramen at the apex of the orbit. The muscles are inserted to the sclera by flat tendons, at various distances from limbus, as follows—
    (a) Superior rectus—about 8 mm.
    (b) Inferior rectus—6.5 mm.
    (c) Medial rectus—5.5 mm.
    (d) Lateral rectus—about 7 mm.

The lines of insertions of the superior and inferior rectus muscles are convex forward and oblique.

The lateral and the medial rectus muscles extend in a strictly anteroposterior direction. But the superior and inferior rectus muscles run forwards and slightly making an angle of 23° with the anteroposterior median (Fig. 99).

Origin and insertion of the oblique muscles

The superior oblique—It takes its bony origin from the upper and inner margin of the optic foramen. It then runs forwards to the upper and inner angle of the orbit, near the junction of the superior and the medial orbital margin, where it ends in a rounded tendon, which passes through a fibrous pulley called trochlea. After passing through the pulley, the tendon is reflected backwards and laterally underneath the superior rectus muscles, and is inserted into the upper and outer part of the sclera behind the equator.

The inferior oblique

It originates from the floor of the orbit near the inner end of the inferior orbital margin, and then passes outwards below the inferior rectus muscle and is inserted into the outer part of the sclera behind the equator and underneath rectus muscle.

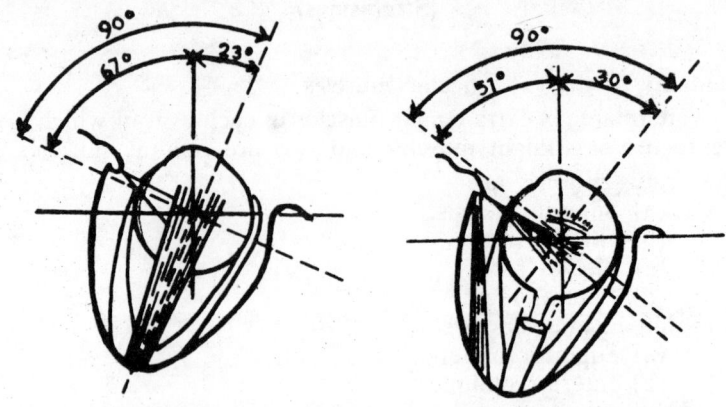

Fig. 99.   The lateral deviation of   F⁄g. 100.   The oblique position of
the right superior rectus.   the reflected tendon of
                                      the right superior oblique.

The reflected tendons of the superior oblique and the inferior oblique musecle make an angle of 51° with the antero-posterior meridian (Fig.100).

The extra-ocular muscles are ensheathed by the fascia of the orbit, which covers the sclera as Tenon's capsule. The fascial sheaths send prolongations to the orbital walls which are known as check ligaments, because they check the movements of the eyeball.

Nerve supply of the extra-ocular muscles

(a) Superior oblique—by the 4th cranial nerve.

(b) Lateral rectus—by the 6th cranial nerve.

(c) Superior, inferior and medial rectus and the inferior oblique—by the 3rd cranial nerve.

Blood supply

By the muscular branches of the ophthalmic artery.

Action of the extra-ocular muscles

The action of extra ocular muscles is to rotate the eye around a centre of rotation situated 12 or 13 mm behind the cornea.

Rotation takes place in the horizontal, vertical or antero-posterior axes. In movement of the eye ball every muscle is involved either with contraction or inhibition, more or less.

1. The laterial rectus—moves the eyeball outwards, *i.e.*, abduction.

2. The medial rectus—moves the eyeball inwards, *i.e.*, adduction.

3. The superior rectus—

Main action

It moves the eyeball upwards, *i.e.*, elevation.

Subsidiary actions

(a) It moves the eyeball inwards, *i.e.*, adduction.

(b) It rotates the eyeball inwards, *i.e.*, intorsion.

4. The inferior rectus—

Main action

It moves the eyeball downwards, *i.e.*, depression.

Subsidiary actions

(a) It moves the eyeball inwards, *i.e.*, adduction.

(b) It rotates the eyeball outwards, *i.e.*, extorsion.

5. The superior oblique—The actions are due to contraction of the reflected portion of the muscle.

Main action

It moves the eyeball downwards, *i.e.*, depression.

Subsidiary actions

It moves the eyball outwards, *i.e.*, abduction.

(b) It rotates the eyeball inwards, *i.e.*, intorsion.

6. The inferior oblique—

Main action

It moves the eyeball upwards, *i.e.*, elevation.

Subsidiary actions

(a) It moves the eyeball outwards, *i.e.*, abduction.

(b) It rotates the eyeball outwards, *i.e.*, extorsion.

These subsidiary action of the vertical recti and the oblique muscles are due to their oblique positions making an angle with the antero-posterior meridian. The rotation of the eyeball is expressed in relation to the vertical corneal meridian, *i.e.*, when this meridian rotates inwards, it is intorsion and when it rotates outwards, it is extorsion.

Conjugate movements of the eyeball

When both the eyes moves together keeping their visual axes parallel, the movements are known as conjugate movements.

Types of conjugate movements
    1. Dextro-version—Horizontally to the right.
    2. Laevo-version—Horizontally to the left.
    3. Dextro-elevation—Upwards and to the right.
    4. Laevo-elevation—Upwards and to the left.
    5. Dextro-depression—Downwards and to the right.
    6. Laevo-depression—Downwards and to the left.

For each of these movements, two muscles take part—one muscle from each eye. These pair of muscles, which work together, are known as synergic or yoke muscles.

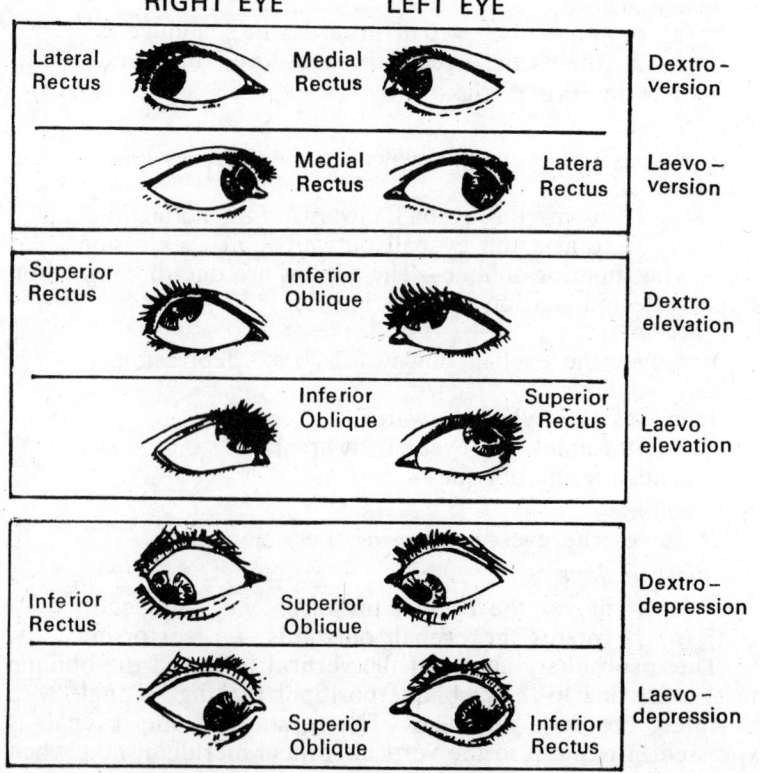

Fig. 101.   Conjugate movements of the eyeball (May and Worth).

The synergic muscles taking part in the conjugate movements are as follows—
    1. Dextro-version—Right lateral rectus and left medial rectus.

2. Laevo-version—Left lateral rectus and right medial rectus.
3. Dextro-elevation—Right superior rectus and left inferior oblique.
4. Laevo-elevation—Left superior rectus and right inferior oblique..
5. Dextro-depression—Right inferior rectus aand left superior oblique.
6. Laevo-depression-Left inferior rectus and right superior oblique.

Similar to the synergists there are antagonists.
The antagonists may be direct or contralateral.

Direct antagonists

(a) The external rectus is directly antagonist to the internal rectus of the same eye and vice versa.
(b) The superior rectus is similarly directly antagonist to the inferior rectus and vice versa.
(c) The superior oblique is also directly antagonist to the inferior oblique and vice versa.

Contralateral antagonists

(a) The right external rectus and the left external rectus.
(b) The right medial rectus rectus and the left medial rectus.
(c) The right superior rectus and the left superior oblique.
(d) The right inferior rectus and the left inferior oblique.
(e) The right superior oblique and the left superior rectus.
(f) The right inferior oblique and the left inferior rectus.

Diplopia (Double Vision)

In general, by diplopia it is meant an object appears double. The diplopia may be binocular, *i.e.,* when both eyes remain open or uniocular, *i.e.,* when only one remains open.

Bonocular diplopia

This type of double vision occurs when the image of an object does not fall on the corresponding parts of the retina in both the eyes. For example, the image of an object falls on the macula in the right eye but not on the macula in the left eye.

Causes of binocular diplopia

1. Paralysis of an extra-ocular muscle–commonest.
2. Displacement of the eyeball as by pressure of the finger or by a space-occupying lesion in the orbit.

3. Restriction of the movements of the eyeball as due to pterygium or symblepharon.

Uniocular diplopia

It occurs when more than one image of the same object falls on different parts of the retina. There may be polyopia due to multiple image.

Cause of uniocular diplopia

1. Subluxation of the lens—when the lens becomes displaced in such a position, that it only covers half the pupillary area, the other half of the pupil remaining aphakic.

2. A double pupil due to a big peripheral iridectomy or due to iridodialysis as a result of injury.

3. Incipient cataract with water-clefts in the lens.

Squint
(Strabismus)

Definition—It is a condition when one eye deviates always from the fixation point (Duke-Elder).

Classification of squint

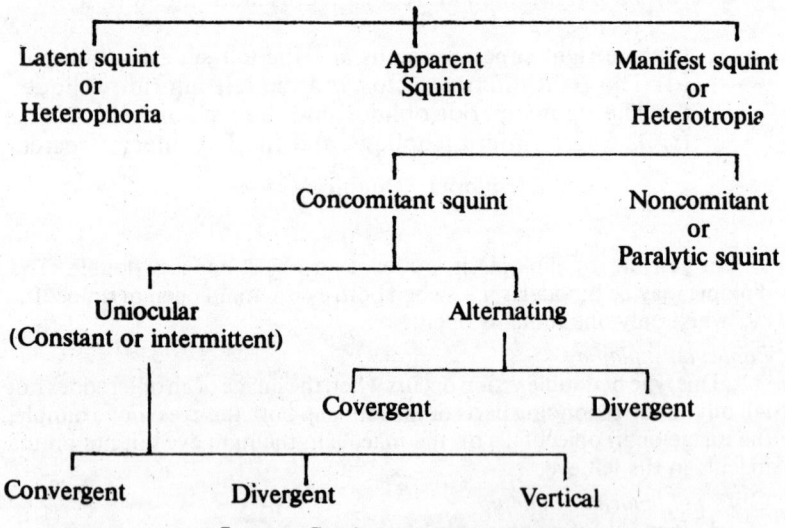

Latent Squint or Heterophoria

If the extra-ocular muscles in both the eye are in perfect equilibrium, so that the eyes retain their normal positional relationships, even when their aactivity is dissociated by the withdrawal of the controlling influence of fusion, the condition is known as orthophoria (Duke-Elder).

Heterophoria

Heterophoria is the condition, when the balance of the extraocular muscles is imperfect due to intrinsic weakness of one or more of the extra-ocular muscles and there is a tendency for the eye to deviate from its normal relative position, as soon as the corrective fusion reflex is withdrawn by dissociating binocular vision. Ordinarily the deviation is not manifest, because the weak muscle is made to overwork in order to maintain normal position for the interest of binocular vision. But the tendency for deviation becomes manifest by dissociation tests.

Types of heterophoria

1. Esophoria—tendency for deviation of the eyeball inwards.
2. Exophoria—tendency for deviation of the eyeball outwards.
3. Hyperphoria—tendency for deviation of the eyeball upwards.
4. Hypophoria—tendency for deviation of the eyeball downwards.
5. Cyclophoria—tendency for rotation of the eyeball round the fixation axis.
5. Anisophoria—deviation of the eyeball varies with the direction of gaze.

Etiology of heterophoria
Predisposing factors

Ill health, fatigue of the eyes due to over work, and certain occupations like watch-making.

Exciting factors

1. Age—
   (a) In infancy, binocular reflexes are weak, so there is a tendency for deviation outwards—exophoria.
   (b) In childhood, accommodation and convergence reflexes are very powerful, so there is a tendency for deviation of the eyeball inwards—esophoria.
   (c) In presbyopic age, as the near point of distinct vision recedes, the convergence becomes weaker and as there is tendency for deviation of the eye outwards—exophoria.

2. Influence of refraction—
(a) In hypermetropia there is tendency for esophoria.
(b) In myopia there is tendency for exophoria.
3. Anatomical defects in the muscles, fascia, ligaments or in the bony orbit.
4. Organic muscular or nervous disease, *e.g.*, neurosyphilis, disseminated sclerosis or myaesthenia gravis.

Symptoms of heterophoria

When the ability to overcome the imbalance of ocular muscles becomes impaired due to ill-health, ocular fatigue, mental worries and anxieties or advancing age, symptoms appear as follows:

1. Headache or aching of the eyes—Such symptoms usually occur following prolonged use of the eyes.

2. Blurring of print or jumbling together of words while reading.

3. Intermittent diplopia due to intermittent squint.

Diagnosis of heterophoria

1. By cover test—One eye is covered and the other eye is made to fix on an object. If there is heterophoria, the eye under cover deviates. The cover is then quickly removed and the eye, which was under cover, is watched. As soon as the cover is removed, the covered eye corrects the deviation and regains its normal position quickly. Cover test should be done with and without spectacles both for near and distant objects.

2. By Maddox rod (Fig. 102)—The patient looks at a light point at a distance of 6 metres. A Maddox rod is now held in front of one of the eyes. The eye with the Maddox rod sees the point light as a red straight line of light at right angles to the axis of the rod. Thus the images of the light point in the two eyes become dissimilar and fusion becomes dissociated. If there is heterophoria, due to deviation of the eye, the line of light becomes separated from the point light by a distance. In orthophoria, although the fusion has been disso-

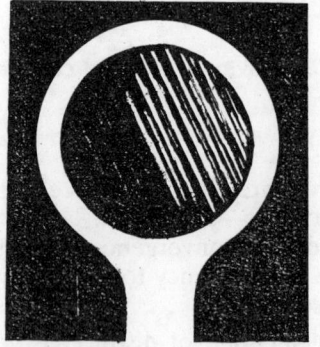

Fig. 102.   Maddox rod.

ciated, as there is no tendency for one eye to deviate, the line of light passes through the point. By placing the Maddox rod in different meridians, eso exo, hypo, or hyperphoria can be detected. Maddox rod test can also be done for near and distance.

3. **By Maddox wing**—Fig. 103).—It is a device to find out heterophoria at a distance of 33 cm. from the eye. Through the two slits of the instrument, one eye sees white numerical numbers in a horizontal line and the other eye sees a vertical white arrow underneath the white numbers. In orthophoria, the white arrow is seen underneath the number 0. But in heterophoria the arrow deviates either outwards or inwards. Similarly there are red numerical numbers in a vertical line and a red horizontal arrow. If there is vertical deviation of the eyes, the arrow is seen either above or below the number 0.

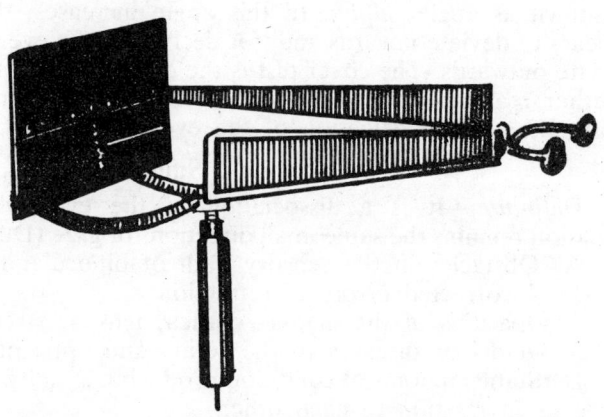

Fig. 103. Maddox wing.

4. By synoptophore—It is a useful instrument particularly to detect all varities of squint and the state of binocular vision (Fig)

Treatment of heterophoria

The refractive error must be corrected.

2. Orthoptic treatment to increase the fusional range and muscle power, is done with synoptophore.

3. Use of prism is no more practised.

4. Operative treatment—By this method, the weak muscle is strengthened or its antagonist is made weaker.

the eyeball, but the eye may appear to be deviated, due to the following reasons—

(a) Configuration of the tissues round the eye, e.g., epicanthus or a broad nose. An epicanthus is a congenital condition, in which a perpendicular fold of skin runs from the root of the nose to the inner end of the lower lid, hiding the medial canthus and caruncle. It gives the appearance of a convergent squint.

(b) Alteration of the angle between the visual axis and the optical axis of the eye, i.e., the angle alpha.

The visual axis is the line joining the fixation point and the fovea and it passes through the nodal point of the eye. The optical axis is the line passing through the centres of the refracting surfaces of the eye. Normally the optical axis and the visual axis are not the same, but the optical axis meets the retina on the nasal side of the macula. So there is an angle between these axes which is known as angle. alpha. In this angle increases, the eyeball appears to deviate inwards and if it decreases, the eye appears to deviate outwards. The cover test is the diagnostic test to find out whether real deviation exists under cover or not. In apparent squint there is no deviation of the eyeball by cover test.

Concomitant Squint

Definition—It is a dissociation of the eyes wherein the deviation remains the same in all directions of gaze (Duke-Elder).

A. Obstacles in the sensory path of binocular .reflex—

1. Uncorrected errors of refraction.
2. Opacities of the media—cornea, lens or vireous.
3. Defets or diseases of the retina and optic nerve.

B. Static anatomical condition producing a faulty position of the eyes in relation to each other—

1. Congenital abnormality of the shape or position of the orbit
2. Space occupying lesion in the orbit.
3. Congenital absence of a muscle, paresis of a musecle or abnormalities of the insertion of a muscle.

C. Decompensation of heterophoria producing manifest squint.

D. Disharmony in the accommodation convergence relationship, as for example, in hypermetropia as more accommodation is exerted to correct the error, there is more convergence and so a convergent squint may develop. Similarly in myopia accommodation does not come into play for correction of the error and so the convergence is weak and there is a tendency for divergent squint.

E. Central causes—

1. Deficient development of the fusion faculty.

2. Mental trauma or hyperexcitability of the central nervous system, *e.g.*, during teething.

Age incidence—Usually concomitant strabismus develop. during the period when reflexes governing binocular vision are established, *i.e.*, within five years of age.

Symptoms of concomitant squint in general

Usually there is no symptom. The squint is detected by the parents or relatives. Although the image of an object does not fall on the macula in the squinting eye, there is no diplopia. The reason is that the image in the squinting eye is automatically suppressed. This suppression develop easily as the concomitant squint usually occurs in the young age. The main feature of the concomitant squint is the failure of binocular vision.

Clinical signs of concomitant squint in general

There are two important signs for the concomitant squint—

1. The primary deviation is equal to the secondary deviation. The primary deviation means the angle of deviation of the squinting eye, when the normal'eye fixes an object. The secondary deviation is the angle of deviation of the normal eye under cover, when the squinting eye is made to fix an object by covering the normal eye.

2. Usually there is no limitation of movements of the eyeball in any direction. The exception is in case of a squint due to congenital weakness or paresis of a muscle.

In case of uniocular concominant squint, the vision in the squinting eye is usually defective.

Types of concomitant squint

A. Uniocular squint—

When one eye always deviates and the normal eye takes up fixation. At the beginning, the squint may be intermittent but later on it becomes constant. An uniocular squint may be convergent, divergent, or vertical.

1. Convergent concomitant squint—This develops typically in the early life before the binocular reflexes are firmly established. One eye always deviates inwards. The usual causes of this type of squint are—

    (a) Excessive use of accommodation as in hypermetropia— The great majority of convergent squint cases come within this group.

(b) Congenital myopia—Due to myopia, the child can only see objects very close to the eye. Naturally he is used to excess of convergence and so a convergent squint develops.

(c) Anatomical conditions—These are asymmetry of orbits, narrow interpupillary distance, enophthalmos or microphthalmos.

(d) Uncompensated esophoria—The esophoria becomes manifest and convergent squint develops.

2. Divergent concomitant squint—In this type one eye deviates outwards while the other eye fixes an object. The causes of this type of squint are as follows—

(a) Inherent neuromuscular incoordination—It is the cause of primary divergent squint. It usuallt starts at the age of 2 to 5 years and is at first intermittent and later on becomes constant.

(b) Refractive error—Uncorrected myopia.

(c) Complete loss of vision—A blind eye, particularly in adults diverges, because that is the position of anatomical rest of the eyeball. This type of squint is known as the secondary divergent squint.

(d) Post-operative cause—Over correction of a convergent squint by operation may lead to a divergent squint. It is known as consecutive squint.

(e) Uncompensated exophoria—The exophoria becomes manifest to produce a divergent squient.

3. Vertical concomitant squint—A true vertical squint is rate. The majority of case are those of hyperphoria in which the vertical deviation becomes manifest.

B. Alternating squint—Convergent or divergent.

Alternating squint means when one eye fixes, the other deviates either inwards or outwards and either of the eyes can take up fixation alternately. One important feature of alternating squint is normal vision in each eye. The image of the deviating eye is completely suppressed in the brain, and so there is no diplopia.

Causes of alternating squint

(a) Congenital paresis of either the external or the internal rectus of each eye. This type is known as paretic alternator. It becomes manifest in very early life, and the fusion faculty never develops in such cases.

(b) Hypermetropia—A minority of cases are due to hyper-metropia and this type is known as iso-ametropic alternator. It usually starts at the age of three years and the child uses one eye at a time either wilfully or indiscriminately.

Investigation of a case of concomitant squint
A. History—

(a) Age of onset of the squint—Usually accommodative squint becomes manifest about the age of 3 to 6 years. The squint due to congenital paresis of muscles appears at a very early age. In general, the older the age of onset and shorter the squinting period, better is the prognosis.

(b) Any history of illness, mental shock or head injury at the time of onset of the squint.

(c) Is the squint intermittent or constant? Does one eye only deviate or there is alternation?

(d) Family history—Is there any history of squint in the family or are there cases of poor eyesight in the family?

B. Examination of the patient—

(1) Inspection—

(a) Which eye is deviated, right or the left?

(b) Is the deviation inwards, outwards, or vertical?

(c) Any opacity in the cornea or lens and reaction of the pupil.

(2) Cover test—This is done to find out whether the squint is uniocular or alternating. In alternating squint, when one eye of fixed the other deviates and both the eyes can take up fixation alternately. But in case of uniocular squint, it is the fixing eye which always maintains fixation.

(3) Movements of the eyeball—Movements of individual eye are tested in all directions to find out any limitation of movement in any direction.

(4) Recording of visual acuity in each eye and to find out any error of refraction by retinoscopy under atropine. The media and the fundus of the eye must also be examined by ophthalmo-scope to find out any cause for the squint.

(5) To find out the state of binocular vision—Normally the binocular vision is of three grades, *i.e.*,simultaneous macular perception, fusion and stereopsis. Actual grade of binocular vision is determined by synoptophore. Usually accommodative squints have the first grade of binocular vision.The alternating squint

cases usually do not possess any grade of binocular vision.

(6) Measurement of the angle of the squint—

The angle of deviation must be measured. This is necessary for operative treatment. The angle may be measured by several methods but the following two methods are simple—

    (a) By noting the position of the image of a light on the cornea—Light from an electric torch is thrown on the eye from the front, when the patient looks towards the light. In the normal eye the image of the light on the cornea is approximately at the centre of pupillary area.If the image of the light is on the pupillary margin in the squinting eye, the approximate angle of squint is 20° and if the image is on the limbus, the approximate angle is 45°.

    (b) By synoptophore—This method is very accurate.

C. Treatment of concomitant squint—

Uniocular squint—

1. Correction of error of refraction by suitable glasses and a squint of minor degree may be corrected.

2. Occlusion to cure amblyopia—If the vision does not become normal with corrected glasses and the squint persists, the normal eye must be kept constantly occluded by a suitable occluder for 3 months.This occlusion makes the squinting eye work with the corrected glasses and vision rapidly improves. Within three months' effective occlusion, the vision in the squinting eye becomes normal. This improvement of vision occurs if the age is within 9 to 10 years, but afterwards the visual improvement takes a longer time to occur. After improvement of vision the occlusion is no longer used and the uniocular squint becomes an alternating squint as the squinting eye now can take up fixation.

3. Operative measure—Following successful occlusion and improvement of vision in the squinting eye, operative procedure is undertaken. By operative procedure, the squinting eye is made straight by the following methods—

    (a) In convergent squint—

        (i) The internal rectus of the squinting eye is recessed, *i.e.,* its insertion to sclera is shifted backwards. One mm. of recession of internal rectus corrects about 3° of the angle of squint. But this recession must not exceed 5 mm. as in that case convergence insufficiency may develop.

        (ii) The external rectus is resected, *i.e.,* a portion of the muscle is removed. Usually 1 mm. of resection of the external rectus corrects 2° of the angle.

Depending on the angle of the squint both the muscles may have to be tackled.

(b) In divergent squint—Similarly the external rectus is recessed and the internal resected.

(c) In vertical squint, the corresponding vertical muscles are tackled.

4. Fusional exercise—When the eyes become straight after the operation, fusional exercise is practised by a synoptophore to improve binocular vision, because if binocular vision is not properly established, the correction of squint becomes only cosmetic and the eye may deviate again later on.

D. Treatment of alternating squint—

As fusion faculty does not develop in this type of squint, the treatment is only for cosmetic purpose. Both the eyes may have to be tackled to correct the deviation. The same procedure, *i.e.*, either recession or resection of the internal or external rectus is followed depending on the type of the squint, *i.e.*, convergent or divergent.

Noncomitant or Paralytic Squint

Definition—Noncomitant squint is a deviation caused by paralysis of extra-ocular muscles and it is a condition in which the deviation of the eye varies in different directions of gaze.

Etiology

1. Any lesion of the cranial nerve supplying the muscle—The lesion may have the following locations—

(a) Lesion of the motor nerve nucleus—
   (i) Congenital absence of the nucleus.
   (ii) Inflammatory lesions affecting the nucleus, *e.g.*, encephalitis, neurosyphilis, disseminated sclerosis.
   (iii) Neoplasms affecting the nucleus.
   (iv) Toxic factors like alcohol or toxins of diphtheria.
   (v) Degenerative and vascular causes affecting the nucleus.

(b) Lesion of the nerve root just beyond the nucleus—
   (i) Inflammation, **e.g.**, encephalitis, neurosyphilis and disseminated sclerosis.
   (ii) Neoplasms.
   (iii) Vascular causes—aneurysm, haemorrhage and thrombosis affecting the arteries supplying the root.

(c) Lesion of the nerve trunk—
   (i) Trauma—Direct injury to the trunk or pressure on the

nerve by a haematoma or stretching of the nerve due to cerebral oedema or intracranial haemorrhage.

(ii) Neuritis of the nerve as in diabetes mellitus, vitamin deficiency or lead poisoning.

(iii) Toxic causes, *e.g.,* alcohol.

(iv) Pressure on the nerve by an aneurysm or a neoplasm.

2. Lesion of the muscle itself—

(a) Congenital absence or maldevelopment of a muscle, *i.e.,* congenital musculo-fascial anomaly.

(b) Injury to the muscle.

(c) Disease of the muscle or myopathy—as in exophthalmic opthalmoplegia in endocrine exophthalmos, thyrotoxic myopathy or ocular myopathy.

Symptoms of noncomitant squint

1. Diplopia—It is the chief symptom. It is most marked in the direction of action of the paralyzed muscle. Diplopia may be crossed or uncrossed. If the eye diverges the diplopia is crossed, but if the eye rotates inwards the diplopia is uncrossed. If the horizontally acting muscles are affected, the two images are seen side by side. If the vertically acting muscles are affected, one image appears at a slightly lower level than the other. If oblique muscles are affected one of the images appears slightly tilted.

2. Vertigo and nausea—these symptoms are due to diplopia.

Clinical signs

Primary deviation

1. Deviation of the eyeball, whose muscle has been paralyzed, in the primary position of the eyes, *i.e.,* when the patient looks straight ahead.

2. The secondary deviation, *i.e.,* the deviation of the normal eye, when the squinting eye is made to fix an object, is much more than the primary deviation. The reason for this difference is due to the fact that the extra motor energy necessary to fix the squinting eye is also shared by the normal eye and so it deviates more.

3. Marked restriction of the movement of the eyeball in the direction of action of the muscles affected.

4. Visual acuity is normal in each eye and there is no amblyopia.

5. Compensatory head tilt to avoid diplopia—This is done in such a way that the eye need not be rotated in the direction of the action of the paralyzed muscle. As for example, if the right external rectus is paralyzed, the head is kept turned towards the right.

6. False orientation—If a person, whose right external rectus is paralyzed, attempts to fix an object situated towards the right with his left eye closed, his finger passes considerably to the right of the object. This sign is known as false orientation or projection.

Sequelae of external ocular muscle palsy

If the paralysis is of some duration, certain changes occur in the muscles. These happen more in cases of affection of the nerve itself than in cases where the muscles are primarily affected. These changes are—

(a) Overaction of the contralateral synergist.

(b) Contracture of the direct antagonist.

(c) Secondary inhibitional palsy of the contralateral antagonist.

Example

(a) In a case of right external rectus palsy there are— over-action of the left internal rectus, contracture of the right internal rectus, and secondary palsy of the left external rectus.

Similarly

(b) In a case of left superior oblique palsy there are— over-action of the right inferior rectus, contracture of the left inferior oblique and secondary inhibitional palsy of the right superior rectus.

Neurogenic palsies

Clinical pictures of extra-ocular muscle paralysis, due to the affection of the motor nerves for those muscles, vary according to the nerve affected. The palsies may be—

(a) Oculomotor palsy—Affection of the 3rd cranial nerve.

(b) Trochlear palsy—Affection of the 4th nerve.

(c) Abducens palsy—Affection of the 6th nerve.

The 3rd nerve may be affected in whole or in part. It may be associated with the affection of the 4th and 6th nerve.

Total ophthalmoplegia

It is a condition, when the entire motor apparatus of the eye, including the intrinsic muscles (ciliary muscle, sphincter and dilator pupilae), the extrinsic muscles and the levator palpebrae, is paralyzed.

External ophthalmoplegia

It is a condition when only extrinsic muscles, including the the levator, are paralyzed.

Clinical signs of total ophthalmoplegia

   (a) Complete ptosis.

   (b) On raising the upper lid, the eye is found to be slightly proptosed and slightly divergent, as it lies in the anatomical position of rest.

   (c) No movement of the eyeball in any direction.

   (d) The pupil is dilated without any reaction to light, accommodation and convergence.

   (e) Complete loss of accommodation.

In bilateral cases of total ophthalmoplegia, there is usually a wide spread lesion, *i.e.,* vascular or inflammatory, in the brain stem. In uniocular cases, the lesion is either in the cavernous sinus or near the superior orbital fissure in the orbit.

Clinical signs of external ophthalmoplegia

The clinical picture is the same as that for total ophthalmoplegia except that pupillary activity and accommodation are normal.

The lesion in such cases is usually nuclear, *i.e.,* the motor nuclei are affected, leaving alone the Edinger-Westphal nucleus which supplies the intrinsic muscles.

Oculomotor Palsy or 3rd Nerve Palsy

Clinical signs

   (a) Ptosis, *i.e.,* drooping of the upper lid.

   (b) The eyeball rotates outwards and slightly downwards due to unopposed action of the external rectus and minimal depressive action of the superior oblique.

   (c) Vertical meridian of the cornea rotates inwards, *i.e.,* intorsion, due to the action of the superior oblique.

   (d) Movement of the eyeball is restricted in all directions except outwards.

   (e) The pupil is dilated and inactive.

   (f) Accommodation is completely lost.

Trochlear Palsy or 4th Nerve Palsy

Clinical signs

These are due to paralysis of the superior oblique.

   (a) The eyeball is deviated upwards and inwards.

   (b) The vertical meridian of the cornea is rotated outwards, *i.e.,* extorsion.

   (c) Downward and inward movement of the eyeball is markedly restricted.

Abducens Palsy or 6th Nerve Palsy

This is the commonest.

Clinical signs

These are due to paralysis of the external rectus.

(a) The eyeball is rotated inwards.

(b) There is marked restriction of the movement of the eyeball outwards.

Investigation of a case of paralytic squint

1. History—Regarding the onset and associated illness which may be a precipitating factor.

2. Ocular posture, *i.e.,* the deviation of the eyeball.

3. Head posture, *i.e.,* any tilting or rotation of the head.

4. Cover test to find out whether the secondary deviation is more than the primary deviation.

5. Ocular movements—Any restriction of the movement in any direction gives an idea of the muscle involved. Movements should be examined for individual eye and both eyes together.

6. Diplopia test—A spectacle containing a red glass for the right eye and a green glass for the left eye is worn by the patient. In the dark room a streak of light—from a specially devised torch, is shown, in the following nine fields—

    (i) up and to the right,

    (ii) straight upwards,

    (iii) up and to the left,

    (iv) straight to the right,

    (v) straight in front,

    (vi) straight to the left,

    (vii) down and to the right,

  (viii) straight downwards,

    (ix) down and to the left.

In the fields where there is diplopia, the patient notices two images of the light—one red and the other green. He is then asked to find out in which field the diplopia is most marked, *i.e.,* the separation of the two images is greatest. Then he is asked to notice which of the images, red or green, in that field is most external. The external image belongs to the eye which has the paralyzed muscle.

There are other methods to find out exactly which muscle is affected like testing by a Hess screen and a Lancaster screen. Synoptophore examination can also be done in different positions of gaze.

Treatment of paralytic squint

1. Treatment of the underlying cause.

2. To avoid diplopia, occulsion of the affected eye may be

done, but the patient should be encouraged to look from time to time in the direction where there is no diplopia, so that binocular vision may be maintained.

3. Injection of vitamin B1, B6, and B12 in heavy doses may be tried as empirical treatment.

4. Operative measure—This should not be done before six months from the onset, as sufficient time must be allowed for recovery. The operative measure consists mainly of tackling the contracture of the direct antagonist and overaction of the contralateral synergist.

CHAPTER XVI

NYSTAGMUS

Definition—Nystagmus means rapid oscillatory movements of the eyes due to disturbance of ocular posture.

General features of nystagmus
  (a) The oscillations are involuntary and they do not affect the normal movements of the eyeball.
  (b) The oscillations are usually horizontal, but may be vertical or rotatory.
  (c) The condition is usually bilateral.

Etiology of nystagmus
  As nystagmus is considered as a disturbance of ocular posture, the etiology consists of the affections of the factors responsible for maintenance of ocular posture, i.e., the visual sensory pathway, the vestibular apparatus, the motor mechanisms which co-ordinate the sensory and the motor functions.
  The following are the etilogical factors (after Duke-Elder)—
  1. Ocular nystagmus (due to defect in maintaining fixation)—
  It may be one of the following types—

A. Physiologically induced nystagmus—
  (a) Deviational nystagmus—It occurs– normally when the eyes are maintained in extreme lateral position.
  (b) Opto-kinetic nystagmus—It occurs if the fixation is confused by a succession of moving objects traversing the visual field. It is visible when a person travels in a train and keeps on looking outside. Or a drum with black and white stripes is rotated in front of eyes.
  (c) Latent nystagmus—It is a condition wherein the nystagums is not present when both the eyes are open, but it becomes manifest on closing either eye. The vision is usually unequal in the eyes. There is either corneal scarring or disease in the fundus in one of the eyes, so that there is formation of a sharp image on the fovea of one eye and its absence on the other.

B. Spontaneous nystagmus—
  a) Amaurotic nystagmus of pendular or jerky type occurring

in infants who are born blind and in whom macular fixation has not developed.

(b) Amblyopic nystagmus—This occurs due to hindrance to the development of macular fixation within the first four to six months life. The vision is poor in each eye. The causes are albinism, macular coloboma, congenital total colour blindness or any anomaly in the ocular media which makes fixation difficult.

(c) Spasmus nutans—This is a type of nystagmus with headnodding movements occurring in young children, particularly females, of the poorer classes brought up in very dim illumination. This condition, which is acquired, is rare.

(d) Miner's nystagmus—This is an occupational disease, confined to the workers in coal mines. The etiological factors are lack of illumination at the coal face and crouched attitude of the miner, which is pendular in type which may be horizontal, vertical or rotatory.

2. Vestibular nystagmus—
   It may be of the following types—

   (a) Labyrynthine nystagmus—It results physiologically by stimulating the labyrynths by heat, rotatory movement or compression. The nystagmus is jerky, fine, rapid and horizontal-rotatory nystagmus towards the sound side. An irritative lesion produces an opposite effect.

3. Central nystagmus—
   The nystagmus is typically jerky. It is most commonly elicited on lateral deviation of the eyes. Spontaneous bilateral and purely vertical nystagmus is always of central origin. The causes are—

   (a) Lesions of the brain-stem, e.g., disseminated sclerosis, epidemic encephalitis, vascular lesions and tumours and abscesses.

   (b) Cerebellar lesions, e.g., tumours and abscesses.

   (c) Spinal lesions—Nystagmus is occasionally seen in disease of the upper part of the spinal cord, due to affection of the spinocerebellar pathway, e.g. tabes and syringomyelia.

   4. Congenital idiopathic nystagmus—It is hereditary and the cause is not known and eyes are usually normal.

Treatment :- It is mostly palliative like correction of refraction, the use of smoked glass or contact lens in albinism and the treatment of any disese. Nystagmus tends to diminish with advancing age.

CHAPTER XVII

ANATOMY AND DISEASES OF THE EYELIDS

Anatomy of the eyelid

The eyelids are mobile tissue curtains, placed in front of the eyeball with protective functions. (Fig. 104).

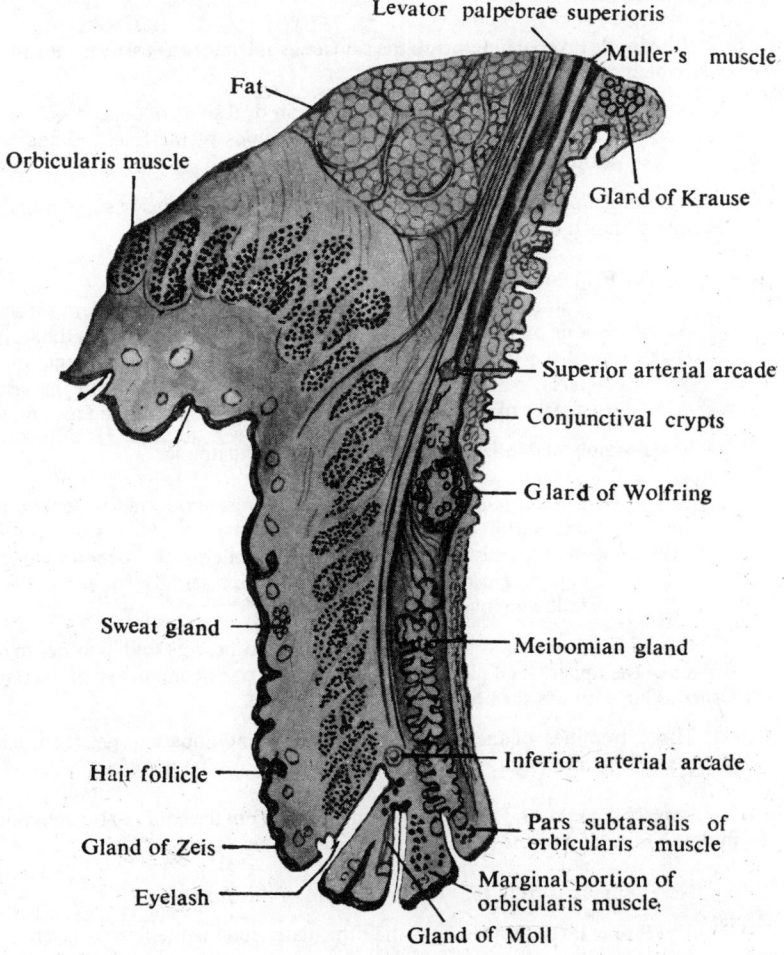

Fig. 104. Vertical section through the upper lid (Parsons).

An eyelid is made of four layers of tissues. These are the following–

Cutaneous layer–It consists of the skin of the eyelid which is extremely delicate and highly elastic. It is covered with fine downy hairs. On looking straight ahead, there is a horizontal fold in the skin of the upper lid which becomes more marked on looking upwards.

Underneath the skin is the loose areolar tissue which does not contain any fat. Due to this areolar tissue, the skin is loosely attached to the underlying muscle and this arrangement permits ready accumulation of oedematus fluid or extravasation of blood underneath the skin.

2. Muscle layer–Underneath the skin and subcutaneous tissue is the muscle layer which consist of–

(a) Orbicularis oculi muscle–This is an oval sheet of concentric muscle fibres, covering the lids and the regions of the forehead and face, around the orbital margins.

By contraction of this muscle, the lids are firmly closed; nerve supply is by the zygomatic branch of the facial nerve.

(b) Palpebral muscles–They are as follows–

(i) Palpebral muscles of Muller–These are sheets of plain muscles, one on each lid. In the upper lid, the muscle arises from the surface of the levator muscle and is inserted to the upper margin of the tarsal plate. The muscle in the lower lid arises from the fascial sheath of the inferior rectus and is inserted into the tarsal plate.

Nerve supply of Muller's muscles–Cervical sympathetic.

(ii) Levator palpebrae superious–It is present only in the upper lid. It arises from the apex of the orbit, above the annulus of Zinn; the muscle belly proceeds forwards just underneath the roof of the orbit and ends in a flat aponeurosis, which is inserted by three parts to the following places–

One part is inserted to the skin of the upper lid near its fold, another to the surface of the upper tarsal plate, and the third part to the conjunctiva of the upper fornix along with the sheath of the superior rectus.

The extremities of the aponeurosis remain tendinous and get themselves attached to the mid-points of the lateral and medial orbital margins.

It raises the upper lid along with the upper fornix of the conjunctiva and causes folding of the skin of the upper lid.

Nerve supply is from the–Upper division of the 3rd nerve.

3. Fibrous layer–Underneath the orbicularis oculi is the fibrous layer.

It consists of

(a) **Septum orbitale**—It is a thin membrane of connective tissue, extending in each lid from the proximal border of the tarsal plate to a thickened line of periosteum around the orbital margin. It is perforated by vessels and nerves entering the lids from the orbit.

(b) **Tarsal Plates**—These are two plates of dense connective tissue, one in each lid. The tarsal plate is larger in the upper than in the lower lid. The extremities of each plate meet at the medial and lateral canthus and are continued to the orbital margin as medial and lateral palpebral ligaments. In the substance of the tarsal plates, disposed in vertical parallel rows, are the meibomian glands.

4. **Mucous layer**—It is formed by the palpebral conjunctiva underneath the fibrous layer.

Glands of the eyelids

There are three types of glands in the eyelids—

(a) **Meibomian glands**—They are situated in vertical rows, embeded in the tarsal plates. They are also known as tarsal glands. They number about 30-40 in the upper lid and 20 to 30 in the lower lid. They are modified sebaceous glands of enormous size, secreting oily secretion and opening on the lid border just in front of its sharp posterior margin.

(b) **Glands of Zeis**—They are sebaceous glands developed as out growths of the epithelial wall of the hair follicle of the eyelash. They are situated on the margin and open into the follicles of the eyelashes.

(c) **Glands of Moll**—These are modified sweat glands. They are tubular in shape and they lie between the cilia on the lid margin. The ducts open either into the ducts of glands of Zeis or directly into the follicles of the cilia or on the surface of the lid margin.

The lid margin—It is a thick border with anterior rounded and posterior sharp margin which lies in close contact with the eyeball. It consists of—

(a) **The eyelashes**—They are stouter than hair and are arranged in 2-3 rows in the upper lid and 1-2 rows in the lower lid, being more in the upper than in the lower lid. The roots of the lashes are deeply embeded in the connective tissue of the lid margin. The upper eyelashes are curved forwards and upwards and the lower ones are directed downwards and forwards. Except in diseases, they never grey even due to age.

(b) **Openings of the ducts of the Meibomian glands**—They are arranged in a single row just in front of the sharp posterior margin.

(c) **Glands of Zeis and Moll**—Which have already been described. Between the anterior edge and the openings of the Meibomian glands is the grey line or intermarginal sulcus. Along this line the lid can be split into two layers—anteriorly skin and orbicularis muscle and posteriorly the tarsal plate and the septum orbitale.

The lid margins unite laterally at an acute angle, forming the lateral canthus. Medially they unite to form the medial canthus, but in between the junction of the lids, there is a rounded space known as lacus lacrimalis which is occupied by a small reddish elevation known as the caruncle.

Arterial supply of the lids is from the following sources :

(a) Lacrimal and palpebral branches of the opthalmic artery.

(b) The facial artery.

(c) The superficial temporal artery.

(d) The infra-orbital artery.

In the upper lid, arterial branches from two arterial arcades—a superior one running along the upper tarsal margin and an inferior one near the free border of the lid. In the lower lid there is only one arch near the free border.

Venous drainage—The veins empty into the

(a) ophthalmic vein.

(b) temporal vein, and

(c) facial vein.

Lymphatic drainage—The lymphatics from the outer half of the lids drain into the pre-auricular lymph glands and those from the inner half to the sub-maxillary lymph nodes.

Sensory nerve supply

(a) Supra-orbital, supratrochlear, infratrochlear and lacrimal branches of the ophthalmic division of the 5th nerve.

(b) Infra-orbital branches of the maxillary division of the 5th nerve.

Congenital Abnormalities of the Eyelids
.1. Coloboma of the eyelid

It is rare. There is a triangular gap in the lid margin with the absence of eyelashes and glands in the affected area.

2. Epicanthus

It is a bilateral condition, which may be associated with ptosis. A more or less vertical fold of skin runs from the root of the nose to the inner end of the lower eyelid, covering the medial canthus and the caruncle.

3. Distichiasis

It is also a rare condition when the Meibomian glands are represented by an extra row of eyelashes which are directed towards the cornea (Fig. 105 C.)

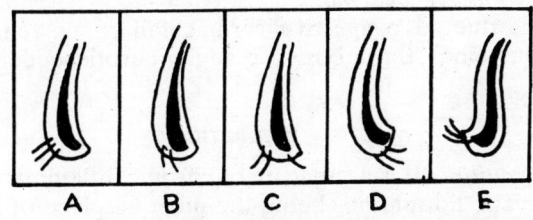

Fig. 105. Section of the upper eyelid showing normal and abnormal positions of tarsus and eyelashes. A—Normal eyelid; B—Trichiasis; C—Distichiasis; D—Entropion; E—Ectropion (May and Worth).

4. Congenital ptosis

It is to be described under ptosis.

Oedema of the Eyelids

Owing to the looseness of the subcutaneous tissues, the lids may be oedematous easily and the oedema may be of a marked degree.

A. *Active oedema or inflammatory oedema*

1. Due oedema to inflammatory condition of eye lid—
   (a) External hordeolum.
   (b) Internal hordeolum.
   (c) Insect bite.
   (d) Dermatitis of the lid.
   (e) Lid abscess or cellulits of the lid.

2. Secondary to inflammation of other neighbouring structures—
   (a) Acute purulent conjunctivitis.
   (b) Acute membraneous or pseudo-membranous conjuctivitis.
   (c) Acute iridocyclitis and panophthalmitis.
   (d) Orbital cellulitis.
   (e) Acute dacryocystitis.
   (f) Facial cellulitis.
   (g) Inflammation of nasal sinuses.

B. *Passive oedema.*

It is due to congestive cardiac failure or renal failure or cavernous sinus thrombosis or angioneurotic oedema.

Blepharitis

Definition—It is a subacute or chronic inflammation of the lid margin. The lid margin, being the meeting place of the skin and the conjunctiva, tends to share in the affections of ether.

Etiology

Predisposing factors—
   (a) Age—Usually common in children but any age group may be affected. It is usually bilateral.
   (b) External irritants—dust, wind, smoke and cosmetics.
   (c) Unhygienic condition.
   (d) Eyestrain due to error of refraction.
   (e) Constitutional factors—
      (i) Nature of the skin, *e.g.,* tendency to seborrhoea.
      (ii) Metabolic disturbances, *e.g.,* excessive carbohydrate diet.
      (iii) Toxic factors, *e.g.,* alimentary auto-intoxication, and septic focus.
      (iv) Allergic factor, *e.g.,* eczematous condition of the skin.
   (f) Inflammation of neighbouring structures—chronic conjunctivitis, chronic dacryocystitis.
   (g) Parasitic infection—Phthiriasis palpebrarum due to infection with the parasite phthirus pubis. The eyelashes are covered with black nits of the pediculis pubis and the lid margin is red and irritable.

Exciting cause–Infection with coagulase positive staphyloicoccus.

PLATE XIV

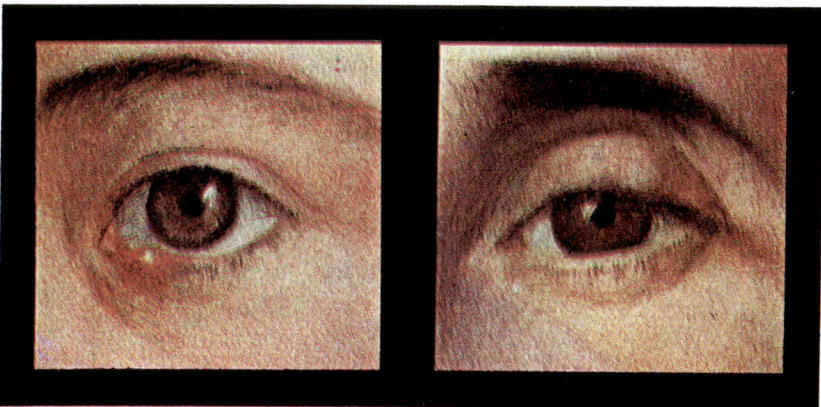

Fig. 1

Fig. 2

Stye (External Hordeolum)

Chalazion (Internal Hordeolum)

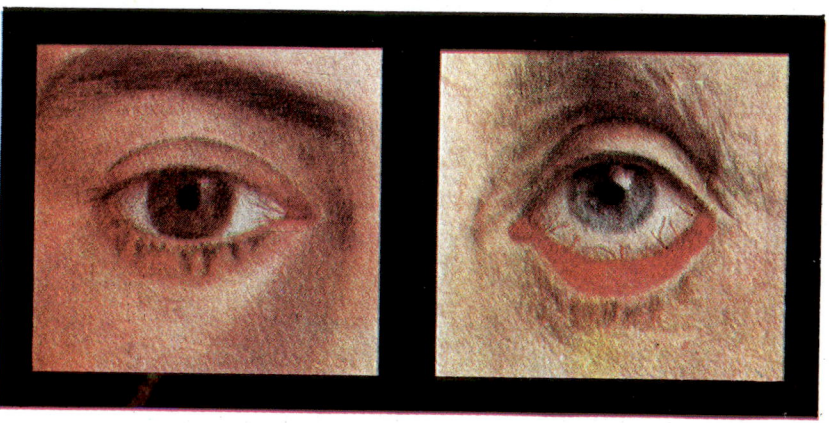

Fig. 3

Fig. 4

Blepharitis.

Ectropion.

(May and Worth)

(To face page 258)

In short, commonest causes are dirt and staphylococcus in children, seborrhoea in adolescents and allergic sensitization in adult life.

Clinically there are two types of blepharitis—1. Squamous type. 2. Ulcerative type.

Squamous Blepharitis

It is not essentially an infective condition. Metabolic causes, hygienic factors, eye strain and seborrhoea of the scalp usually lead to the development of this condition.

Symptoms

(a) There is no pain but there may be discomfort in the eyes.

(b) In untreated cases, epiphora develops due to anatomical changes in the lid margin—the sharp posterior border tends to be rounded.

Clinical signs

(a) Accumulation of white scales like dandruff on the lid margin.

(b) On removing the scales, the lid margin appears hyperaemic but there is no ulceration.

(c) Falling of eyelashes, but they are replaced quickly without distortion.

(d) The lid margin may be thickened.

Ulcerative Blepharitis

This condition is due to infection of the lid margin with coagualase positive staphylococcus, superimposed on predisposing conditions. There is suppurative inflammation of the ciliary follicles along with the glands of Zies and Moll.

Symptoms–(a) Soreness of the lid margin. (b) Lacrimation, itching and photophobia.

Clinical signs

(a) Yellow crusts are deposited at the roots of the eyelash by which the lashes are glued together.

(b) On removing the crusts, small ulcers appear around the base of the lashes which bleed freely.

(c) Falling of the eyelashes, which are either not replaced or when replaced become misdirected.

Sequelae of ulcerative blepharitis

If not treated energetically, the following sequelae may occur—

(a) Madarosis—scanty eyelashes due to destruction of the roots of the cilia.

(b) Trichiasis—misdirection of the eyelashes.

(c) Tyloisis—hypertrophy of the lid margin due to development of cicatricial tissue which causes drooping of the lid.

(d) Ectropion—eversion of the lid margin due to contraction of cicatricial tissue at the lid margin. This condition leads to constant epiphora.

Treatment of blepharitis—both types

A. General treatment—

1. Improvement of general health in children.

2. Judicious and balanced diet with vitamins, particularly vitamin A.

3. Removal of septic focus like bad tonsils.

4. Correction of any error of refraction.

5. Treatment of seborrhoea of scalp.

6. Treatment of associated condions like chronic conjunctivitis, chronic dacryocystitis or louse infection.

B. Local treatment—

1. Removal of scales and crusts from the lid margin with 3% sodibicarb lotion.

2. Application of broad spectrum antibiotic ointment to the lid margin like gentamycine or chloromycetin ointment 3 times a day.

3. After healing of the ulcers, hydrocortisone ointment 1% has to be applied to the lid margin 3 times a day to remove congestion and any allergic factor.

4. Treatment for trichiasis and ectropion (*see* under trichiasis and entropion.

External Hordeolum or Stye

Definition—It is a suppurative inflammation of the follicle of the eyelash including the glands of Zies.

Treatment

A. Predisposing factors—

1. Age—It can occur in any age but common in young adults.

2. Metabolic factors—diabetes, debility and excessive intake of carbohydrate.

B. Causative agent—coagulase positve staphylococcus.

Symptoms—Acute pain in the lid margin with a sense of heaviness and heat.

Clinical sings
  (a) Swelling, redness and marked oedema of the affected lid.
  (b) Marked tenderness at the point of fnflammation on the lid margin.
  (c) Chemosis of the bulbar conjuctiva may occur.
  (d) Finally a white pus point becomes visible on the lid margin in relation to the root of a cilia.
  (e) Enlargement of the corresponding pre-auricular lymph gland.
  Course—The pus point bursts outside and pain and swelling subsides.

Treatment
  (a) Hot compress 2-3 times a day.
  (b) Genticyn eye drop 4 times daily. Genticyn eye oint at bed time.
  (c) Ampicillin 250 mgm. 4 times a day by mouth for 5 days.
  (d) When the pus points, the pus should be drained either by pulling out the affected eyelash or by a tiny horizontal incision with a knife.

Chalazion or Tarsal Cyst or Meibomian Cyst

Definition–It is a chronic inflammatory granuloma of the Meibomian gland.

Pathology–A low grade infection, usually staphylococcal, enters through a duct of the Meibomian gland. As a result of the low grade infection, there is infiltration of the wall of the duct with leucocytes as well as proliferation of the epithelium of the duct. Thus the duct gets blocked and the Meibomian secretion accumulates and causes enlargement of the gland. The secretion, which is fatty in nature, acts like an irritant and causes inflammation and granuloma formation. More than one gland may be affected cuasing multiple chalazia.

Histology of a chalazion–A chalazion consists of sebaceous material in the centre, surrounded by giant cells, epitheliod cells and lymphocytes.

Age incidence–In the young and young adults.

Symptoms–Depending on the size of the chalazion, there is sense of heaviness in the lid and mild irritation.

Clinical signs

(a) Small, cystic or hard swelling of the size of a pea on the lid, a little distance away from the lid margin. In multiple chalazia, there is more than one swelling.

(b) The swelling is fixed to the tarsus, with the skin freely moving over it and it is not tender.

(c) No sign of any inflammation.

(d) On everting the lid, the tarsal conjunctiva over the swelling appears velvety red or purple.

(e) The regional glands are not palpable.

Course of a chalazion

(a) A very small chalazion may undergo resolution.

(b) It may remain as it is.

(c) The chalazion may burst either on the skin surface or on the conjunctival surface, with granulation tissue protruding.

(d) The granuloma may protrude through a duct of the Meibomian gland on the lid margin, when it is called a marginal chalazion.

(e) The chalazion may be secondarily infected forming an internal hordeolum.

(f) The chalazion may be calcified.

(g) In the old people, recurrent chalazion may lead to the development of Meibomian carcinoma.

Treatment

(a) A course of antibiotic ointment like chloromycetin oint may be applied to expect a resolution.

(b) Bigger chalazia should be incised vertically through the tarsal conjunctiva, after application of local anaesthesia and the granulation tissue should be scooped out.

Internal Hordeolum

Definition—It is the suppurative inflammation of a Meibomian gland due to staphylococcus. It is also often called a suppurating chalazion. Sometimes it may be also due to secondary infection of a chalazion.

Etiology—It is same as for external hordeolum.

Symptoms—They are same as for external hordeolum but are more intense.

Clinical signs—The point of maximum tenderness is away from the lid margin. Other clinical signs are similar to those for external hordeolum, but the pus points on the tarsal conjunctiva and not on the root of an eyelash.

Treatment

(a) Hot compress and board spectrum antibiotic by mouth as in case of a stye.

(b) Incision on the tarsal conjunctiva in a vertical direction to drain the pus.

Anomalies in the Position of Eyelashes and Lids Trichiasis

Definition—This is a condition, where the eyelashes are misdirected backwards, so as to rub against the cornea. A few or all the cilia may be misdirected (Fig. 105 B).

Causes of trichiasis

A. Congenital—known as districhiasis. (*See* under congenital abnormalities of the lids).

B. Acquired—

1. Trachoma stage IV.
2. Ulcerative blepharitis.
3. External hordeolum.
4. Membraneous conjunctivitis.
5. Any operation or injury on the lid margin.

Symptoms

(a) Foreign body sensation in the eye.

(b) Lacrimation.

(c) Pain.

Clinical signs

(a) Ciliary congestion.

(b) Reflex blepharospasm.

(c) Superficial opacities and vascularization of the cornea.

(d) Corneal ulcer.

Treatment

(a) Isolated misdirected cilia may be removed by epilation forceps. But the cilium grows again as the root is not destroyed by this method of epilation. The ideal method of epilation is electrolysis epilation, by which a weak galvanic current from cathode is passed to the root of the eyelash by a fine platinum needle and the root is destroyed due to the liberation of hydrogen gas. 3 mv of current for 30 seconds is usually needed.

(b) If many cilia are affected, plastic operation on the lid margin is necessary.

Entropion

It is a condition in which the lid margin rolls inwards (Fig. 105 D).

Causes of entropion

A. Congenital—It is rare and is usually associated with microphthalmos and anophthalmos (absence of the eyeball).

B. Acquired—

1. *Spastic entropion*—It develops typically in a case of blepharospasm due to any cause, particularly chronic irritative corneal condition. It also occurs after prolonged bandaging of the eye. The lower lid is usually affected. Both the children and the adults may be affected.

2. *Mechanical entropion*—It occurs due to lack of support of the lids, as due to phthisis bulbi, enophthalmos or lack of orbital fat. The lower lid is usually affected.

3. *Senile entropion*—It is the commonest type usually affecting the lower lid. There is lack of support of the eyelid due to disappearance of orbital fat and also due, to atrophic and inelastic condition of the skin in senility. These factors, along with a reasonable tone of the orbicularis muscle, are responsible for the entropion. Bandaging of the eye in old age invariably causes entropion of the lower lid.

4. *Cicatricial entropion*—The entropion occurs due to contraction of the conjunctival scar as in trachoma stage IV, membraneous conjunctivitis and burns. The upper lid is usually affected.

Symptoms of entropion—They are similar to those for trichiasis.

Treatment of entropion—The spastic entropion is cured when the cause of blepharospasm is treated. The senile entropion can be treated by keeping the lower lid pulled downwards by a strip of adhesive plaster. If bandaging is the cause, it should be discontinued. Senile entropion which is not cured by application of adhesive plaster, should be treated by plastic operation. Simplest operation is "Skin muscle" operation. Here an eliptical area of loose skin & the underlying orbicularis oculi muscle are resected.

Ectropion

It is a condition in which the lid margin rolls outwards *i.e.,* becomes everted (Fig. 105 E). It may occur in various degrees.

Causes of ectropion

1. *Spastic ectropion*—It occurs due to powerful contraction of the orbicularis muscle, when the skin is elastic and the eyeball is prominent or slightly proptosed. It is commonly seen in children, during an attempt to separate the lids for the examination of the eyeball.

Both the lids may be affected.

2. *Senile ectropion*—The lower lid is affected in old age due to laxity of the tissues of the lid and due to loss of tone of the orbicularis muscle.

3. *Paralytic ectropion*—It occurs as a result of weakness of the orbicularis muscle due to paralysis of the facial nerve.

The lower lid is only affected.

4. *Mechanical ectropion*—It is caused by the weight of a mass in the eyelid, *e.g.*, a tumour or by pressure on the eyelid from behind, as in proptosis. The lower lid is usually affected.

5. *Cicatricial ectropion*—It follows burns, ulcers, trauma or skin diseases of the eyelid. Both the eyelids may be affected.

Symptom of ectropion—The commonest symptom is epiphora.

Clinical signs

(a) Chronic conjunctivitis due to exposure.

(b) In long continued cases, the conjunctiva becomes dry and thickened.

(c) Corneal ulcer may develop due to exposure.

Treatment—In case of spastic ectropion the cause of blepharospasm has to be treated. For other types of ectropion, plastic operation is needed.

Symblepharon

It is a condition in which the lid becomes adhered to the eyeball,due to adhesion between the palpebral and bulbar conjunctiva (Fig 106). This adhesion usually occurs in case of the lower lid.

There are two types of symblepharon—

(a) Anterior symblepharon—In this conditon the addition is situated more anteriorly as in the picture (Fig. 106). Due to constant movement of the eyeball the area of fusion may be stretched to an elongated strap.

(b) Posterior symblepharon—In this condition the conjunctival surfaces are entirely adhered togehter.

Cause–Any rawness of the conjunctival surfaces of the palpebral and bulbar conjunctiva causes adhesion. This may occur in burns due to heat, chemical burns, and ulcerative condition as in membranous conjunctivitis.

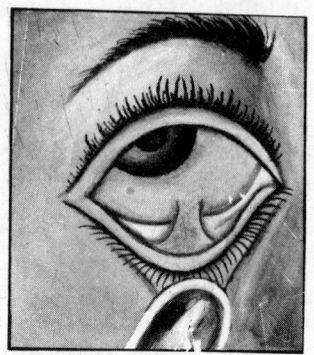

Symptoms–Pronounced adhesion may cause diplopia due to limitation of movements of the eyeball. The lids may not be closed properly and in that case consequences due to exposure may occur.

Fig. 106. Symblepharon.

Treatment–Prevention is most important. A soft contact lens should be used which covers the eyeball and prevents the adhesion. When the condition is already established, operative procedure is necessary.

Ankyloblepharon

It is a condition wherein the lid margins adhere together. The adhesion may be complete or partial and is usually associated with symblepharon.

Cause—Either congenital or acquired due to burn.

Treatment—Separation of lid margins by operation.

Lagophthalmos

It is a condition in which the eyelids cannot be closed properly when the eyes are shut.

Cause

(a) Congenital deformity of lid.
(b) Acquired causes—paralysis of the orbicularis, weakness of the muscle as in deep coma, cicatricial contraction of the lids or proptosis.

Exposure keratitis may develop in this condition. Usually the lower part of the cornea is affected.

Treatment

(a) Application of a bland ointment or liquid paraffin during sleep to keep the cornea moist.

(b) Operative procedure in the form of tarsorraphy, by which the palpebral aperture is narrowed by uniting the margins of the lids on the lateral side. Even a central tarsorrpapy may be done.

Blepharospasm

It is a condition in which the lids are firmly closed, due to forcible contraction of the orbicularis muscle. The spasm of the muscle is involuntary and may last for a few moments to a few weeks or months.

Effects of blepharospasm

(a) Persistent epiphora due to spasmodic closure of the canaliculi.
(b) Eczematous condition of the skin of the lower lid due to constant watering.
(c) Oedema of the lids due to constant pressure on the palpebral veins.
(d) Spastic entropion or ectropion of the lower lid.

Causes of blepharospasm

1. Reflex sensory stimulation through the branches of the trigeminal nerve—commonest—
   (a) Phlyctenular keratitis.
   (b) Interstitial keratitis.
   (c) Foreign body, ulcer or erosion of cornea.
   (d) Membranous and psedo-membranous conjunctivitis.
   (e) Severe iritis and iridocyclitis.
2. Excessive stimulation of retina–Exposure to dazzling light.
3. Stimulation of the facial nerve.
4. Hysteria.

Treatment—treatment of the cause.

Blepharophimosis

It is a condition in which the palpebral fissure is diminished in extent, without adhesion of the lid margins. The condition is usually congenital.

Ptosis or Blepharoptosis

It is a condition in which there is drooping of the upper lid below its normal position. The condition may be unilateral or bilateral and partial or complete.

Causes of ptosis

A. Congenital ptosis—
1. Simple ptosis due to maldevelopment of the levator muscle.
2. Ptosis associated with congenital weakness of the superior rectus.
3. Ptosis associated with deformities of the lid like epicanthus.
B. Acquired ptosis—
1. Paralytic ptosis—this is the commonest.
   (a) Due to partial or complete 3rd nerve palsy affecting the levator.
   (b) Due to lesion of the cervical sympathetic and paralysis of the Muller's muscle—the Horner's syndrome.
2. Lack of support of the upper lid—as in case of microphthalmos, shrunken eyeball and enophthalmos.
3. Mechanical ptosis—due to increased weight fo the upper lid as a result of oedema, inflammation, hypertrophy or tumour formation. This type of ptosis is also known as pseudo-ptosis.
4. Myogenic ptosis—
   (a) Trauma to the levator muscle.
   (b) Muscular dystrophy of the levator muscle as in ocular myopathy.
   (c) Myasthenia gravis.
Symptoms of ptosis—There is no symptom, if the pupil is not covered by the lid. Otherwise there is visual disturbance.

Clinical signs
   (a) The margin of the upper lid covers more of the cornea than normal.
   (b) Palpebral fissure is narrower than normal.
   (c) There is no fold, in the skin of the upper lid.
   (d) On an attempt to elevate the upper lid, there is elevation of the eyebrow and wrinkling of the skin of the forehead due to hyperaction of the frontalis muscle.
   (e) Head is tilted backwards so as to draw the lid upwards beyond the pupillary area.
   (f) If the patient is asked to look upwards while firm pressure is applied on the eyebrow, there is very little or no action of the levator—provided the ptosis is due to weakness of the levator.

Treatment
   (a) For the acquired ptosis the cause must be treated.
   (b) For the congenital ptosis, operative procedures are necessary for correction of the deformity. The underlying principles for operation are—

(i) If there is some action of the levator, this muscle is shortened.

(ii) If there is no action of the levator but the superior rectus is normal, a part of this latter muscle is attached to the arterior surface of the upper tarsal plate, so that the upper lid becomes elevated along with the action of the superior rectus.

(iii) If both the levator and the superior rectus are inactive, the frontalis muscle is utilized by suturing it to the tarsal plate by strips,of fascia lata and so contraction of the frontalis elevates the lid.

Tumours of the Eyelids

They may be benign or malignant.

Benign tumours of the lid are—
  (i) Papilloma.
  (ii) Angioma.
  (iii) Naevus.
  (iv) Xanthelasma or Xanthoma.
  (v) Neurofibroma.

Malignant tumours of the lid are—
  (i) Rodent ulcer.
  (ii) Epidermoid carcinoma.
  (iii) Malignant melanoma.

Benign Tumours

1. Papilloma

It is the commonest tumour of the eyelid. It appears as a warty growth which may be sessile or pedunculated. There are papillae on the surface. Histologically, a papilla consists of a fibrous tissue core with blood vessels covered by proliferated epithelium. The basement membrane of the epithelium remains intact.

2. Angioma

It may occur as a localized capillary or cavernous angioma or the lid may be affected along with the facial angioma as in Sturge-Weber's syndrome.

3. Naevus

This is a benign pigmented tumour, composed of pigment producing cells, usually affecting the lid margin. It originates either from sensory nerve end-organ or from the basal layer of epidermis.

4. Xanthelasma or Xanthoma

It is a slightly raised yellow plaque, commonly situated in the skin of the upper and lower lid near the inner canthus and may be bilateral. These tumours are more frequent in females and sometimes are associated with diabetes and excessive blood cholesterol.

5. Neurofibroma

Usually the plexiform type of neurofibroma affects the lid, mostly the upper one. The lid becomes hypertrophied and droops down and hypertrophied nerves can be felt through the skin. Along with the upper lid, the temporal side of the face also may be affected.

Malignant Tumours

1. Rodent Ulcer or Basal-Celled Carcinoma

It is the commonest malignant tumour of the lid. It originates either from the basal layer of the epidermis or from the epithelium of the hair follicles and glands of the skin. The commonest site of the tumour is the lower lid, near the inner canthus (Fig. 107).

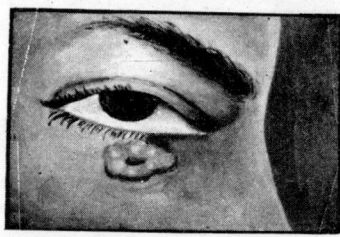

FIG. 107.—Rodent ulcer of lid

(Parsons)

It starts as a small pimple which ulcerates and the edges of the ulcer become raised and indurated. The ulcer grows very slowly destroying the lid, orbital structures and even bone. It is locally malignant and the regional glands are not involved. Histologically, the tumour consists of of the epidermis. There are no down-growths of the basal layer prickle cells or cell nests.

2. Epidermoid Carcinoma or Squamous-Celled Carcinoma

It originates from the epidermis, at places where the character of the epithelium changes, as for example the lid margin. It starts as a nodule which ulcerates very soon. It is much more destructive than the rodent ulcer and the regional lymph glands become affected. Histologically, the tumour consists of cells of all the layers of the epidermis, invading the subepithelial tissue, and cell nests are common.

Both the rodent ulcer and the epidermoid carcinoma occur in elderly persons.

3. Malignant Melanoma

It is a rare malignant pigmented tumour, usually originating from a naevus. Its course is like the malignant melanoma elsewhere in the body.

Treatment of tumours of the lid

1. Benign tumours are removed by surgical operation.

2. Malignant tumours may be removed in the early stages by surgical method. In advanced stages, a rodent ulcer and epidermoid carcinoma should be treated with radium or deep X-ray. But the malignant melanoma is not susceptible to any radiational therapy.

CHAPTER—XVIII

ANATOMY AND DISEASES OF THE LACRIMAL GLAND AND LACRIMAL PASSAGE

Anatomy of the lacrimal gland—It is a serous gland, situated at the upper and outer angle of the orbit, just within the orbital margin, in a depression of the orbital plate of the frontal bone known as the fossa for the lacrimal gland. Anteriorly the gland is deeply divided into two parts by the lateral expansion of the aponeurosis of the levator muscle—the upper orbital part and the lower palpebral part.

The ducts of the lacrimal gland which are about 12 in number, pass through the plpebral lobe of the gland and open into the conjunctival sac, 4.5 mm. above the upper border of the tarsal plate of the upper lid.

The minute structure of the lacrimal gland is similar to that of a serous acinous gland, resembling a salivary gland.

Accessory lacrimal glands—These are very small glands of exactly the same structure as the lacrimal gland. There are two types—

1. Glands of Krause—They number about 20 in the upper lid and 8 in the lower lid, and are deeply situated within the substantia propria of the conjunctiva, near the fornix particularly on the lateral side.

2. Glands of Wolfring—They are few in number situated in the conjunctiva, near the upper border of the tarsal plate.

Blood supply of the lacrimal gland

1. Arterial supply—By the lacrimal branch of the ophthalmic artery and the infra-orbital branch of the maxillary artery.

2. Venous drainage—By the lacrimal vein which opens into the superior ophthalmic vein.

Lymphatic drainage—The lymph vessels join the conjunctival and palpebral lymphatics and pass to the pre-auricular lymph nodes.

Nerve sypply of the lacrimal gland

1. Sensory supply—By the lacrimal branch of the ophthalmic division of the 5th nerve.

2. Sympathetic supply—From the carotid plexus of cervical sympathetic.

3. Secreto-motor fibres—These are derived from the facial nerve in the following manner—

The superior lacrimal nucleus in the brain-steam—nervus intermedius of the facial nerve-greater superficial petrosal **nerve-nerve** of pterygoid canal—sphenopalatine ganglion—Zygomatic branch of the maxillary nerve-anastomosis with the lacrimal nerve—lacrimal gland. (Duke-Elder).

Anatomy of the lacrimal passage

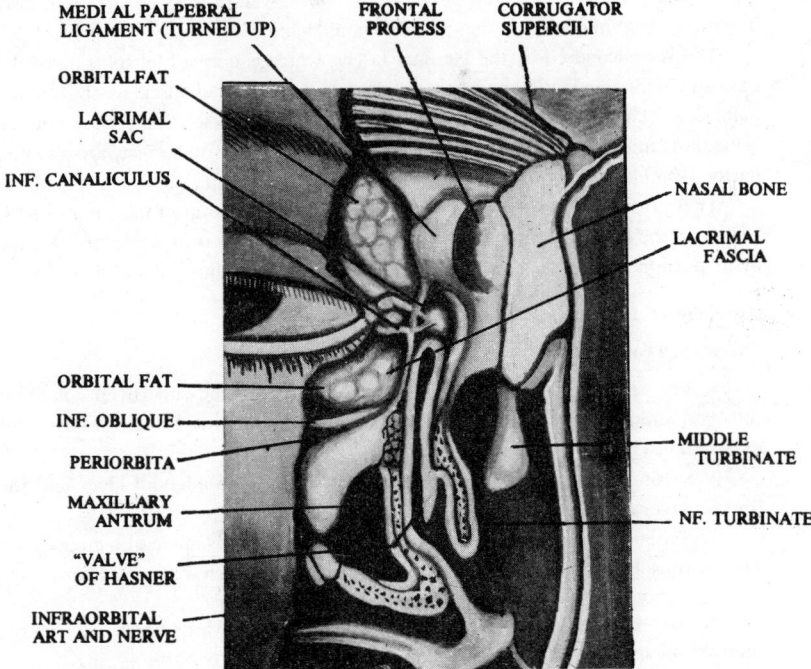

Fig. 108. Lacrimal passage.

The lacrimal passage consists of (Fig. 108)—
1. Lacrimal puncta (2 in number).
2. Canaliculi (2 in number).
3. Lacrimal sac.
4. Naso-lacrimal duct.

1. Lacrimal puncta—These are two small openings, each of which is siutated on a small elevation known as lacrimal papilla, about 6 mm. from the inner canthus on each lid margin. The puncta are visible only when the lids are slightly everted.

2. Canaliculi—These are two in number and they start from the puncta as narrow tubular passages to end in the lacrimal sac. Each canaliculus consists of a short vertical portion about 1 to 2 mm. long and a long horizontal portion, the

length of which is 6-7 mm. They are lined by stratified squamous epithelium.
The two canaliculi may open into the lacrimal sac separately or they may join
to form a common canaliculus (sinus of Mair) before opening into the sac.

3. **Lacrimal sac**—It is about 13 mm. long vertically and 5 to 6 mm wide,
situated in the lacrimal fossa formed by the lacrimal bone and the frontal process of
the maxilla. The two canaliculi open on the lateral wall of the sac and inferiorly
the sac is continuous with the naso-lacrimal duct.

The sac is covered by the lacrimal fascia, which is derived by splitting of the
periosteum of the lacrimal fossa. Anterior to the lacrimal fascia is the medial
palpebral ligament and the fibres of the orbicularis muscle. Some fibres of the
orbicularis muscle, which originate from the posterior lacrimal crest, are situated
partly behind the sac and are known as Horner's muscle.

That portion of the sac, which is above the opening point of the canaliculi, is
known as the fundus. It lies slightly above the medial palperbral ligament. But the
main portion of the sac lies behind and below the medial palpebral ligament.

Histology of the lacrimal sac

The sac wall consists of–

1. The epithelium—It consists of 2 layers of cells—the superficial columnar
cells containing goblet cells and the deeper flattened cells resting on a basement
membrane.

2. Substantia propria —It consists of two layers—the adenoid layer and the
fibrous layer.

The adenoid layer lies underneath the epithelium and is made of lymphocytes
The fibrous layer contains many elastic fibres and a rich venous plexus.

4. **Naso-lacrimal duct**—It is the continuation downwards of the sac to the
inferior meatus of the nose. It may be divided into two parts—

(a) An intra-osseous part, situated within the bony naso-lacrimal canal
which is about 12 mm. long.

(b) An intra-meatal part extending beyond the termination of the bony canal
and situated within the mucous membrane of the lateral wall of the
nose. This is about 5 mm. long.

The histology of the wall of the duct is the same as that of the sac, although the
substanitia propria is much thinner.

1. Arterial supply is derived from—

(a) Palpebral branches of the ophthalmic artery.

(b) Angular branch of the facial artery.

(c) Infra-orbital and and spheno-palatine branches of the internal maxillary
artery.

2. **Venous drainage—**

(a) Above into the **angular** and infra-orbital veins.

(b) Below into the pterygoid plexus and internal maxiallry vein.

Lymphatic drainage—The lymphatic vessels drain into the submaxillary lumph glands.

Nerve supply of the lacrimal passage

1. Sensory nerves—The canaliculi, the sac and the upper part of the naso-lacrimal duct are supplied by the infratrochlear branch of the nasociliary nerve. The lower part of the duct is supplied by the anterior superior alveolar **nerve,** derived from the maxillary division of the 5th nerve.

2. Sympathetic **supply—from** the sympathetic nerves in the orbit.

Tears

It is the **secretion** from the lacrimal gland. It is slightly alkaline and consists mainly of water and minute quantities of salts, particularly sodium chloride, sugar, urea and protein. It also contains an enzyme known as lysozyme, which has definite anti-bacterial property. The **secretion** of tears does not begin before 3-4 weeks after birth.

Drainage of tears—There are many theories regarding the **mechanism** of drainage of tears. But it is accepted, that both capillary action and muscular contraction during blinking, help to propagate the tears along the canaliculi, sac and duct, to the nose from where it is evaporated.

Watering of the Eye

Two terms are used in connection with watering of the eye—epiphora and lacrimation.

Epiphora denotes watering due to obstruction to outflow of tears.

Lacrimation denotes watering due to excessive secretion of tears.

Causes of watering of the eye

A. Obstruction to outflow of tears–

1. Stenosis of the punctum, particulary the lower one—congenital or acquired.

2. Eversion of the lower punctum due to **laxity** of the orbicularis muscle as in senility, facial paralysis and ectropion.

3. Obstruction in the lower canaliculus due to calculus or infection by the fungus streptothrix.

4. Obstruction in the sac, as due to tumour of the sac or following removal of the sac.

5. Obstruction in the naso-lacrimal duct, e.g., chronic dacryocystitis, nasal polyp, and maxillary antrum tumour pressing on the duct.

B. Excessive secretion of tears—

1. Reflex causes—

(a) Due to sensory stimulation of the structures of the eyeball, e.g., corneal foreign body, corneal ulcer, keratitis, or exposure to cold wind, dust, smoke or irritant gases.

(b) Due to stimulation of the optic nerve, e.g., exposure to very bright light.

(c) Due to stiumulation of the sensory nerves of the eye muscles, e.g., eye strain.

(d) Due to stimulation of the nasal mucous membrane as in nasal catarrh.

2. Action of parasympathomimetic drugs like pilocarpine and physostigmine.

3. Diseases of the lacrimal gland as in early stage of Mikulicz's syndrome characterized by symmetrical enlargement of the lacrimal and salivary glands.

4. Central causes, e.g., emotionl and psychical effects.

Dryness of the Eye

The eye does not become dry even if the entire lacrimal gland is removed, because the secretions from the accessory lacrimal glands and the mucous glands of the conjunctiva are sufficient to keep the eye moist.

Causes of dryness of the eye—

1. In advanced stage of vitamin A deficiency.

2. Trachoma stage IV, when there is marked scarring.

3. Kerato-conjunctivitis sicca known as Sjogren's syndrome, which is accompanied by lack of secretion of the salivary glands and polyarthritis.

4. Following Stevens-Johnson's Syndrome.

Diseases of the Lacrimal Gland
Acute Dacryo-Adenitis

Definition

It is the acute inflammation of the lacrimal gland. It is rare. It occurs in association with mumps and gonorrhoea.

PLATE XV

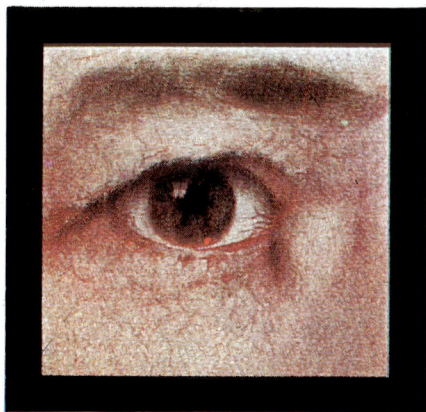

Fig. 1

Chronic Dacryocystitis
with Mucocele of the
lacrimal Sac.

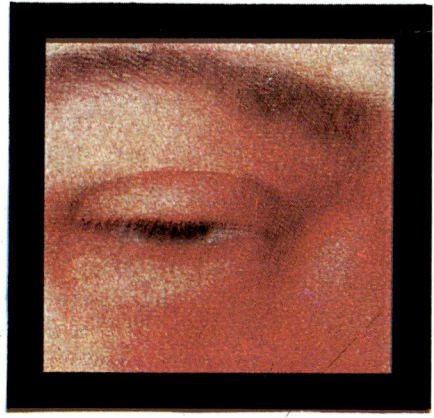

Fig. 2

Acute Dacryoystitis.

(May and Worth)

(To face page 276)

Symptoms

Pain in the upper and outer angle of the orbit and watering.

Clinical signs—

(a) Painful swelling at the upper and outer angle of the orbit.
(b) The gland becomes enlarged and tender.
(c) Congestion and chemosis of the conjunctiva.

Treatment

(a) Hot compress.
(b) Antibiotic drugs by mouth.
(c) Incision, if the gland suppurates.

Dacryops

Definition—It is a cystic swelling of the gland due to retention of lacrimal secretion, as a result of blockage of one of the lacrimal ducts.

Tumours of the Lacrimal Gland

The commonest tumour is pleomorphic adenocarcinoma. It is slowly growing but locally infiltrative tumour. It occurs in middle aged persons.

Symptoms

There may be mild pain and transient diplopia.

Clinical sings

(a) A hard tumour mass at the upper and outer angle of the orbit.
(b) The eyeball is proptosed and displaced downwards and medially and movement of the eyeball is restricted upwards and laterally.

Treatment—Surgical removal.

Disease of the Lacrimal Sac
Dacryocystitis

Definition—It is the inflammation of the lacrimal sac.

Classification of dacryocystitis

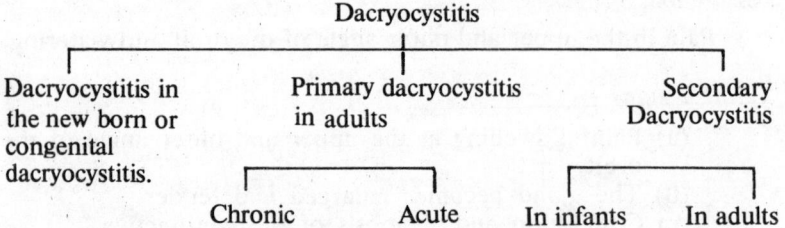

Dacryocystitis

Dacryocystitis in the new born or congenital dacryocystitis.	Primary dacryocystitis in adults	Secondary Dacryocystitis
	Chronic Acute	In infants In adults

Congenital dacryocystitis or dacryocystitis in the new born

Cause—This condition arises due to failure in canalization of the naso-lacrimal duct, the lumen being blocked by epithelial debris. The condition may be bilateral.

Clinical signs

(a) It starts with epiphora and purulent discharge at the inner canthus.

(b) By pressure on the sac there is regurgitation of mucopurulent matter.

(c) The purulent matter is at first sterile but very soon becomes infected.

(d) Acute attacks are extremely rare.

Treatment

Sharp pressure over the Sac area may force the contents down thus the patency of the nasolacrimal duct is achieved, probing of the naso-lacrimal duct cures the condition. It is unwise to wait beyond the age of 2–6 months. Delay in treatment causes complete cicatricial obliteration of the duct.

Chronic Dacryocystitis (Primary)

Etiology

1. Age—Usually adults over middle age.
2. Sex—75% in females.
3. Bilaterality—May be unilateral or bilateral.
4. Social incidence—Common in the lower middle class group.
5. Predisposing factor—Stricture of the naso-lacirmal duct due to narrowness of the bony canal chronic inflammation of the nasal mucosa, hypertrophied inferior turbinate, extreme deviation of the nasal septum or by the pressure of a nasal polyp.
6. Exciting factor—Infection of the stagnated sac contents by bacteria, most commonly by pneumococcus but also by streptococcus and staphylococcus aureus.

Pathology—There is stagnation of the sac contents due to stricture of the naso-lacrimal duct. The contents become infected, usually by the penumococcus and the sac wall becomes chronically inflammed. The epithelium of the sac wall multiplies to form several layers, and the adenoid layer becomes infiltrated with plasma cells and large mononuclear cells in addition to the lymphocytes. The vascularity of the wall increases and the sac wall becomes atonic. The contents of the sac which are at first watery, later on become mucoid due to excessive secretion of mucous by the goblet cells and afterwards mucopurulent due to exudation of pus cells.

Sympotms—The commonest symptom is epiphora.

Clinical signs—They may be described in three stages—

1. In catarrhal stage (early stage) :
   (a) Persistent watering of the eye.
   (b) Mild conjunctival hyperaemia at the inner canthus of the affected side.
   (c) Very little or no regurgitation of any fluid matter through the punctum on pressure on the sac.
   (d) **On** syringing the sac, fluid regurgitates through the upper punctum, mixed with flakes of mucous.
   (e) No local swelling over the sac area or tenderness.

2. In mucocele stage (next stage) :

   (a) In addition to watering, there is swelling over the sac area below the medial palpebral ligament which is not tender.
   (b) On pressure over the sac, mucoid material regurgitates through the punctum.
   (c) Sometimes both the canaliculi may be blocked, when there is no regurgitation on pressure and the condition is known as encysted mucocele.
   (d) Conjunctival hyperaemia at the inner canthus remains the same as in catarrhal stage.

3. In the pyocele stage or suppurative stage (final stage) :

   (a) Conjunctival hyperaemia at the inner canthus becomes more pronounced.
   (b) Similar swelling over the sac area below the medial palpebral ligament, which is not tender. Also there is no redness of the skin over the swelling.
   (c) On pressure over the sac, there is **regurgitation** of

mucopurulent matter through the punctum.

(d) Watering of the eye remains as before.

N.B.—Sometimes if the stricture of the naso-lacrimal duct is not complete, in the mucocele or pyocele stage the sac contents on pressure may evacuate into the nose.

Complications of chronic dacryocystitis

(a) Acute dacryocystits.

(b) Development of a corneal ulcer, which is known as hypopyon ulcer or ulcus serpens of cornea, as the causative agent is pneumococcus derived from the sac.

(c) Chronic conjunctivitis.

Acute Dacryocystitis

Definition—It is the acute suppurative inflammation of the lacrimal sac.

Etiology

It occurs usually as an acute exacerbation of chronic dacryocystits. Rarely it may start spontaneously without any history of epiphora.

Causative agent—Usually superimposed infection of streptococcus haemolyticus. But pneumococcus and staphylococcus aureus may also take part.

Pathology—The sac becomes filled with frank pus with abundant polymorphonuclear leucocytes. The anterior sac wall give way and inflammation spreads to the tissues surrounding the sac, causing pericystitis. Finally an abscess is formed known as lacrimal abscess, which usually bursts on the skin surface below the medial palpebral ligament, forming a lacrimal fistula. As soon as the pus drains out, the inflammation subsides and the sac ultimately becomes shrunken and fibrous.

Symptoms

(a) Severe pain and sensation of heat over the sac area. radiating over the frontal region.

(b) Fever

(c) Watering

Clinical signs

(a) Marked swelling and redness of the skin over the sac area.

(b) Oedema of the skin of the lids and of the side of the nose.

(c) Skin over the sac is markedly tender and hot.

(d) No regurgitation through the puncta at this stage, as the canaliculi become blocked due to oedema of the surrounding tissues.

(e) Slight congestion or chemosis of the conjunctiva.

(f) Enlargement of the sub-maxillary lymph glands.

(g) When lacrimal abscess is formed, fluctuation can be elicited.

(h) When the abscess bursts on the skin surface, a fistula is formed and the signs and symptoms of acute inflammation subside.

If the condition is not treated properly and left as it is, the fistula may close later on and there may be further attacks of acute dacryocystitis.

Complications of acute dacryocystitis

(a) Osteomyelitis of the lacrimal bone which may be eroded and an internal lacrimal fistula may be formed opening into the nose.

(b) Orbital cellulitis, due to spread of the inflammation into the orbit.

(c) Facial cellulitis due to the spread of inflammation into the face.

(d) Cavernous sinus thrombosis due to spread of infection along the angular vein.

Secondary Dacryocystitis

1. *In infants*—It is rare and usually originates from tuberculous or syphilitic affections of the surrounding bones.

2. *In adults*—The secondary dacryocystitis may be due to—

(a) trachoma,

(b) tuberculous and syphilitic affections of the surrounding bones, and

(c) leprosy.

These are of course rare conditions.

Treatment

A. *Chronic dacryocystitis*

1. Probing of the naso-lacrimal duct and syringing of the sac–This may be tried in the early stage to open up the duct and to control infection by syringing with penicillin 50,000 units in one c.c. of distilled water. But this method invariably fails as the patency of the duct cannot be restored.

2. Removal of the sac by dacryocystectomy operation—As the sac is a local source of infection, it must be removed to avoid development of corneal ulcer. The operation is easy but the end result is troublesome, as there is life-long epiphora.

3. Nasal drainage or dacryocystorhinostomy operation—By this operation, the medial wall of the sac is anastomosed with the mucous membrane of the middle meatus of the nose. If successful, the condition is cured and there is neither epiphora nor regurgitation.

B. *Acute dacryocystitis*

1. Before abscess formation and localization of inflammation—

(a) Hot compress over the sac area.

(b) Injection of crystalline penicillin 500,000 units daily for five days.

(c) Broad spectrum antibiotic like Amoxycilline 250 mgm. 4 times a day for 5 days, by mouth.

(d) Analgesics like aspirin.

2. When the inflammation has localized and fluctuation can be elicited—

(a) A vertical incision over the sac to drain the pus.

(b) Removal of the sac, when inflammation completely subsides. Dacryocystorhinostomy is not easy after an acute attack, as the sac shrinks and becomes fibrous.

3. When a lacrimal fistula has formed—Excision of the fistulous passage and removal of the sac. However excision of the fistulous passage and a dacryocystorhinostomy may also be tried.

Tumours of the Lacrimal Sac

They are extemely rare. The common tumours are papilloma, carcinoma or sarcoma.

CHAPTER XIX

ANATOMY AND DISEASES OF THE ORBIT

Anatomy of the orbit—The two orbits are two bony cavities, one on either side of the midline of the skull. They are roughly pyramidal in shape—the base, which is represented by the orbital margin, is directed forwards, laterally and slightly downwards and the apex is represented by the optic foramen.

The walls of the orbit—(Fig. 109)—

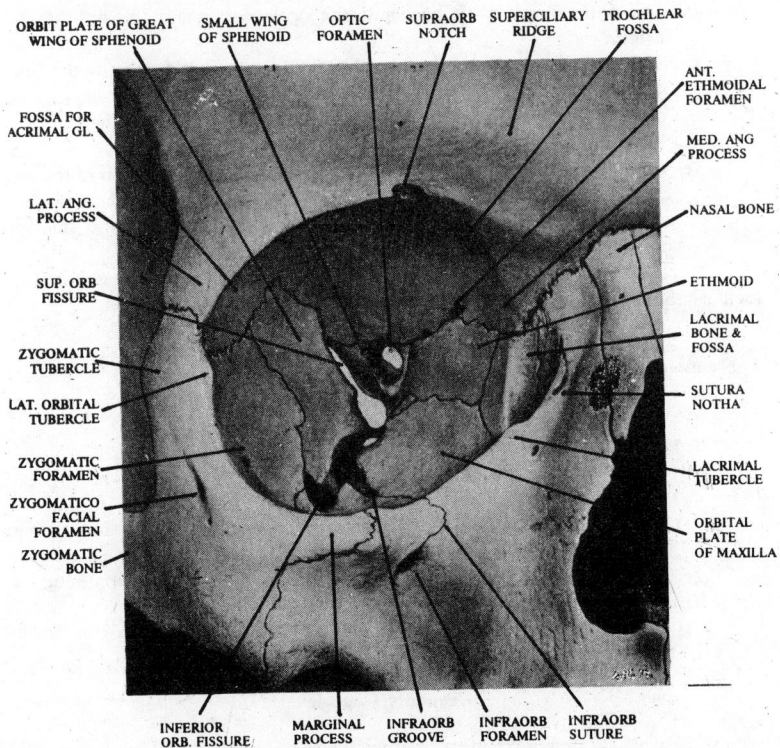

Fig. 109. The right orbit (Wolff).

The roof—It is formed largely by the orbital plate of the frontal bone in front and by the lesser wing of the sphenoid behind.

The medial wall—The bones forming this wall from before backwards are—

(a) Frontal process of the maxilla,

(b) Lacrimal bone,

(c) Lamina papyracea of the ethmoid,

(d) A small part of the body of the sphenoid.

The floor—It is formed by the following bones—

(a) Orbital plate of the maxilla,

(b) Orbital surface of the zygomatic,

(c) Orbital process of palatine bone.

The lateral wall—It is formed by two bones—

(a) Posteriorly by the orbital surface of the greater wing of the sphenoid.

(b) Anteriorly by the orbital surface of the zygomatic bone.

The posterior portion of the orbit presents three openings—

(a) **The optic foramen**—It transmits the optic nerve and the ophthalmic artery.

(b) **Superior orbital fissure or the sphenoidal fissure**—It transmits the 3rd, 4th and 6th cranial neres, first division of the 5th cranial nerve, the ophthalmic vein, the recurrent lacrimal artery and sympathetic fibres from the cavernous sinus to the ciliary ganglion.

(c) **The inferior orbital fissure**—It transmits the maxillary division of the 5th cranial nerve, the infra-orbital artery, the zygomatic nerve, the branches of the spheno-palatine ganglion, and the branches from the inferior opthalmic vein to the pterygoid venous plexus.

The orbits are surrounded by nasal fossae and by the accessory nasal sinuses such as the frontal, sphenoidal, ethmoidal and maxillary air sinuses.

The contents of the orbit are as follows—

(a) The eyeball and the intra-orbital part of the optic nerve.

(b) The Tenon's capsule.

(c) The extra-ocular muscles.

(d) The lacrimal gland and the lacrimal sac.

(e) The ophthalmic artery with its branches.

(f) The third, fourth and sixth cranial nerves and the first and second divisions of the 5th nerve.

(g) Branches from the carotid and cavernous plexus of sympathetic.

(h) The ciliary ganglion.

(i) The orbital fat and fascia.

Tenon's Capsule

It is a layer of fascia which covers the eyeball from the limbus to the attachment of the optic nerve. It is attached loosely to the sclera and anteriorly it merges into the subconjunctival tissue and posteriorly with the sheath of the optic nerve. The extra-ocular muscle pierce this fascia before their insertion to the sclera. This capsule forms a socket in which the eyeball moves.

Surgical Spaces in the Orbit

There are four spaces in the orbit, which are important from surgical point of view, as an inflammatory process may remain localized in any one of them. The spaces are—

1. **The subperiosteal space**—Underneath the periosteum of the orbital walls.

2. **The peripheral orbital space**—It lies between the orbital periosteum and the extra-ocular muscles, which are joined by fascial connections.

3. **The central space**—It lies inside the muscle cone formed by the four rectus muscles.

4. **Tenon's space**—Around the eyeball underneath the tenon's capsule.

Orbital Cellulitis

It is the purulent inflammation of the cellular tissues of the orbit.

This condition should not be taken lightly, as it carries danger with it not only to vision but also sometimes to life.

Etiology

1. Age and sex—Any age or sex may be affected.

2. Commonest cause is extension of infection from the nasal sinuses and the teeth.

3. Penetrating injury with or without retention of a foreign body in the orbit.

4. Postoperative infection as following enucleation operation.

·5. Other causes are—Extension of inflammation from intraorbital structures, *e.g.,* in panophthalmitis or in suppurative dacryoadenitis

6. Facial erysipelas is a rare cause.

7. Systemic conditions like pyaemia, meningitis or infective fevers also may cause orbital cellulitis.

Symptoms

1. Severe pain in the orbit, particularly on any attempt to move the eyeball.

2. Lacrimation.

3. Photophobia.

4. Diplopia due to limitation of movement of the eyeball.

5. Visual acuity may not be impaired at the beginning, but there may be dimness of vision later on, due to retrobulbar neuritis.

6. Feverish feeling or actual rise of body temperature.

Clinical signs
1. Marked swelling of the lids.
2. Congestion and chemosis of the conjunctiva.
3. Eyeball slightly proptosed and tender to touch.
4. Marked limitation of the movements of the eyeball.
5. Ophthalmoscopic examination shows congestion of retinal veins, and signs of papillitis due to optic neuritis or papilloedema due to compression of the central retinal vein. Later on, there are signs of optic atrophy.

Course

(a) The inflammation may subside after proper treatment.
(b) An abscess may be formed which may point somewhere on the skin near the orbital margin or may burst into the conjuctival sac.

Complications
1. Panophthalmitis.
2. Optic atrophy.
3. Purulent meningitis.
4. Cerebral abscess.
5. Cavernous sinus thrombosis.

TABLE XII

Differential diagnosis of orbital cellulitis

Orbital cellulitis.	Panophthalmitis.	Cavernous sinus thrombosis.
1. Unilateral.	1. Unilateral.	1. At first unilateral but soon becomes bilateral.
2. Vision not affected in the early stage.	2. Complete loss of vision from the onset.	2. No affection of vision in early stage.
3. Cornea, anterior chamber, lens and vitreous are clear.	3. All the media are hazy due to pus formation.	3. Media are clear.
4. Marked limitation of movements of eyeball.	4. Limitation of movements to some extent.	4. Complete limitation of movements due to complete paralysis of extra-ocular-muscles.

5. No oedema over the mastoid process.	5. No oedema over the mastoid process.	5. Oedema over the mastoid process due to thrombosis of the emissary vein.
6. General symptoms are mild, e.g., fever.	6. General symptoms are mild, e.g., fever.	6. General symptoms are marked like fever with rigorvomiting and severe supraorbital pain.

Treatment
1. Hot compress.
2. Broad spectrum antibiotic like ampicillin 250 mgm 4 times daily or administration of antibiotic drugs like injection of crystalline penicillin 500,000 units twice daily for 5 days.
3. Analgesics like aspirin by mouth.
4. If an abscess points—incision and drainage.

Other inflammatory conditions of the orbit are—
1. Periostitis.
2. Tenonitis.

Orbital Periostitis

It is not very common. The causes are—
1. Injury.
2. Extension of inflammation from adjacent parts.
3. Tuberculosis particularly in children.
4. Syphilis in adults.

Orbital periostitis may affect the orbital margin or it may be deep-seated.

A. When margin is affected

Clinical signs and symptoms
    (a) Swelling, pain and tenderness over the margin.
    (b) If abscess is formed, it bursts on the skin surface.
    (c) In tubercular cases a fistula may be formed.

B. When periostitis is deep-seated

Clinical signs and symptoms
    (a) Deep-seated pain.
    (b) Proptosis with shifting of the eyeball to the opposite side.

(c) If the apex of the orbit is involved, various oculomotor palsies may develop.

Treatment

(a) Antibiotic drugs.
(b) Drainage of pus when abscess is formed.
(c) Treatment of the cause.

Tenonitis

Definition

It is the inflammation of the Tenon's capsule.

Causes

(a) Gout and rheumatism.
(b) Severe iridocyclitis.
(c) Panophthalmitis.

Clinical signs and symptoms

(a) Pain on any attempt to move the eye.
(b) Oedema of the lids and chemosis with congestion of conjunctiva.
(c) Slight axial proptosis with limitation of movements of the eyeball.

Treatment

(a) Antibiotic drugs.
(b) Hot bathing of the eyeball.
(c) Atropine sulph 1% drop.
(d) Analgesics by mouth.
(e) Drainage of pus if it forms.

Thrombosis of Cavernous Sinus

It may be of two types—
1. Primary thrombosis of the cavernous sinus—

Etiology

(a) Occurring at the extremes of life—in wasted, marasmic infants or in cachectic elderly persons suffering from tuberculosis or carcinoma.
(b) In anaemia, in increased coagulability of blood, in dehydration and in low blood pressure favouring stagnation of circulation.

2. Secondary thrombosis due to thrombophlebitis of cavernous sinus—

Etiology

It is due to spread of infection to cavernous sinus in the following condtions—

(a) orbital cellulitis,

(b) mastoiditis,

(c) facial cellulitis.

Clinical signs and symptoms of both the groups are more or less the same. They are as follows—

(a) Severe supra-orbital pain due to affection of the ophthalmic division of the 5th nerve.

(b) General symptoms like fever, rigor, and vomiting are more common in the thrombophlebitis group.

(c) Affection is at first unilateral, but in 50% of cases it becomes bilateral.

(d) The most important sign is the oedema over the mastoid process of the temporal bone of the affected side.

(e) Other clinical signs are similar to those in orbital cellulitis, but the exceptions are—

   (i) complete paralysis of extra-ocular muscles,

   (ii) anaesthesia of the cornea,

   (iii) proptosis is not so marked.

   Prognosis for the thrombophlebitis group is very grave.

Treatment

Massive doses of antibiotic drugs with anticoagulant therapy.

Proptosis (Exophthalmos)

Definition

It means forward displacement of the eyeball, which may be straight forward (axial) or to one side. Proptosis has to be differentiated from pseudo-proptosis. Pseudo-proptosis is a condition in which the eyeball appears to be proptosed but actually there is no forward displacement.

Causes of pseudo-proptosis are—

(a) Buphthalmos.

(b) High degree of axial type of myopia.

(c) Anterior staphyloma.

(d) Any cause producing retraction of the lids.

Proptosis may be unilateral, bilateral, acute, intermittent or pulsating.

Unilateral Proptosis

Causes

1. Inflammatory lesions—
   (a) Acute—orbital cellulitis, dacryoadenitis, panophthalmitis.
   (b) Chronic—osteo-periostitis, tuberculoma, gumma, pseudotumour.
2. Circulatory disturbances—
   (a) Oedema of orbital tissues.
   (b) Haemorrhage in orbit. Sometimes caused by retro bulbar injection.
   (c) Varicosity of orbital veins.
   (d) Aneurysm of blood vessels.
3. Cysts or tumours of the orbit
   (a) Dermoid or parasitic cysts.
   (b) Benign tumours of orbital tissues like osteoma, haemangioma, lymphoma, neurofibroma or fibroma.
   (c) Malignant tumours of orbital tissues like lymphosarcoma or adenocracinoma of the lacrimal gland.
   (d) Tumours from the optic nerve like glioma or meningioma of the optic nerve.
   (e) Tumours extending from the eyeball as retinoblastoma or malignant melanoma.
   (f) Metastic deposits in the orbit or extension of malignant tumours from neighbouring structures, like maxillary antrum carcinoma or naso-pharyngeal carcinoma.
4. Systemic disease—
   (a) Cellular deposits in leucaemia, both myeloid and lymphoid.
   (b) Endocrine disturbance as Grave's disease and thyrotropic exophthalmos.
5. Paralysis of extra-ocular muscles as in complete ophthalmoplegia.

Bilateral Proptosis

Causes

1. Endoctrine exophthalmos, both thyrotoxic and thyrotropic.
2. Developmental anomalies of the skull and orbit as in oxycephaly.
3. Cavernous sinus thrombosis.
4. Neoplasms like lymphosarcoma, and mlaignant tumour of

naso-pharynx affecting both the orbits.

5. Xanthomatosis of orbits as in Hand-Schuller-Christian syndrome.

Acute Proptosis

Causes
1. Orbital emphysema due to fracture of the medial wall of the orbit.
2. Orbital haemorrhage.

Intermittent Proptosis

Causes
1. Orbital, *i.e.,* varicose condition of the orbital veins.
2. Highly vascular neoplasms causing intermittent proptosis due to periodic congestion.
3. Recurrent orbital haemorrhages.

Pulsating Proptosis

Causes
1. Carotico-cavernous aneurysm in which there is a communication between the internal carotid artery and the cavernous sinus.
2. Saccular aneurysm of the ophthalmic artery.
3. Cerebral pulsation transmitted to the orbit, due to erosion of the orbital roof as in neurofibromatosis.

How to measure proptosis
1. By an exophthalmometer (Fig. 110) which is placed tightly on the lateral orbital margin and the level of the apex of the cornea is read from the scale, and the reading is compared with the other eye. Normally the apex of the cornea lies about 16 mm. in front of the plane of the lateral orbital margin.

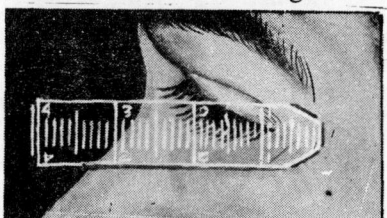

Fig. 110. Exophthalmometer.

2. By clinical observation— The patinet is made to sit in front of the surgeon, with his back towards the surgeon and his head slightly tilted backwards with the eyes looking slightly downwards. The surgeon bending over the patient's head raises the upper lids of both the eyes of the

patient and compares the position of the apex of each cornea for any forward displacement of the eyeball.

Investigations :

Besides the routine laboratory investigations like TC. DC. ESR, blood surgur, cholesterol, stool urine etc. the following special investigations may be necessary. The are T_3 T_4 TSH of blood, orbital venography, Xray skull CAT, scan, ultrasonography etc.

Enophthalmos

Definition

It is a condition in which the eyeball is displaced inwards. It is rare.

Causes of enophthalmos

1. Absorption of orbital fat as in old age or after a severe illness.

2. Horner's syndrome due to paralysis of cervical sympathetic.

3. Trauma, particularly fracture of the floor of the orbit ; blowout fracture.

4. Smallness of the eye, *e.g.,* microphthalmos and phthisis bulbi.

CHAPTER XX

EYE CHANGES IN SYSTEMIC DISEASES

1. Vitamin Deficiencies

A. Deficiency of vitamin A

The symptom-complex, developing in the eyes due to deficiency of vitamin A, is known as Xerophthalmia.

Causes of vitamin A deficiency

    (a) Reduced consumption of vitamin A which may be due to—

        (i) Prolonged defective absorption of vitamin A, owing to digestive disturbance like chronic diarrhoea and helminthiasis.

        (ii) Prolonged diminished intake of vitamin A with diet — daily requirement of vitamin A for a child is 3000-4000 International units.

    (b) Excessive utilization of the vitamin which may happen in rapid growth or in serious debilitating illness.

Stages of keratomalacia (Xerophthalmia)

The vitamin A deficiency manifests itself in both the eyes in several stages. Age incidence is usually 1 to 3 years, occurring more in males than in females.

Stage 1.—The earliest symptom is night-blindess without any other clinical sign in the eye. The child collides with objects, while moving about in dim light. This night-blindness is due to defective regeneration of the visual purple in darkness. Normal cycle of regeneration of visual purple is known as Wald's cycle—

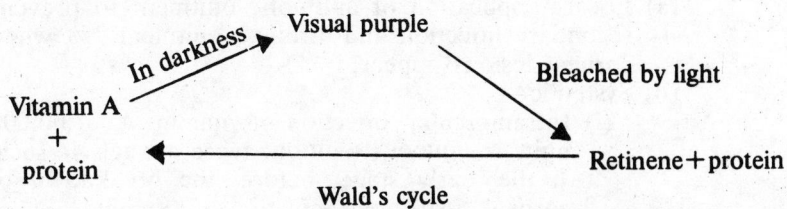

Stage 2.—The conjunctiva becomes dry and lustureless and may be wrinkled and pigmented. Bitot's spots appear on the bulbar conjunctiva, a little away from the limbus in the horizontal meridian usually on the temporal side first. These are whitish, raised, foamy and triangular spots, with the base towards the limbus. These changes collectively are known as xerosis of the conjunctiva or xerophthalmia.

N.B. Bitot's spot may also occur in adults without vitamin A deficiency due to excessive Meibomian secretion or due to exposure, drying and actinic stimulation of the conjunctiva. They have also been seen in patients suffering from pellagra.

Stage 3.—The pre-xerotic stage of the cornea—The cornea becomes dull and lustureless. The window reflex on cornea appears hazy. Corneal sensation is diminished.

Stage 4.—Greyish spots of infiltrations appear either in the central or in the peripheral part of the cornea.

Stage 5.—The areas of infiltration break and ulcers form. Associated with this change, there is photophobia and marked blepharospasm. But the most characteristic feature is the complete absence of any sign of inflammation and so there is no ciliary congestion. This condition, of course, only holds true provided there is no secondary infection.

Stage 6.—The cornea either perforates through the ulcerated areas or the whole of the cornea sloughs off and so either adherent leucoma or an anterior staphyloma is the end result.

Associated with these eye changes, there are some general features in the form dry skin with phrenoderma, thin lustureless hair and dry mouth.

Pathology—Dryness of the cornea and conjunctiva is due to hyperplasia and metaplasia of the epithelium. The Bitot's spots also show metaplasia of epithelium with collection of Meibomian secretion on it, which is the cause of the foamy appearance. A scraping from the Bitot's spot shows xerosis bacilli on culture. Corneal ulcer is due to necrosis of corneal substance.

Treatment

(a) Local—application of antibiotic ointment to prevent secondary infection and atropine ointment 1% when corneal lesions appear.

(b) Systemic—

(i) Intramuscular injection of vitamin A, 1,00,000 units in aqueous solution, twice a week 4 such. In the early stage, before the breakdown of corneal tissue, one injection of vitamin A saves the eye and the cornea becomes bright again. But once corneal tissue has undergone necrosis, the condition is irreversible.

(ii) Treatment of gastro-intestinal disturbance.

(iii) Administration of vitamin A containing diet by mouth specially dark green leafy vegetable (DGLV).

Prophylactic treatment :

2 lac units of Vitamin A in oil is now a days given to children below 5 years of age every 6 months to protect them from Xerophthalmia.

B. Deficiency of vitamin B complex

1. *Vitamin B 1 deficiency*

This condition leads to—

(a) Diminution of corneal sensation due to affection of the trigeminal nerve.

(b) Optic neuritis involving mainly the papillo-macular bundle of nerve fibres, producing pallor of the temporal half of the optic disc and central scotoma with dimness of vision.

2. *Riboflavin deficiency*

This condition leads to—

(a) Burning sensation in the eyes and photophobia due to conjunctival irritation.

(b) Vascularization of the cornea.

C. Deficiency of vitamin C

This condition may cause—

(a) Proptosis as seen in infantile scurvy due to orbital haemorrhage.

(b) Haemorrhage in the conjunctiva, lids, anterior chamber or retina.

D. Deficiency of vitamin D

This condition leads to hypocalcaimia and the eye changes are—

(a) Cataract formation.

(b) Increased lacrimation.

(c) Papilloedema may occur in association with tetany.

II. Common Infections

The eye signs in different infections ae as follows—

1. *Septic abortions*

(a) Endophthalmitis

(b) Orbital cellulitis

2. *In measles*—

(a) Conjunctival hyperaemia or subconjunctival haemorrhage.

(b) Koplik's spots may occur in the conjunctiva & xerosis.

(c) Acute muco-purulent conjunctivitis.

(d) Optic neuritis with dimness of vision.

3. *In diphtheria*—

(a) Membranous conjunctivitis.

(b) Paralysis of accommodation.

(c) Paralysis of extra-ocular muscles particularly the external rectus.

4. *In typhoid fever*—

(a) Corneal ulcer due to lagophthalmos.

(b) Optic neuritis.

5. *In whooping cough*—

(a) Subconjunctival haemorrhage.

(b) Rarely orbital haemorrhage leading to proptosis.

6. *In mumps*—

(a) Acute dacryoadenitis.

(b) Uveitis.

7. *In meningococcal meningitis*—

(a) Metastatic conjunctivitis.

(b) Dilatation and loss of reaction of pupil to light.

(c) Paresis of extra-ocular muscles.

(d) Metastatic endophthalmitis or panophthalmitis.

(e) Complete loss of vision due to optic neuritis or due to
affection of the occipital cortex.

8. *In tuberculosis*—

(a) Any structure of the eyeball may be affected, *e.g.*,
tubercular conjunctivitis, interstitial keratitis, iritis or
iridocyclitis and chorio-retinitis may occur.

(b) Tubercular meningitis may lead to optic atrophy due to
arachnoiditis of the optic chiasma.

(c) Intracranial tuberculoma may produce papilloedema
due to increased intracranial tension.

9. (i) *In syphilis (acquired)*—

(a) Primary stage—chancre of the conjunctiva and conjunctivitis.

(b) Secondary stage—iritis, iridocyclitis and nodules on iris.

(c) Tertiary stage—chorio-retinitis, gummata in the orbit.

(d) Quarternary stage—Argyll Robertson pupil, primary optic atrophy and ocular palsies.

(ii) *In syphilis (congenital)*—

(a) Interstitial keratitis.

(b) Iritis and iridocyclitis.

(c) Chorio-retinitis.

10. *In leprosy*—

(a) Cutaneous nodules on the skin of the eyelids.

(b) Falling of hairs of eyebrows and eyelashes.

(c) Conjunctivitis.

(d) Superficial punctate and interstitial keratitis.

(e) Pannus formation, keratitis and leucoma.

(f) Lepromatous nodules in the sclera.

(g) Granulomatous uveitis.

(h) Dacryocystitis.

III Parasitic Infection

The eye changes are the following—

1. *In malaria*—

(a) Dendritic ulcer of cornea.

(b) Embolism of retinal artery by parasites.

2. *In toxoplasmosis*—necrotizing chorio-retinitis particularly in infants.

3. *In taenia echinococcus infection*—

(a) Hydatid cyst in the orbit.

(b) Intracranial cyst formation may produce papilloedema.

4. *In taenia solium infection*—

(a) Cysticercus cyst in retina and vitreous.

(b) Cyst formation in the orbit & conjunctiva.

IV. Metabolic Diseases

The eye signs are—

1. *In gout and rheumatism*—

(a) Episcleritis and scleritis.

(b) Uveitis.

2. *In diabetes mellitus—*

(a) Changes in refraction—hypermetropia when blood sugar falls and myopia when blood sugar rises.
(b) Haemorrhagic iritis and new blood vessels on the iris.
(c) Diabetic cataract, particularly in juvenile diabetes.
(d) Diabetic retinopathy—microaneurysms in retina, retinal haemorrhage and hard waxy exudate.
(e) Lipaemia retinialis—in juvenile diabetes with marked acidosis, when the retinal vessels appear as if filled with milk.
(f) Palsies of extra-ocular muscles.
(g) Optic neuritis.

V. Diseases of the Kidney—Nephritis

The eye changes are—

(a) Passive oedema of eyelids.
(b) Renal retinopathy similar to hypertensive retinopathy, *i.e.,* flameshaped retinal haemorrhages and woolly exudates in retina.

VI. Toxaemia of Pregnancy

The eye signs are—

(a) Sudden black out of vision due to spasm of retinal arteries.
(b) Retinopathy similar to hypertensive retinopathy, with added signs of detachment of the retina, due to transudation in the subretinal space.

VII. Cardio-vascular system

The changes occur mainly in the retina which have already been described under retinopathy of hypertension.

(a) Benign and Malignant Hypertension
(b) Cardiac vegetation from mitral valvular diseases may cause central retinal artery occlusion- mostly of left side.

VIII. Blood Diseases

1. *In leucaemia—*

(a) Dilatation of retinal vessels.
(b) Retinal haemorrhages with central white areas.
(c) Subconjunctival haemorrhages.

2. *In purpura and haemophilia*—Subconjunctival, retinal, and orbital haemorrhages.

3. *In pernicious anaemia*—retinal haemorrhages with central white spots.

IX. Intracranial Lesions

1. *In subdural haematoma*—papilloedema.

2. *In subarachnoid haemorrhage*—

    (a) Subhyaloid haemorrhage in retina.
    (b) Proptosis.
    (c) Ocular palsies.

3. *Intracranial tumours are associated with*—

    (a) Papilloedema.
    (b) Ocular palsies if cranial nerves are affected.

In pituitary tumour there is bi-temporal hemianopia, *i.e.,* loss of temporal field in each eye and later on optic atrophy. There is no papilloedema so long as the tumour remians within sella turcica.

4. *In head injury*—

    (a) Contraction of the pupil of the same side as the injury.
    (b) In the next stage, if there is rise of intracranial pressure, this pupil dilates and does not react to light (Hutchinson's pupil.) If the pressure rises still further, the other pupil also dilates.
    (c) Paralysis of extra-ocular muscles if the base of the skull is involved.
    (d) Injury to the optic nerve is followed by optic atrophy.
    (e) Subconjunctival haemorrhage, if the roof of the orbit is fractured.
    (f) Field defects, if the visual pathway is affected

5. *In intracranial aneurysms*—

    (a) Aneurysms in the vessels of circle of Willis—ocular palsies.
    (b) Aneurysm of the internal carotid artery outside the cavernous sinus—optic atrophy due to pressure on optic chiasma.
    (c) Aneurysm of the internal carotid inside the cavernous sinus—
        (i) Oculomotor palsies.

(ii) Pulsating exophthalmos—If a communication is made between the anerurysm and the cavernous sinus.

X. Demyelinating Diseases

1. *In disseminated sclerosis—*

(a) Nystagmus.
(b) Dimness of vision due to retrobulbar neuritis.
(c) Paralysis of extra-ocular muscles.

2. *In neuromyelitis optica—*

(a) Sudden blindness due to papillitis.
(b) Dilatation of pupil due to loss of visual acuity.

XI. Diseases of the Muscles

1. *In myasthenia gravis*—ptosis, and defect in eye movements due to weakness of muscles.

XII. Endocrine Disorders

1. *In thyrotoxic or Grave's disease*—due to excessive thyroxin secretion.

(a) Bilateral exophthalmos which is not very marked but reducible on pressure.
(b) Retraction of the upper lid.
(c) Lid-lag, i.e., on attempt to look down, the upper lid does not follow the eyeball but lags behind it.
(d) Weakness of convergence.
(e) Sometimes pigmentation of the skin of the upper lid.

2. *In thyrotropic exophthalmos*—due to excessive secretion of the thyrotropic hormone of the anterior pituitary.

(a) Marked proptosis of both the eyes which is irreducible on pressure.
(b) Marked chemosis of the conjunctiva and oedema of the lids.
(c) Due to exposure, the cornea may be ulcerated.
(d) External ophthalmoplegia—at first the movements of elevation and abduction are affected, but later on all the movements are hampered.

CHAPTER XXI

SYMPTOMATIC DISTURBANCES OF VISION

Amblyopia

Definition—Amblyopia means partial loss of vision.
It may be due to—
  (a) Suppression of macular function—when it is known as amblyopia *ex anopsia*. It is associated with squinting eye in the child.
  (b) Disuse of the macula as in a case of uncorrected high error of refraction or due to opacity of the media, e.g., corneal opacity or cataract.

Amaurosis

Definition—Amaurosis means complete loss of eyesight.
Causes of unilateral amaurosis of sudden onset—
1. In children—
  (a) Acute iridocyclitis or exudative choroiditis.
  (b) Acute retrobulbar or optic neuritis.
  (c) Thrombosis of the central retinal vein.
  (d) Neuromyelitis optica or Devic's diseases—although blindness starts in one eye, the condition becomes bilateral very soon.
  (e) Accidental injury as by pen knife, darts, arrows or bombs.

2. In young adults—
  (a) Vitreous haemorrhage as in Eale's disease.
  (b) Acute exudative choroiditis.
  (c) Detachment of the retina.
  (d) Thrombosis of the central vein of the retina.
  (e) Acute retrobulbar neuritis as in disseminated sclerosis.
  (f) Occlusion of the central artery of the retina due to embolism.
  (g) Industrial injury.

3. In elderly persons—
  (a) Acute congestive glaucoma.
  (b) Vascular accidents like thrombosis of the central retinal vein or occlusion of the central retinal artery.
  (c) Detachment of the retina.
  (d) Massive vitreous haemorrhage as in diabetic retinopathy.
  (e) Industrial injury.

Amaurosis Fugax

Definition—It means sudden but temporary complete loss of vision.

Causes

(a) Effect of gravity as on rising suddenly from sitting position or 'black out' experienced by the pilot of a plane reaching high altitude.

(b) Due to spasm of retinal arteries as in migrane, papilloedema, Raynaud's disease or toxaemia of pregnancy.

(c) In uraemia and in cerebrospinal meningitis due to spasm of cerebral vessels.

Night-Blindness (Nyctalopia)

Definition—It means poor vision in feeble illumination, so that a person cannot move about freely in such an illumination and collides with objects.

Causes

A. Congenital and hereditary conditions—

Congenital and hereditary night-blindness with other anomalies in the retina as in Oguchi's disease usually occurring in Japan.

B. Diseases of the eye—

1. Retinitis pigmentosa or pigmentary degeneration of the retina.

2. Peripheral chorio-retinitis.

3. Myopic degenerative changes in the periphery of the retina.

4. Chronic simple glaucoma with marked contraction of the visual field.

5. Retinal detachment.

C. Systemic diseases—

1. Vitamin A deficiency.

2. Pathological changes in the liver, e.g., cirrhosis of liver and occasionally in jaundice.

The night-blindness is mainly due either to the damage to the rods or due to deficient regeneration of visual purple. It can be detected by an instrument known as adaptometer.

Day-Blindness (Hemeralopia)

Definition—It means that vision is poor in bright light but better in dim light. In dim light, the pupil dilates and so the peripheral retina is used for vision.

Causes

(a) Pathological changes in the macula.

(b) Central opacity of cornea or lens.

(c) Congenital condition when it is usually associated with total colour blindness.

Colour Blindness

Definition—It means inability to recognize colour.

Causes

A. Congenital causes.

Usually they are hereditary. The colour blindness is from birth, bilateral and is incurable. The congenital colour blindness may be of two types—

(a) Partial colour blindness—

It means that the person cannot recognize green, red, or blue colour. Green-blindness is the commonest.

(b) Total colour blindness.

In this condition, a person cannot recognize any colour and sees everything grey.

B. Acquired causes—

These are diseases of the macula and optic nerve, e.g., toxic amblyopias and macular affections in various diseases.

CHAPTER XXII

INJURIES

The injuries of the lids and eyeball can be placed under the following categories—
A. *Mechanical injuries.*
  I. Contusional injuries.
  II. Perforating or penetrating injuries.
  III. Retained foreign bodies.
B. *Chemical burns.*
C. *Thermal injuries.*
D. *Electrical injuries.*
E. *Radiational injuries.*

A. Mechanical injuries

1. Contusions caused by blunt instruments—
Lids—Contusions of lid cause swelling and ecchymosis of the lids, a condition known as 'black-eye'.

Conjunctiva—The conjunctive may be lacerated and there is usually subconjunctival haemorrhage.

Cornea—The cornea may be affected in the form of abrasions or rupture of the Descemet's membrane, causing deep corneal opacity. Rupture of cornea is extremely rare.

Sclera—The sclera may be ruptured usually at its weakest part, in the vicinity of the canal of Schlemm. There may be associated prolapse of uveal tissue, or even of vitreous through the rupture and profuse intra-ocular haemorrhage, depending on the severity of the injury.

Anterior chamber—There may be bleeding in the anterior chamber due to rupture of vessels of the iris or ciliary body. If this condition is associated with rise of intra-ocular tension, blood-staining of cornea may result, in which the cornea takes up a reddish brown colour. The colouration clears up from the periphery, but it may take several months for the central part to clear.

Iris and pupil—
  (a) The pupil may constrict— traumatic miosis—due to irritation of the nerves. This may be accompanied by spasm of accommodation causing temporary myopia.

(b) The pupil may dilate and remain immobile—traumatic mydriasis—due to paralysis of pupillomotor fibres. The pupil may remain moderately dilated permanently.

(c) The sphincter pupillae may rupture causing irregularly dilated pupil.

(d) Iridodialysis–The iris may be torn from its attachment to the ciliary body and so a 'D' shaped biconvex black area is visible at the periphery.

(e) Anti-flexion of the iris–If the iridodialysis is extensive, there may be rotation of the detached portion of the iris, so that the posterior surface of the iris becomes anterior.

(f) Traumatic aniridia–The entire iris may be torn off from the ciliary body. The iris contracts to form a globular mass and sinks into the bottom of the anterior chamber.

Lens—

(a) Vossius's ring on anterior lens capsule—already described in the chapter on traumatic cataract.

(b) Concussion cataract—The cataract is due mainly to the damage to the capsule, either a rupture or an alteration of its semi-permeability, and entrance of aqueous humour into the lens. Usually the thin posterior capsule is the site of the damage. The cataract may appear in various forms, but the most typical appearance is a rosette shaped cataract, which usually appears in the posterior cortex (*See* under traumatic cataract).

(c) Subluxation or dislocation of the lens—The lens may be subluxated, when only a few fibres of the suspensory ligament are torn but it remains in the pupillary area.

If all the fibres of the ligament are torn, the lens is dislocated either in the anterior chamber or in the vitreous.

Vitreous—

(a) Disorganization of vitreous and formation of opacities may take place. If the injury is very severe, the vitreous may liquify.

(b) Haemorrhage may occur in the vitreous. The entire vitreous becomes full of blood, usually from the ruptured ciliary vessels. The blood may be completely absorbed in course of time, leaving behind a few opacities. But sometimes organized fibrous tissue may develop in the vitreous, a condition known as retinitis proliferans.

Retina—

(a) Commotio retinae or Berlin's oedema—As a result of a blow on the eye, retinal oedema appears at the posterior pole, in the form of milky-white cloudiness. The oedema disappears after sometime but the central vision remains defective due to chorioretinal degeneration.

(b) Formation of a macular hole—The oedematous change may cause cystic degeneration of the retina and the rupture of a cyst causes a macular hole.

(c) Retinal haemorrhage—This may occur of any degree due to the rupture of retinal vessels.

(d) Detachment of the retina—This happens due to a tear in the retina.

Choroid—

(a) Rupture of the choroid—This happens as a result of a severe contusion. Immediately after the injury, there is extravasation of blood. After the blood gets absorbed, the rupture is seen as two curved white streaks, concentric with the disc margin, and situated usually on its temporal side.

(b) Choroidal haemorrhage—It appears as a dark red patch, underneath the retinal vessels due to rupture of choroidal vessels.

Optic nerve—In very severe injuries there may be avulsion of the optic nerve which is however extremely rare.

Alteration of intra-ocular pressure—As a result of concussion, there may be hypotony of traumatic glaucoma due to vasomotor reaction. Usually there is initial vasoconstriction followed by intense vasodilation.

Treatment of contusional injuries

The treatment of contusional injuries is mainly expectant and is done on conservative lines. For the 'black eye', an immediate cold compress is useful. Subconjunctival hemorrhage usually disappears within two to three weeks and local eye drop like 5% argyrol and assurance to the patients are all that are necessary.

A rupture of cornea and sclera may require suturing. Suturing with 8/o virgin silk has saved many eyes.

In case of a hyphaema with rise of tension, paracentesis to drain out the blood is essential. Atropine 1% drop may be instilled to give rest to the eye, if there is no glaucoma. Steroid drops locally are also used.

In case of an iridodialysis, if there is diplopia, the torn iris may be anchored with a silk suture into a scleral incision just behind the limbus.

A concussion cataract, if it impairs vision to a marked extent, should be removed, either by suction evacuation or by extraction, depending on the age of the patient.

A dislocated lens should always be removed. In case of subluxation, the vision may be improved by correction with glasses.

Vitreous haemorrhage, retinal and· choroidal haemorrhages require rest to the eye and expectant treatment.

Traumatic glaucoma may be treated with miotics and diamox tablets by mouth. An angle recession glaucoma may be treated with trabeculotomy.

II. Penetrating injuries, perforating injuries or wounds

This type of injury is caused by sharp objects, small bodies travelling at a high speed or blunt objects striking with a great momentum. Apart from the actual trauma, there is always the risk of introduction of infection with disastrous results.

Wounds of the lids—Either the lid margin or the substance of the lid away from the margin, may undergo an incised wound or laceration. A cut wound in the direction of the orbicularis does not gape, but in vertical wounds the margins separate. A wound on the lid margin produces a notch—traumatic coloboma of the lid margin.

Wounds of the conjunctiva—There may be incised or lacerated wounds in the conjunctiva associated with subconjunctival haemorrhage.

Wounds of the cornea—They may be linear or lacerated and may be situated anywhere in the cornea or on the limbus. If the wound is slanting and valvular, there is not much of drainage of aqueous. But in a straight wound, the aqueous may be entirely drained out and if the wound is not exactly at the centre of the cornea, iris invariably prolapses through the wound or gets adherent to the wound. The margins of a corneal wound swell, due to imbibition of fluid from the aqueous humour and the wound becomes sealed. A penetrating corneal wound always leaves behind an opacity after healing. There is always a chance of fall of intra-ocular tension immediately following the injury.

Wounds of the sclera—A penetrating injury through the sclera is recognized by prolapse of the uveal tissue. If the injury is deep, vitreous also comes through the wound. If uveal blood vessels are damaged, the injury is also acccompanied by intra-ocular haemorrhage,

Wounds of the lens—They cause traumatic cataract. If the wound is very small as by a needle, the punctured capsule may be sealed up leaving a tiny opacity in the lens. This opacity may remain stationary, but usually it spreads in the form of a rosetteshaped cataract similar to concussion cataract. If the lens swells along with the opacity, secondary glaucoma may develop.

If the wound is big enough lens matter may protrude in the anterior chamber as flocculent grey masses, which very soon become opaque white.

Effect of infection—If infection is introduced along with the injury, severe iritis, iridocyclitis with hypopyon formation or panophthalmitis may develop with disastrous results.

Risk of sympathetic ophthalmia—A penetrating wound in the ciliary region with prolapse of uveal tissue is a serious condition, as there is a real danger of development of sympathetic ophthalmia in the other eye. (Described under special types of iridocyclitis.)

Treatment of penetrating injuries

1. Injuries of lids—The lid injuries must be carefully repaired in layers, *i.e.*, tarsal plate, orbicularis muscle and the skin have to be sutured separately.

Injury to the lid margin requires special attention. Because if the cut margins are not accurately apposed, a notch develops which may be the cause of future epiphora, particularly if the injury affects the lower lid. Moreover a vertical injury usually produces a cicatrix even after proper repair, and this cicatrization leads to ectropion formation and epiphora if the injury is in the lower lid.

2. Management of a penetrating injury to the eyeball—
    (a) As a preliminary measure, the first thing to do is to make a thorough examination of the eye to assess the exact extent of the damage. For this purpose a lid retractor may have to be used with the help of local

anaesthetic drops or even general anaesthesia has to be applied, particularly in case of children.

(b) If it is found that the injury is very severe which has led to total disorganization of the globe and there is no chance of any useful vision, the eye should be excised.

(c) But if the injury is such that there is every chance of retaining useful vision, following immediate measures have to be adopted—

(i) Removal of obvious dirt if any, by normal saline wash given very gently.

(ii) Separation of entangled intra-ocular tissue, like iris or uveal tissue from the wound as far as possible. As a rule prolapsed iris tissue should not be reintroduced into the eyeball, but after it is freed from the wound, it should be excised, because replacement may carry infection inside the eye.

(iii) Proper repair of the wound—
It should be attempted only when there is no evidence of infection, as when the injury is attended immediately after occurrence. In presence of infection, the repair work should be done later on, after the infection has been controlled, The scleral and corneal wounds are to be repaired by suturing. A slightly gaping corneal woumd with incarcerated iris is best repaired by cauterizing the wound with thermocautery and covering it with conjunctival flap.

(iv) Rest to the eye is done by instillation of atropine sulph 1% drops with eye bandage and post-traumatic inflammation is minimized by application of 1% cortisone ointment, provided there is no infection.

(v) Effect of any exogenous infection to be combated by subconjunctival injection of gentamycin and by broad spectrum antibiotics like chloramphenicol capsules 250mg. 3 times a day by mouth.

(d) Delayed treatment—
(i) A traumatic cataract causing a marked disturb-

ance of vision should be removed either by suction evacuation or by extraction, depending on the age of the patient.

(ii) If glaucoma develops along with the cataract, temporarily the tension may be reduced by diamox tablet 250 mg. twice daily by mouth, and when tension becomes normal the cataract has to be removed,

(iii) Corneal opacity may be tackled by keratoplasty.

(vi) Adhesions of iris to the corneal scar should be separated by synecheotomy to avoid the risk of future secondary glaucoma.

III. Retained foreign bodies

They may be of two varieties—
(a) Extra-ocular foreign bodies impacted in the conjunctiva or cornea.
(b) Intra-ocular foreign bodies with perforating wound in the eyeball.

(a) Extra-ocular foreign bodies

In the conjunctiva–The usual foreign bodies are particles of coal dust, iron, emery, husk of paddy and wings of insect, the common sites are the middle of the subtarsal sulcus in the upper lid, the fornix and the bulbar conjunctiva. There is immediate discomfort and watering. But if the foreign body is lodged in the subtarsal sulcus, there is pain and blepharospasm due to rubbing of the foreign body against cornea, which is very sensitive.

In the Cornea–The usual foreign bodies are particles of iron, dust or emery and coal. The particle is usually embedded in the corneal epithelium or in the substantia propria. There is sudden onset of discomfort, watering and blepharospasm. As there is no kinaesthetic sensation in the cornea, the exact situation of the foreign body cannot be located by the patient and it is very often referred to the tarsal conjunctiva of the upper lid against which the foreig4 body rubs. There may be ciliary congestion due to reflex irritation.

A corneal foreign body carries a greater risk to the eye than a conjunctival foreign body, because if infected the foreign body leads to corneal ulceration.

Treatment of extra-ocular foreign body

Both the conjunctival and corneal foreign bodies require removal.

The conjunctival foreign body is easily removed by a sterile swab stick, after application of local anaesthetic drops. If it is embedded in the conjunctiva, it can be removed by snipping off a tiny piece of conjunctiva along with the foreign body.

The corneal foreign body should also be removed with a spud or with a foreign body needle and antibiotic ointment has to be applied after removal. (Details given in the chapter on instruments and operations.)

(b)   *Intra-ocular foreign bodies with perforating wound in the eyeball.*

The foreign bodies, which commonly penetrate the eye, are particles of iron, stone, glass, copper, lead or spicules of wood.

The effects of a foreign body entering into the eye can be considered under three headings–

(i)   Mechanical effects.
(ii)   Introduction of infection.
(iii)   Specific side reaction caused by a particular type of foreign body.

(i)   Mechanical effects

It has to be remembered that the mechanical effects produced by a foreign body entering into the eye depend largely on its size and velocity. A big-size foreign body may so severely damage the eye, that the eye has to be excised.

Usually the foreign bodies are small and travel at a high speed.

On penetrating the cornea or sclera, it may remain in the anterior chamber.

It may penetrate into the lens, either through the iris, when a hole is formed in the iris or through the pupil. Penetration of the cornea may be accompanied by entanglement of the iris in the cornea. Injury to the lens causes traumatic cataract.

If it penetrates the eyeball further posteriorly, it may lie in the vitreous or may rest on the retina. These happenings may be associated with haemorrhage in the virteous or in the retina and also with degenerative changes in the vitreous and retina.

(ii) Introduction of infection

Similar to other perforating wounds, introduction of infection along with the foreign body is a real danger to the eye. Fortunately, small flying metallic particles are sterile, due to their high speed and the heat generated on their emission. But chips of wood or pieces of stone are notorious for introducing infection. Once intra-ocular infection is established, there is every possibility that it will end either in endophthalmitis or panophthalmitis.

(iii) Side reactions produced by the foreign body

An intra-ocular foreign body can stimulate the following possible reactions—

(i) If inert—no reaction. Glass, plastics, porcelain or silicon are inert substances which cause no reaction. Stone, depending on its composition may be inert also.

(ii) Local irritation and formation of fibrous tissue to encapsulate the foreign body e.g., lead and aluminium stimulate local reaction and fibrosis.

(iii) A suppurative reaction e.g., pure copper is highly irritant and causes suppurative inflammation.

(iv) Specific degenerative changes e.g., iron produces specific degenerative changes known as siderosis and alloy of copper leads to deposition of copper in various tissues and the condition is then called chalcosis.

Siderosis—If an iron particle remains inside the eye, the metal undergoes electrolytic dissociation and then dessemination of the metal take place throughout the tissues. The epithelial structures are usually most affected and they undergo degenerative changes.

The earliest sign is deposition of iron in the epithelium of the anterior lens capsule, in the form of rusty deposits. This leads eventually to the development of cataract. The iris, ciliary body and retina are also affected. There is pigmentary degeneration of the retina, resembling that in retinitis pigmentosa, leading to defective vision and nightblindness. Secondary glaucoma is a delayed complication.

Chalcosis—In this condition, copper from an alloy undergoes electrolytic dissociation and is deposited on membranous structures. As for example, in the cornea it is deposited in the peripheral part of the Descemet's membrane producing a golden-brown ring known as Kayser-Fleischer ring. In the lens, it is deposited under the capsule at the posterior pole, being aggregated in radiating formations like the petals of a flower with a golden-green sheen, when it is called a sun-flower cataract. But unlike siderosis, there is not degenerative changes in the cells.

Management of a case of intra-ocular foreign body

(1) The first step is to ascertain whether the foreign body has acutally penetrated the eyeball or not. To come to a correct diagnosis following steps are to be taken—

(i) History has to be taken very carefully.

(ii) A thorough examination of the eyeball, if necessary even with the help of a slit-lamp has to be done to find out the wound of entry. If the foreign body is very minute, the wound of entry may not be always visible. A tiny opaque spot in the cornea, a spot of subconjunctival haemorrhage or a tiny hole in the iris gives clue for the entrance.

(iii) A straight X-ray of the corresponding orbit to find out any radio-opaque shadow.

(2) If the foreign body is found to have entered into the eye, all the structures have to be carefully examined to find out the amount of damage.

(3) The third step is to localize the foreign body. This localization can be done by clinical examination with lens and lope or by an ophthalmoscope to find out the location of the foreign body, *i.e.*, in the anterior chamber, on the iris, in the lens, in the vitreous or on the retina.

If the foreign body cannot be detected by clinical methods, a special radiographic technique is followed. After application of local anaesthetic drops, a silver ring, half a mm. thick and with a diameter of 12 mm. is stitched to the limbus of the corresponding eye. Then by asking the patient to look straight ahead, skiagrams the skiagram is properly taken, in the antero-posterior view the ring appears as a circle but in the side view as a straight vertical line. From these pictures, the distance of the foreign body from the ring which represents the limbus, and also the meridian in which the foreign body lies, are found out.

(4) Removal of the foreign body—After a correct localization, the foreign body has to be removed as soon as possible.

Removal of Magnetic Foreign Bodies

This is fairly easy. If the foreign body is in the anterior

chamber or on the iris, it can be removed either by a forceps through a limbal incision or by introducing the point of a hand-magnet into the anterior chamber through a similar incision. If the particle is entangled in the iris, a narrow portion of the iris has to be removed along with the particle.

If in the lens and if there is a cataract, the foreign body is easily removed along with the extraction of the lens.

A foreign body, either in the ciliary body, in the vitreous or in the retina, is best removed by a giant electromagnet, by the posterior route. By this method, the conjunctiva and sclera over the foreign body are incised after applying diathermy points on the sclera. Then the choroid and the retina are also incised, and the narrow point of an electro-magnet is introduced into the vitreous and the magnet at once attracts the foreign body. If any one of the extra-ocular muscles comes in the way of approach to the foreign body, this is also incised between preplaced sutures before incising sclera. Finally the scleral and conjunctival wounds are closed by sutures.

Removal of non-magnetic foreign bodies

This is not always easy. If a foreign body is inert like glass, it may be left alone. If the approach to the foreign body is easy, as when it lies in the anterior chamber, attemptsf may be made to remove it with forceps introduced through a limbal incision. If a non-magnetic foreign body rests in the vitreous it may be removed with endoscope or vitrectomy apparatus.

B. Chemical Burns

The chemical injuries to the eyes are usually due to external contact with the chemical in the form of solid, liquid, powder or dust, occurring in private houses, in chemical laboratories or in industry.

In general, chemical burns comprise two main groups—the alkali burns and the acid burns; besides these thousands of chemicals industry may damage the eyes.

Alkali Burns

These are much more dangerous than acid burns. Usually lime, caustic potash or caustic soda, liquid ammonia or ammonium hydroxide are responsible agents. Most harmful of all these is the liquid ammonia.

Changes in the ocular tissues when they come in contact with an alkali are as follows—

(1) Unlike inorganic acids, the alkalis do not cause instant coagulation of proteins of cells, but the proteins are converted into gel-like alkaline proteinates.

(2) There is destruction of the cell membrane due to conversion of the fatty matter of the membrane into soaps.

(3) The lipoids of the cells are converted into soluble compounds, which are soft and gelatine like.

The end result of all these changes is the power of penetration of the chemical agent deep into the tissues. So the prognosis in a case of alkaline burn must always be guarded.

The ocular lesions are—

(a) Conjunctiva—There is marked congestion, oedema, widespread necrosis and profuse purulent discharge. Later on symblepharon is formed.

(b) Cornea—There is destruction of the epithelium followed by corneal opacity and new vessel formation. In severe cases cornea may slough out, causing anterior staphyloma to form.

(c) Iris—Iris becomes violently inflammed and in worst cases both the iris and the ciliary body may be replaced by granulation tissue. The lens becomes cataractous and the eyeball atrophies.

Acid Burns

Inorganic acids like sulphuric, hydrochloric and nitric acids are the common agents.

Changes in the ocular tissues

With strong acids, there is instant coagulation of all the proteins with the formation of insoluble proteinates. The cellular death is immediate with coagulative necrosis. The coagulated protein acts as a barrier, so that there is no penetration of the chemical in the deeper tissues and thus the lesion becomes sharply limited.

The ocular lesions are—

(a) Conjunctiva—There is necrosis followed by sloughing of tissues are fibrosis and later on symblepharon forms.

(b) Cornea—It may slough out completely and staphyloma forms.

Treatment of chemical burns

(1) The first and immediate measure is a thorough wash of the conjunctival sac with plain water or normal saline, whichever is available. No time must be spent searching for neutralizing solutions whose effieciency is doubtful.

(2) If any particle is left behind, particularly in case of lime, it must be carefully removed with swab sticks.

(3) Any necrotic tags of conjunctiva should be excised.

(4) Atropine, steroids and antibiotic ointment may be freely used to make the inflammation subside, and to create a suitable condition for repair.

(5) Care must be taken to prevent symblepharon formation. Sweeping a glass rod round the fornices once a day is an old method and is totally replaced by soft contract less application.

C. Thermal Injuries

These are usually caused by contact with hot bodies like glowing coal or molten metal and hot fluids. The ocular lesions depend on the size and temperature of the hot body or fluid. Very hot bodies can cause severe damage to cornea and conjunctiva.

Treatment of such lesions is on general lines, *i.e., atropine, steroids and antibiotics.*

D. Electrical Injuries

The passage of a high tension electric current, through the head near the orbit, can cause ocular lesions.

The usual eye lesions are–
- (a) Conjunctiva–Both ciliary and conjunctival type of congestion.
- (b) Cornea–Punctate or diffuse interstitial opacities.
- (c) Iris and ciliary body–Iritis and iridocyclitis.
- (d) Retina and optic nerve—Retinal haemorrhage and optic neuritis.

But the most important lesion is the development of electric cataract. The cataract takes on the average two to four months to appear as punctate opacities both in the anterior and in the posterior cortex. Ultimately the entire lens becomes opaque. Younger the patient more liable he is to this type of lental change.

Treatment—The cataract can be treated as an ordinary cataract. The other lesions of the eye are treated on general lines with atropine, steroids and antibiotics. The damage to the optic nerve, if severe, remains permanent.

E. Radiational Injuries

Any radiation, only when absorbed by a tissue, can cause change. The common radiational injuries are—

1. Thermal lesions—produced by infra-red rays, when the energy is converted into heat.

2. Abiotic lesions—produced by ultra-violet rays which cause photo-chemical and photo-electrical effects.

3. Ionizing lesions—as produced by roentgen rays and gamma rays from radium.

1. *Thermal lesions*—These occur either due to sudden release of a large amount of radiations as in exposure to arc-lights or due to long continued exposure to small amount of radiations. The second variety is more common, when a cataract develops as in glass-workers or furnace-workers due to infra-red rays.

The glass-worker's or the furnace-men's cataract takes several years to develop. The cataract starts as a saucer-shaped opacity in the posterior cortex and in course of time the entire lens becomes opaque.

2. *Abiotic lesions*—These are the effects of exposure to ultra-violet rays which occur in workers engaged in oxy-acetylene or arc-welding.

The clinical condition which develops is known as *photophthalmia*. After a latent period of 6-8 hours, the first symptom is a marked foreign body sensation in both the eyes. This is accompanied by pain, lacrimation and blepharospasm. The conjunctiva becomes congested and the cornea when stained with fluorescein shows minute stained areas. The lens is not affected. Usually the symptoms disappear within 48 hours.

3. *Ionizing lesions*—These types of lesions are commonly seen in workers who deal with radio-active luminizing paints for coating the figures on the dials of clocks or as a result of deep X-ray therapy or radium therapy to the tumours of the lids or eyeball.

Before the lesions appear, there is a long latent period of several months. The most susceptible tissues are the hair follicles of eye-lashes and eyebrows and the lens which becomes cataractous.

Treatment of radiational injuries

(a) Adequate measures are to be taken to prevent the radiotional injuries. Ordinary dark glasses can prevent lesions by infra-red and ultra-violet rays. Ionizing rays can be prevented by lead sheets of 2 mm. thickness.

(b) Glass-workers' and furnace-men's cataract can be extracted like ordinary senile cataract. The cataract due to ionizing rays is also amenable to treatment.

(c) For photophthalmia—cold compress, a drop of xylocaine 4%, atropine and steroid drops with pad and bandage relieve the symptoms.

CHAPTER XXIII

OPHTHALMIC INSTRUMENTS

1. EYE SPECULUM

There are two types—universal and guarded.

(a) Universal eye speculum (Fig. 1, a)—It is called universal because it can be used for either eye. It has a spring and two limbs to keep the eyelids separate.

Use—It is used to keep the eyelids separate during any operation on the eyeball.

Advantage of the instrument—

(i) As there is no guard, more space is obtained during operation.

(ii) It can be used for both the eyes.

Disadvantage—As there is no guard to cover the eyelashes of the upper lid, the lashes protrude into the field of operation.

(b) Guarded speculum (Fig. 1. b)—There are two such instruments—one for the right eye and the other for the left eye. Each one has a spring and two limbs. The upper limb has a guard to keep the eyelashes of the upper lid covered during operation.

It is seldom used now a days.

2. FIXATION FORCEPS

Usually there are 2×3 teeth in the limbs of the forceps (Fig. 2). But the number of the teeth may vary and may be 3×4 or 4×5.

Use—For fixation of the eyeball through the conjunctiva and the episcleral tissue during an operation on the eyeball.

3. Von Graefe's CATARACT KNIFE

It has a long, narrow, thin and straight blade with a sharp point and a sharp cutting edge (Fig. 3).

PLATE 1

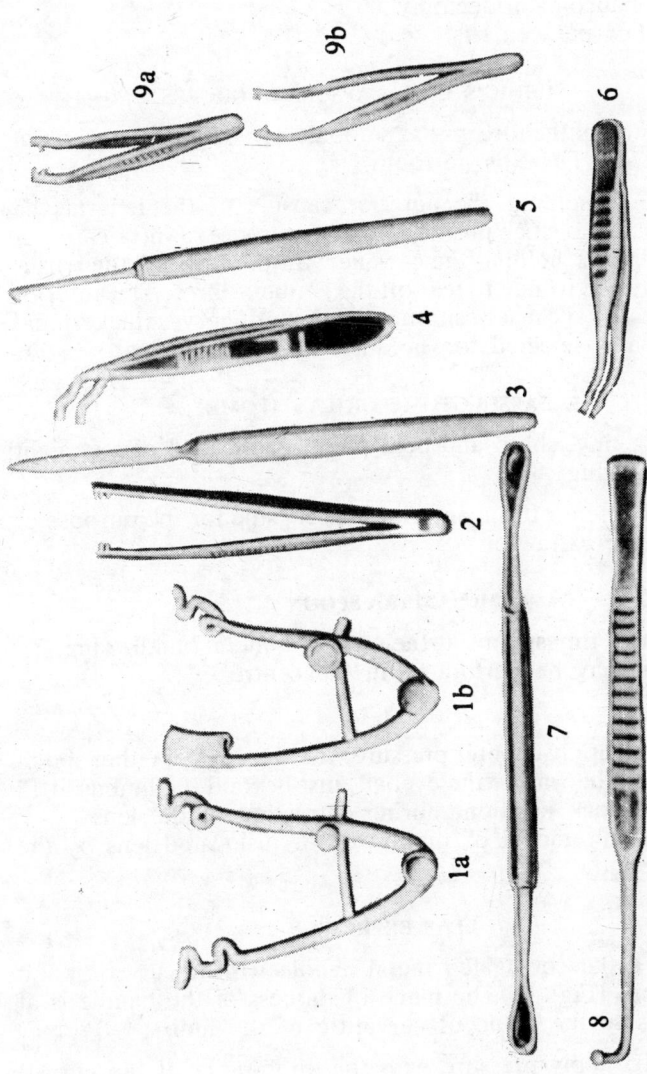

Fig. 1a. Universal Eye Speculum. Fig. 1b. Guarded Eye Speculum. Fig. 2. Fixation Foreceps. Fig. 3. Von Graefe's Cataract Knife. Fig. 4. Elschnig's Intra-Capsualr Forceps. Fig. 5. Capsulotome or Cystitome. Fig. 6. Capsule Forceps. Fig. 7. MacNamara Spoon. Fig. 8. Lens Expressor. Fig. 9a. Iris Forceps—Angular, Fig. 9b. Iris Forceps—Curved.

Use—

(a) For making section for cataract operation.
(b) For making section for optical iridectomy or for glaucoma iridectomy.
(c) For paracentesis.

4. ELSCHNIG'S INTRACAPSULAR FORCEPS

Each limb of the forceps has a dobule curve, ending on a blunt point (Fig. 4.) There is no tooth.

Use—For holding the anterior capsule of the lens at the lowest part, at 6 o'clock position, for the purpose of intra-capsular extraction. After holding the capsule with the forceps, the lens is moved from side to side to tear off the zonular fibres. The anterior lens capsule at 6 o'clock position near the periphery is thickest and so that area is selected for holding with the forceps.

5. CAPSULOTOME OR CYSTITOME

It has a tiny, sharp and bent point, at the end of a straight narrow limb (Fig. 5).

Use—To tear off the anterior lens capsule for the purpose of extra–capsular extraction.

6. McNAMARA SPOON

It has two tiny spoons at the ends of a metal handle (Fig. 7). The spoons may be perforated in the centre.

Use—

(a) To apply counter pressure with the edge of either spoon on the wall of the eyeball, just beyond the limbus at 12 o'clock position, during extraction of the lens.
(b) For removal of subluxated or dislocated lens by the spoon.

7. LENS EXPRESSOR

It has a flat corrugated metal handle with a curved knob pointed limb. (Fig. 8). The plane of flatness of the handle is at right angles to the plane of curvature of the limb.

Use—To apply pressure with the knob-point of the curved limb on the limbus and on the neighbouring part of the cornea at 6 o'clock position during extraction of the lens.

PLATE II

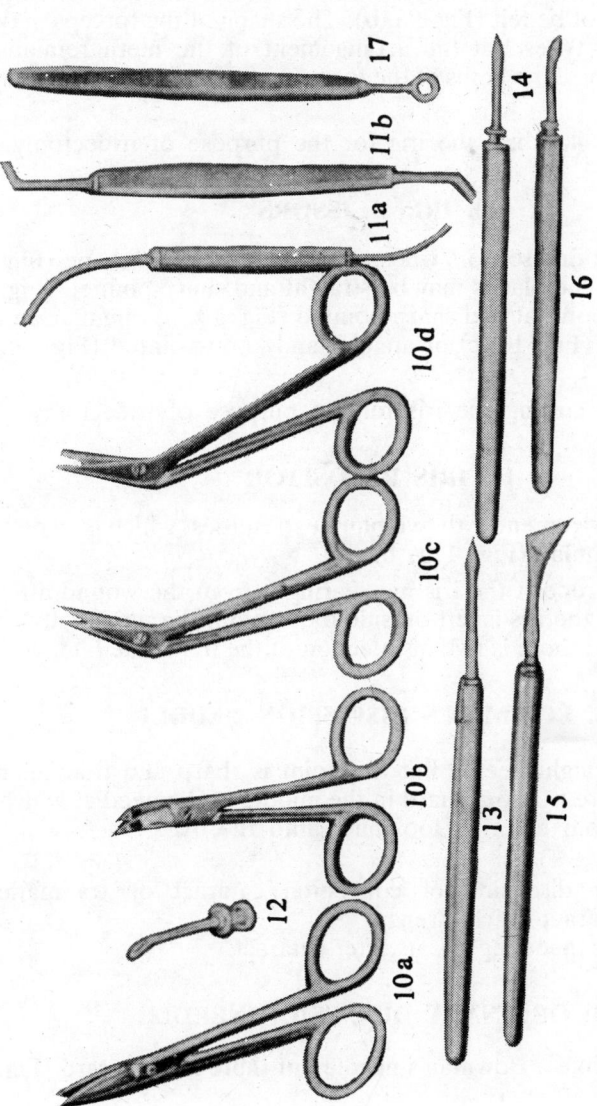

Fig. 10a. Iris Scissors—Straight and Sharp-pointed. Fig. 10b. Iris Scissors—Curved on flat and sharp-pointed. Fig. 10c. Iris Scissors—Angular and sharp-pointed. Fig. 10d. Iris Scissors—Angular and Knob-pointed. Fig. 11a. Iris Repositor—'S' shaped. Fig. 11b. Iris Repositor—Angular. Fig. 12. Anterior Chamber Washing canula. Fig. 13. Bowman's Discission Needle. Fig. 14. Ordinary Discission Needle. 15. Keratome. Fig. 16. Zeigler's Knife. Fig. 17. Vectis

9. IRIS FORCEPS

These are tiny forceps, with fine limbs, carrying 1 × 2 teeth on the inner side of the limbs, so that when the limbs are closed, the teeth cannot be felt (Fig. 9a, b). The shape of the forceps may be of various types but the arrangement of the teeth remians always the same. The limbs of the forceps may be straight, angular or curved.

Use—For holding the iris for the purpose of iridectomy.

10. IRIS SCISSORS

These are fine scissors whose blades may vary in shape (Fig. 10a, b, c, d). The blades may be straight and sharp-pointed (Fig. 10, a), curved on flat and sharp-pointed (Fig. 10, b), angular and sharp-pointed (Fig. 10, c) or angular and knob-pointed (Fig. 10, d).

Use—For cutting the iris for the purpose of iridectomy.

11. IRIS REPOSITOR

It is an instrument with two blunt extremities, which may be S shaped or angular (Fig. 11a, b).

Use—To reposit the iris by clearing it from the wound after iridectomy. If the iris is left outside the wound, the pupil will not be circular and there is risk of infection of the iris tissue later on.

12. BOWMAN'S DISCISSION NEDDLE

It is a straight needle but the point is sharp and triangular (Fig. 13). There is also a guard in the middle of the needle, which prevents it from entering too much into the eye.

Use—
    (a) For discission of congenital cataract or traumatic cataract in children.
    (b) For needling of an after-cataract.

13. ORDINARY DISCISSION NEEDLE

It is just like a Bowman's needle but there is no gurard (Fig. 14).

Use—Same as for the Bowman's needle.

14. KERATOME

It has a triangular blade with a sharp point and sharp cutting edges and the blade is bent at an angle to the handle (Fig. 15).
Use—
  (a) For corneal incision for curette and evacuation operation.
  (b) For making limbal incision for glaucoma iridectomy or optical iridectomy.
  (c) For paracentesis.

15. ZEIGLER'S KNIFE

It has a tiny curved blade with a sharp point at the end of a narrow limb, attached to a handle (Fig. 16).
Use—For incising the after-cataract in the pupillary area.

16. VECTIS

It is a loop of wire at the end of a narrow limb attached to a handle (Fig. 17).
Use—For removal of subluxated or dislocated lens.

17 TOOKE'S KNIFE

It has a short elongated blade attached to a handle, with a semicircular cutting edge, bevelled on both the surfaces (Fig. 18).
Use—For splitting the cornea during Elliot's sclero-corneal trephining operation. Splitting of cornea is necessary so that the blade of the trephine may cover half of corneal tissue and half of scleral tissue.

18. ELLIOT'S SCLERO-CORNEAL TREPHINE HANDLE WITH BLADE

The blade is cylindrical with a sharp circular cutting edge, fitted to a bigger cylindrical handle. The diameter of the blade may be 1.5 or 2 mm. and the length is more than 1 inch (Fig. 19).

Use—For punching a hole in the wall of the eyeball at the sclero-corneal junction at 12 o'clock position during trephine operation.

19. DISC-HOLDING FORCEPS

It is a small and fine forceps with 1 × 2 teeth at the end of the limbs, hanging downwards (Fig. 20).

Use—For catching the disc of sclero-corneal tissue made by the trephine blade.

20. BROAD NEEDLE OR PARACENTESIS NEEDLE

It has a lance-shaped blade, about 3/4 inch long, with a sharp point and sharp cutting edges, at the end of a metal handle (Fig. 21).

Use—For paracentesis to drain out aqueous humour to lower the intra-ocular pressure temporarily in cases of secondary glaucoma, *e.g.*, secondary glaucoma due to iridocyclitis. (For other indications *see* under operations.)

21. THERMO-CAUTERY

The cautery is a metallic knob or a metallic ball and a point, at the end of a handle. The cautery is heated in the flame of a spirit lamp and then applied (Fig. 22).

Use—
   (a) For cauterizing tiny iris prolapse.
   (b) For cauterizing the progressive margin of a croneal ulcer, when the ulcer is not responding to medical treatment.
   (c) For cauterizing any bleeding point during an operation on the eyeball.

22. EPILATION FORCEPS

It is a small forceps with stout limbs which have no tooth. The opposite surfaces of the limbs are flat (Fig. 23).

Use—For epilation of the offending eyelashes in a case of trichiasis. The eyelash is held by the forceps and pulled out. This is not the ideal method for epilation, as the root is not destroyed and the lash grows again. The ideal method for epilation is electrolysis epilation, when a weak galvanic current is applied for 30 seconds to the root of the eyelash by a fine platinum needle and thereby the root is destroyed.

23. DESMARRE'S UPPER LID RETRACTOR

The retractor is a saddle-shaped appliance folded on itself, at the end of a metal handle (Fig. 24).

Use—
   (a) For examination of the eye in a child.

PLATE III

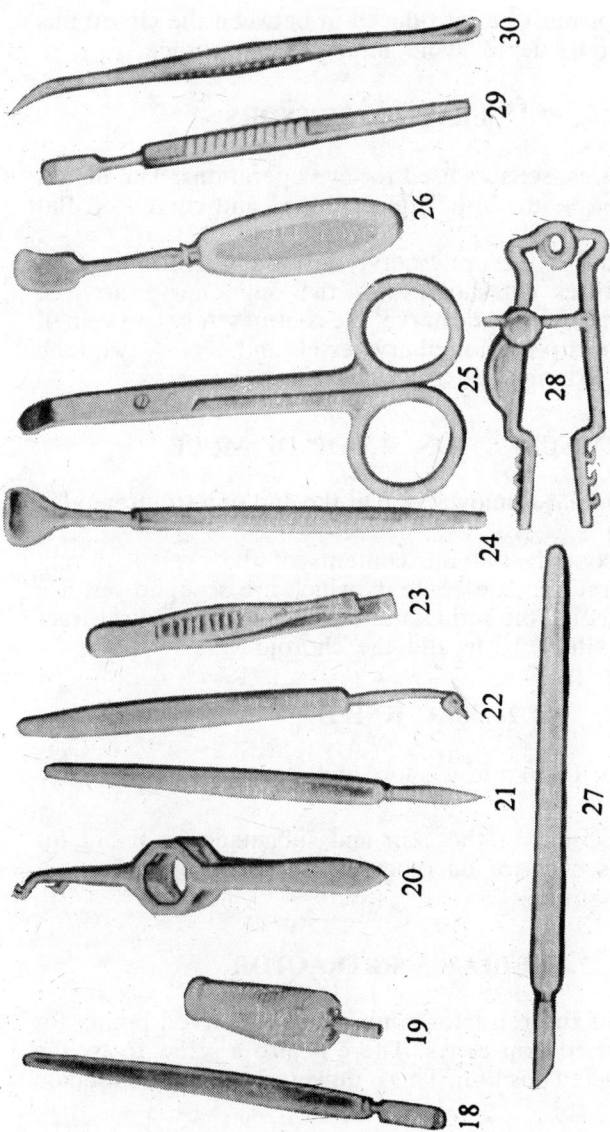

Fig. 18. Tooke's Knife. Fig. 19. Elliot's Sclero-Corneal Trephine Handle with Blade. Fig. 20. Disc-Holding Forceps. Fig. 21. Broad Needle or Paracentesis Needle. Fig. 22. Thermo-Cautery. Fig. 23. Epilation Forceps. Fig. 24. Desmarre's Upper Lid Retractor. Fig. 25. Enucleation Scissors. Fig. 26. Evisceration Scoop of Mule. Fig. 27. Sac Knife. Fig. 28. Muller's Retractor. Fig. 29. Rougine. Fig. 30. Lang's Dissector with Scoop.

(b) For examination of the eyeball when there is marked blepharospasm.

This retractor must be introduced in between the closed lids from the temporal side to avoid injury to the cornea.

24. ENUCLEATION SCISSORS

It is the stoutest scissors used for eye operations. The blades of the scissors are stout, broad, blunt-ended and curved on flat (Fig. 25).

Use—For cutting the optic nerve during enucleation operation. The structures cut along with the optic nerve are the meningeal sheaths of the optic nerve, the central artery and vein of the retina, the short posterior ciliary vessels and nerves, two long posterior ciliary arteries and two long ciliary nerves.

25. EVISCERATION SCOOP OF MULE

It is a rectangular shallow scoop at the end of a stout metallic handle (Fig. 26).

Use—For scooping out the contents of the eyeball during evisceration operation. The contents which are scooped out are the lens, the vitreous, the retina and the whole of the uveal tract comprising iris, ciliary body and the choroid.

26. SAC KNIFE

The blade of this knife is short and stout, the cutting edge being straight (Fig. 27).

Use—For incision of the skin and subcutaneous tissue for removal of the sac or for dacryocystorhinostomy operation for chronic dacryocystitis.

27. MULLER'S RETRACTOR

Each limb of the retractor contains three curved points for engaging the incised skin edges. There is also a screw to fix the limbs in the retracted position. This is universal and can be used on either side (Fig. 28).

Use—For retraction of the incised skin edges during dacryocystectomy or dacryocystorhinostomy operation.

28. ROUGINE

It has a corrugated metal handle and a small rectangular blade with a curved cutting edge, bevelled on one surface, at the end of a narrow limb (Fig. 29).

Use—For separating the lacrimal sac from the lacrimal fossa during an operation on the sac.

29. LANG'S DISSECTOR WITH SCOOP

At one end of a metal handle is a tiny oval, scoop and at the other end is a pointed dissector (Fig. 30).

Use—Following the removal of the sac, the scoop is used to scrape off the epithelium from the upper end of the naso-lacrimal duct for drainage purpose.

30. NETTLESHIP'S PUNCTUM DILATOR

It has a corrugated cylindrical handle with a conical point (Fig. 31).

Use—
(a) For dilatation of the punctum in case of congenital or acquired stenosis of the punctum.
(b) For dilatation of the lower punctum for the purpose of testing the patency of the sac.
(c) It can also be used for marking the sclera by dipping the point in gentian violet during squint or detachment operation.

For dilatation of the punctum, the dilator must be introduced first vertically and then horizontally following the direction of the canaliculus.

31. LACRIMAL CANULA

It is a slightly bent needle with a blunt point, which can be fitted to a glass syringe containing a coloured liquid or even normal saline. (Fig. 32.)

Use—To test the patency of the sac, the canula is introduced through the lower punctum into the sac. The coloured fluid is then injected into the sac and if the sac and naso-lacrimal duct are patent, the coloured fluid comes out of the nose. But if there is a block, the fluid comes out through the upper punctum.

PLATE IV

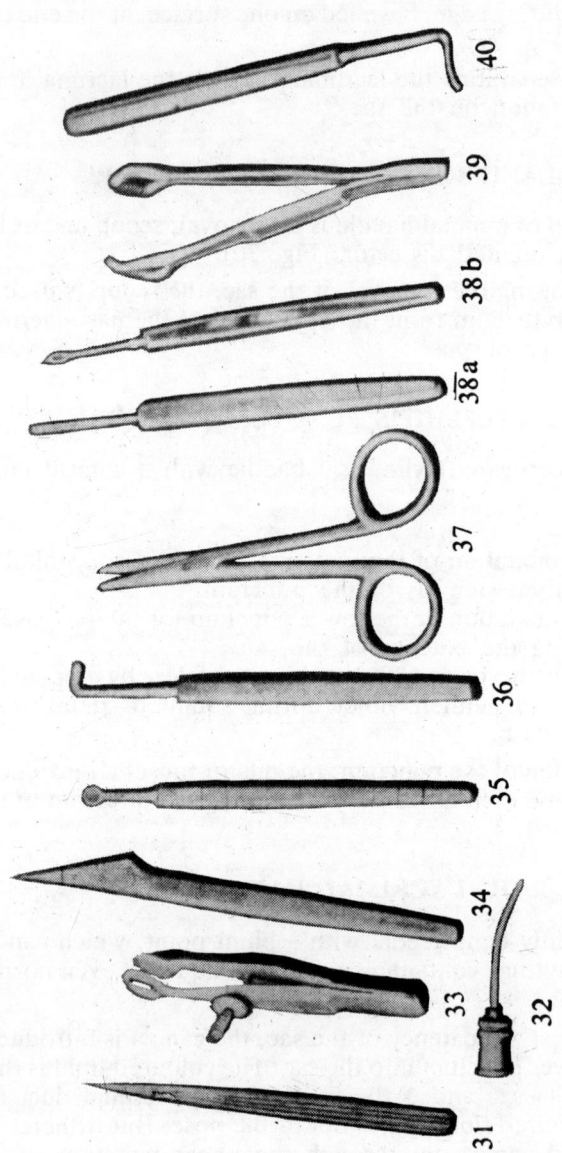

Fig. 31. Nettleship's Punctum Dilator. Fig. 32. Lacrimal Canula, Fig. 33. Chalazion Forceps. Fig. 34. Beer's Knife. Fig. 35. Chalazion Scoop. Fig. 36. Strabismus Hook or Squint Hook. Fig. 37. Strabismus Scissors. Fig. 38a. Foreign Body Spud. Fig. 38b. Fireign Body Needle. Fig. 39. Knapp's Roller Forceps. Fig. 40. Sinclair's Cyclodialysis Spatula.

32. CHALAZION FORCEPS

One limb of the forceps carries a solid blade and the other limb is fenestrated. There is also a screw for fixing the limbs like a clamp and thereby causing haemostasis also (Fig. 33.)

Use—For fixing the chalazion during an operation for chalazion. The solid blade is applied on the skin of the lid, and the fenestrated blade is applied to the tarsal conjunctiva encircling the chalazion. The screw is then tightened and the lid, thus fixed, is everted to expose the chalazion.

33. BEER'S KNIFE

The blade of the knife is big-sized and triangular with a sharp point and sharp cutting edge (Fig. 34).

Use—For incising a chalazion. The incision is vertical to avoid injury to the neighbouring Meibomian glands.

34. CHALAZION SCOOP

It is a tiny scoop with a sharp edge (Fig. 35).

Use—For scooping out the granulation tissue of the chalazion after incision with a beer's knife.

35. STRABISMUS HOOK OR SQUINT HOOK

It has a handle and a curved limb which may or may not be knob-pointed. The handle is not corrugated and the plane of the handle is the same as the plane of curvature of the limb (Fig. 36).

Use—For catching the extra-ocular muscles during squint operation, enucleation operation or operation for detachment of the retina.

36. STRABISMUS SCISSORS

The blades are straight and blunt pointed (Fig. 37).

Use—For cutting the extra-ocular muscles during the operations mentioned above.

37. FOREIGN BODY SPUD AND NEEDLE

They may be separate instruments or they may be incorporated in one instrument, being placed on both ends of a handle.

The spud is a blunt instrument and the needle has a tiny scoop like depression just proximal to the point (Fig. 38a, b).

Use—Both of them are used for removal of corneal foreign body. If the foreign body is superficial the spud is used, but if it is embedded within the corneal substance, the needle has to be used.

38. SINCLAIR'S CYCLODIALYSIS SPATULA

It is a narrow slightly curved spatula about 1 cm. long attached at right angles to a handle (Fig. 40).

Use—To separate the ciliary body from its attachment to the scleral spur during cyclodialysis operation for aphakic glaucoma.

CHAPTER XXIV

EYE OPERATIONS

Cataract Operation

It is of two types—
A. Extraction of lens—Extra-capsular or intra-capsular.
B. Discission operation or needling of the lens with suction evacuation.
C. Lensectomy through' anterior route or pars plana.

A. Extraction of Lens

Indications

(a) Mature and hypermature cataract in elderly persons.
(b) Immature cataract in elderly persons, when the vision becomes so reduced that he cannot carry on his day-to-day work.
Always one eye is operated at a time.

Investigations for extraction of lens—

1. *History*—The following points are to be elicited—
 (a) Duration of defective vision and its progress—rapid progress of defective vision followed by cataract formation, may be due to some serious affections of retina and choroid.
 (b) Any trauma or any history of previous inflammation of the eye.
 (c) Any high myopia—in high myopia the vitreous is usually degenerated and liquid. So there is risk of vitreous loss during extraction of lens.
 (d) Any history of diabetes or high blood pressure.

2. *Local investigations*—
 (a) Conjunctival swab to be cultured to detect the presence of any harmful organism in the conjunctival sac, which can cause infection of the wound after operation. If the culture report is no growth, diphtheroids or coagulase negative staphylococcus, an operation may be undertaken. But if any harmful organism like pneumococcus, coagulase positive staphylococcus or streptococcus

haemolyticus is detected, the conjunctival sac has to be made free from organisms, by suitable antibiotics, before any operative undertaking.

(b) Condition of the lacrimal sac—

If there is a frank regurgitation from the sac, the sac has to be removed, and a sufficient time has to be allowed for the conjunctival sac to be free from organisms by using proper antibiotics.

If there is epiphora and if on testing the patency of the sac a block is detected in the naso-lacrimal duct, removal of the sac is mandatory.

(c) Condition of the peripheral retina—

As an ophthalmoscopic examination is not possible due to the opacity of the lens, the function of the peripheral part of the retina is detected by throwing light into the eye from various directions. If the patient has good perception and sense of projection of light, the periphery of the retina is normal.

(d) Condition of the macula—

The function of the macula has to be tested to find out whether the patient has any chance of regaining his central vision after operation. This is necessary because in senility, there may be degenerative changes in the macula which are not visible because of the cataract.

Macular function test may be done by two methods—

(i) Cardboard test—The patient is taken in a dark room. Three or four tiny holes are made in a cardboard, which is held in front of the eye to be tested, the other eye remaining closed. A light is then thrown on the cardboard and the holes become illuminated. If the patient can detect the illuminated holes, his macula is normal.

(ii) Colour vision test—Three primary colours, i.e., red, green and blue are thrown into the eye, keeping the other eye closed. As cones are responsible for perception of colour and as the cones are present in large numbers in the macula, recognition of the colours by the patient proves that his macula is normal.

With a Maddox rod if an unbroken red line is seen then the macula is presumed healthy.

(e) Condition of intra-ocular tension—

The tension must be normal. But if the tension is raised due to accompanying chronic simple glaucoma or due to any secondary glaucoma, the tension has to be lowered either by operation or by medication, before cataract operation is done.

(f) Signs of old inflammation like presence of K.P. or posterior synechia—

If such signs are present, it has to be kept in mind that there may be inflammatory flare up following operative trauma.

(g) Condition of the lens itself—

The stage of the cataract, *i.e.*, immature, mature, intumescent or hypermature and type of the cataract have to be carefully noted, because the operative procedure to be undertaken depends on the nature and type of the cataract. Also one has to be sure that there is no subluxation of the lens.

4. *Systemic investigations*—

(a) Focal sepsis anywehere in the body, has to be removed, if possible.

(b) Evidence of diabetes mellitus—needs critical attention.

In uncontrolled diabetes, there is chance of post-operative infection and delayed wound healing.

(c) Evidence of hypertension—

In the presence of hypertension, the blood pressure has to be reduced to systolic 170 mm. of Hg and diastolic 100 mm of Hg. If operation is done in uncontrolled hypertension, there is a grave risk for expulsive haemorrhage immediately after the section is made for cataract operation.

(d) Evidence of chronic strain—

It may be manifested in the form of asthma, chronic bronchitis, emphysema, enlarged prostate or chronic constipation. If such conditions are present, they should be treated before the operation, just to minimize the strain. Because a strain of any kind invariably leads to post-operative complication like blood in the anterior chamber or prolapse of the iris.

(e) Any tendency for bleeding—

This is detected by examining the bleeding time and coagulation time.

Preparation of the patient before operation for extraction of lens

1. Tranquiliser like diazepam. 1 tablet by mouth in the night before operation.
2. Light breakfast.
3. The tablet siquil 10 mg.—one hour before the operation.
4. Eyelashes of both the upper and lower lids are to be trimmed.
5. The pupil has to be dilated with homatropine hydrobromide solution 1% by instilling every half an hour 3 times.
6. In the operation theatre—surface and block anaesthesia are to be given as follows—

   (a) Surface anaesthesia—by instilling a 4% solution of xylocaine every 5 minutes 6 times.
   (b) block anaesthesia 2% xylocaine with few drops of hyalase.
      (i) Facial block by O'brien's method 5 c.c. of 2% xylocaine injected on the neck of the mandible just below the condyle. The facial nerve becomes paralyzed, so that the patient is unable to squeeze his eyelids during operation due to paralysis of the orbicularis muscle which is supplied by the zygomatic branch of the facial nerve.
      (ii) Ciliary block—to paralyze the ciliary ganglion, 1 c.c. of 2% xylocaine is injected into the neighbourhood of the ciliary ganglion, situated near the apex of the orbit, by puncturing the skin with the injection needle, at the junction of the middle third and the lateral third of the inferior orbital margin and pushing the needle upwards, backwards and medially towards the apex of the orbit, where the xylocaine is injected. The patient must be asked to look upwards during the injection

   By ciliary block, two purposes are served, *i.e.,* lowering of intra-ocular pressure and anaesthesia of deeper structures like iris, so that no pain is felt during iridectomy.
7. Cleaning of the skin of the eyelids, lid margin and the conjunctival sac—

   (a) The skin of the lids and that over the side of the nose are cleaned by application of rectified spirit with a swab stick.
   (b) The conjunctival sac is cleaned by washing the sac with sterlie normal saline contained in a undine. After the

wash, the water on the skin is wiped off by sterile cotton-wool pellets.

8. Application of a face mask with a central circuclar hole which keeps only the eyeball exposed but covers the rest of the face.

9. Application of lid stitches and the patient is ready for operation. If stitches are applied, two lid stitches with black silk through the skin on either side of the middle of the upper lid, near the lid margin, are given and one similar stitch is applied at the middle of the lower lid. The lids are thus kept separate by pulling on the stitches. By this method, the unwanted pressure of the speculum on the eyeball is avoided.

Instruments

1. Artery forceps for the lid stitches
2. Fixation forceps.
3. von Graefe's cataract knife.
4. Elschnig's intra-capsular forceps—for intra-capsular extraction.
5. Capsulotome or capsule forceps for extra-capsular extraction.
6. McNamara spoon.
7. Lens expressor.
8. Iris forceps.
9. Iris scissors.
10. Iris repositor.
11. Needle holder, black silk and suturing needle.

Steps of operation for extraction pf lens :

The surgeon stands or sits on the head end of the patient. The globe is fixed at 6 o'clock position at the limbus and the section is made with the right hand for right eye and left hand for left eye. The section extends from 9 o'clock to 3 o'clock region at the limbus. At present more & more surgeons are using blade breaker with broken razor blade instead of cataract knife. With blade breaker and corneal scissors equally good sections are possible.

At 12 o'clock position, a preplaced 8—0 virgin silk corneoscleral stitch is given and the loop is left loose. Two peripheral iridectomies are done at 10 o'clock and 2 o'clock position.

Anterior capsule of the lens is then pinched near the lower pole with an intracapsular forceps and an upward pull is exerted with a slight side to side zigzag movement. This process is assisted with the pressure of the lens expressor over the ciliary region near the lower pole of the lens. This pull with the intracapsular forceps and push with the expressor help breaking the zonules and the lower pole of the lens tumbles and is delivered first. With further pull the whole of the lens is delivered.

Instead of intracapsular forceps a cryoprobe may be used to pull out the lens when its tip adheres due to ice formation.

Iris is reposited with iris repositor and the wound margins are brought into apposition. Sclero corneal stitch at 12 o'clock is tied. Two more interrupted stitches one at 10 o'clock and the other at 2 o'clock are applied. However more stitches or a continuous stitch may also be applied. Air is injected to reform the anterior chamber.

An antibiotic ointment is applied and the ends of the uper lid stitch is fixed on the cheek to close the eye before pad & bandage.

The application of a miotic like pilocarpine after the intracapsular operation is no longer the practice now a days as the wound in well secured with sutures.

In case the lens capsule breaks during the process of extraction the operation is completed extra capsular. In such cases the anterior chamber wash may remove the cortical matter and the left over capsule may be removed with intra capsular forceps.

Atropine drop 1% after extra capsular cataract operation is a must.

TABLE XIII

Advantages and disadvantages of intra-capsular and extra-capsular extraction of lens.

	Intra-capsular	Extra-capsular
1. Suitability	1. Immature cortical, nuclear, posterior cortical and hypermature sclerotic cataract are suitable, particularly in old people, in whom the zonule is weak.	1. Mature cortical and hypermature Morgagnian cataract are suitable.
2. Visual result.	2. Very good and the eye becomes quiet soon.	2. May not be very good due to presence of tags of capsule.

PLATE XVI

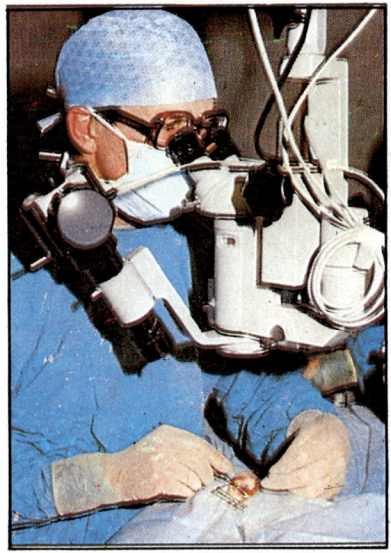

General operation view

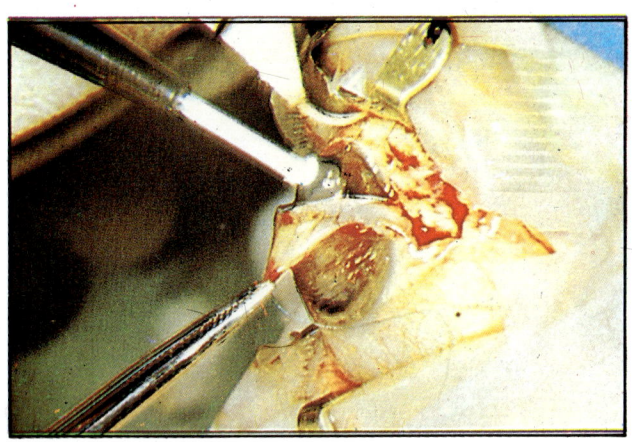

Eye Operation

(To face page 336)

| 3. Chance of after-cataract formation. | 3. Nil. | 3. Always there is a chance of after-cataract formation and consequently the necessity for a second operation of needling may arise. |
| 4. Risk during operation. | 4. Risk of vitreous loss. | 4. No risk of vitreous loss, because the intact posterior capsule protects the vitreous. |

Post-operative management after extraction of lens

First dressing is done after 24 hours. A drop of anti biotic and 1% atropine sulph is instilled into the operated eye, no matter whether the operation is by intra-capsular or by extra-capsular method. This daily instillation of atropine drop continues for one month. The operated eye is again bandaged with pad, but the other eye is kept open. Patient is allowed normal food and can walk upto the toilet.

Daily dressing and bandaging continues for seven days and after that period, limbal stitches are removed on the 10th day and dark glasses are prescribed, to avoid glare.

Bowels may be moved by enema if and when necessary.

Sponging is allowed without disturbing the operated eye.

Aphakic glasses are prescribed five weeks after the day of operation, if everything is favourable.

Complications Following Extraction of Lens

A. *Immediately during operation*

1. *Vitreous loss*—This complication occurs during intra-capsular extraction, particularly when the facial and ciliary blocks are not perfect. Any excessive pressure on the eyeball also leads to vitreous loss.

2. *Expulsive haemorrhage*—This complication is not very frequent. But it may occur as soon as the section for the cataract operation is completed, usually in the arteriosclerotic and hypertensive subjects. The sudden lowering of tension following section causes rupture of choroidal blood vessels and massive haemorrhage. The lens and vitreous are expelled along with the haemorrhage and the eye is lost.

B. *In the post-operative period*

1. *Blood in the anterior chamber*—The bleeding is from the conjunctival flap due to trauma or strain. This frequently gets

absorbed in a weeks time. If not then a paracentesis will be necessary.

2. *Iris prolapse*—A portion of the iris comes out of the wound due to strain or trauma. Very small prolapse may be treated with thermocautery or trichlor acetic acid cautery. A big prolapse needs abscission.

3. *Delayed formation of the anterior chamber*—This occurs if the wound margins ae not properly apposed or if aqueous escapes due to strain. Another frequent cause of delayed formation of the anterior chamber is detachment of the choroid. Bandaging should not be tight. Atropinisation and Diamox by mouth may help.

4. *Infection leading to iritis, iridocyclitis or panophthalmitis*— The infection may be exogenous or endogenous. Routine steroid will control iritis. Panophthalmitis should be prevented by s/c genticyn and systemic antibiotic. Once there is definite infection the prognosis is gloomy and even evisceration may be necessary.

5. *Striate keratitis*—It appears as white double lines in the cornea. This appearance is due to folds in the Descemet's membrane and occurs when there is damage to the endothelial layer of the cornea, during the extraction of the lens.

C. *Delayed complications*

1. *Aphakic glaucoma*—This complication occurs when due to prolonged delay in formation of the anterior chamber, peripheral anterior synechia are formed, thereby closing the angle of the anterior chamber. This complication also takes place when there is vitreous in the anterior chamber. A trabeculectomy may be necessary. Cyclocryo or diathermy may help.

2. *Detachment of the retina*—This occurs due to degenerative changes in the peripheral retina.

3. *Cyst formation in the anterior chamber*—A cyst forms in the anterior chamber, if by chance, conjunctival or corneal epithelium is left in the anterior chamber during operation, due to faulty reposition of the flap. This cyst formation invariably leads to secondary glaucoma which is very difficult to treat.

B. *Discission Operation or Needling of the Lens suction evacuation.*

Indications

    (a) Congenital cataract.

    (b) Traumatic cataract in children.

    (c) Any cataract below the age of 24 years.

Discission is done upto the age of 24 years, because by that age the nucleus of the lens does not become sufficiently hard for extraction. The soft lens matter is aspirated with a wide bone needle bent in the fashion of an iris repositor.

Investigations for discission operation—Conjunctival swab for culture and other local investigations as done before extraction of lens.

Instruments

1. Eye speculum.
2. Fixation forceps.
3. Bowman's discission needle or ordinary discission needle.
4. Suction syringe and aspiration needle.

Complications following discission operation

1. Secondary glaucoma—The rise of tension is due to blockage of the angle of the anterior chamber by lens matter.
2. Iritis—It is due to irritation with the lens matter or due to infection.
3. Detachment of the retina is a possibility after several years. Lensectomy through anterior route or through pars plana

Complications

(a) Vitreous may be disturbed and it may come into the anterior chamber.
(b) Infection causing iritis or iridocyclitis.
(c) Detachment of retina later on but rare.

Needling of After-Cataract

Indication—Presence of after cataract blocking the pupillary area following extra-capsular extraction of lens.

Investigation, preparation and anaesthesia

Local preparation, investigation of the eye, and anaesthesia are the same as for cataract operation, but no block anaesthesia is neccessary and the pupil is dilated with 1% atropine ointment. This operation is usually done 5-6 weeks after cataract operation when the eye becomes completely quiet.

Instruments

1. Eye speculum
2. Fixation forceps.
3. Zeigler's knife or discission needle.

Operation—The lids are separated with universal speculum. The eye is fixed with a fixation forceps and either a Zeigler's knife or a discission needle is introduced into the anterior chamber through the limbus from the temporal side. A gap is made in the after-cataract, in its central region, with the point of the needle or the knife, care being taken not to disturb the vitreous. Atropine and antibiotic ointment are applied and the eye is bandaged with a pad.

Post-operative treatment—The bandage is replaced after twenty four hours with dark glasses. 1% atropine drop is used for 1 week and then aphakic glasses are prescribed, when the eye becomes quiet.

Complication—Iridocyclitis due to traction on the ciliary body in the attempt to make a hole in the after-cataract.

Iridectomy Operations

Types of iridectomy

1. Peripheral button-hole iridectomy—

It is done during extraction of the lens and glaucoma operations to prevent iris prolapse in the immediate post-operative period.

2. Iridectomy dialysis or glaucoma iridectomy—

Indication—It is done in case of acute congestive glaucoma when medical treatment fails to control the tension within twenty four hours.

Investigation, preparation of the patient and anaesthesia—They are same as for cataract operation but the pupil is not dilated with homatropine drop. An injection of 100 mg. of pethidine before operation makes the operation painless.

Instruments

   1. Eye speculum.
   2. Fixation forceps.
   3. Keratome or cataract knife or broken razor blade.
   4. Iris forceps.
   5. Iris scissors.
   6. Iris repositor.

Operation—The eye is fixed with a fixation forceps at the limbus at 6 o'clock position and a small limbal section is made from 10 o'clock to 2 o'clock position with a cataract knife or with a keratome. The iris is pulled out at one end of the section with the iris forceps and the iris is divided from the pupillary margin upto its root. Then the cut margin of the iris is caught with iris forceps and $1/4$th of the circumference of the iris is torn off from its attachment to the ciliary body. The torn iris is then removed from

EYE OPERATIONS 341

the rest of the iris by iris scissors. The wound is made free from any tag of iris by an iris repositor. Atropine and antibiotic ointments are applied and both the eyes are bandaged with pad.

Post-operative treatment—It is the same as for cataract operation.

Complications

(a) A cataract may develop if the lens capsule becomes injured during iridectomy.
(b) Infection of the wound.
(c) Blood in the anterior chamber.

3. Optical iridectomy—

Indication

It is done to improve vision in case of central corneal opacity. The visual improvement is however not very marked.

Investigation, preparation of the patient and anaesthesia

They are the same as those for cataract operation, but the pupil is dilated with atropine.

Instruments

1. Eye speculum.
2. Fixation forceps.
3. Keratome or cataract knife.
4. Iris forceps.
5. Iris scissors.
6. Iris repositor.

Operation

After fixing the eyeball with fixation forceps, a small limbal incision is made, either with a keratome or with a cataract knife, at a downward and inward position. If clear cornea is not available in that area, the section may be made on the temporal side. With the iris forceps, a narrow segment of the iris is taken out and removed by an iris scissors. The cut margins of the iris are replaced by an iris repositor. Thus an artificial coloboma is made in the iris in the form of a false pupil. 1% atropine ointment and antibiotic ointment are applied and both the eyes are bandaged with pad.

Post-operative treatment—The operated eye is bandaged daily with pad, after application of atropine for seven days. Thereafter dark glasses are used upto one month, with daily application of atropine.

Complications

(a) Blood in the anterior chamber.
(b) Infection.
(c) Cataract formation if the capsule is injured.

4. Complete iridectomy—

Indication—It is done during extraction of the lens, if the pupil fails to dilate properly with homatropine. After the section is made, a narrow segment of the iris is removed at 12 o'clock position, with the help of an iris forceps and iris scissors. By this way the pupillary area is increased, so that the lens may be easily removed.

5. Iridectomy in the form of excision of prolapsed iris—

Indications

(a) Iris prolapse following a penetrating injury to cornea.

(b) Iris prolapse occurring as a complication following cataract operation.

The prolapsed iris should be removed, because if left outside, the highly vascular iris tissue may be infected.

Investigation, preparation of the patient and anaesthesia—They are on the same lines as for cataract operation but the pupil need not be dilated with homatropine. In case of children, general anaesthesia is preferable.

Instruments

1. Eye speculum.
2. Fixation forceps.
3. Iris forceps.
4. Iris scissors.
5. Thermo-cautery.
6. Needle holder.
7. Black silk and suturing needle.

The prolapsed iris is held with the iris forceps and removed by iris scissors. The wound is cauterized with a thermo-cautery and stitched with interrupted 8/0 virgin silk.
Atropine and antibiotic oinment are applied and the eye is bandaged.

6. Iridectomy to remove a foreign body entangled in iris—

It is not easy to remove a foreign body entangled in iris. In that case a narrow piece of iris along with the entangled foreign body is removed with iris forecps and iris scissors through a limbal incision with a keratome.

7. Iridectomy to remove a cyst or a tumour of iris—
A tumour or a cyst of iris is easily removed along with the portion of the iris which lodges the cyst or the tumour. This is also done through a small limbal incision as in case of a foreign body on the iris.

Operations for Glaucoma

The following operations are done for various types of glaucoma—
1. Paracentesis—a temporary measure for secondary glaucoma.
2. Trabeculectomy operation—for chronic simple glaucoma, chronic congestive glaucoma and buphthalmos.
3. Iridencleisis—for chronic simple glaucoma and for acute congestive glaucoma.
4. Cyclodialysis— for aphakic glaucoma.
5. Glaucoma iridectomy or iridectomy dialysis—for acute congestive glaucoma (already described under iridectomy operations).
6. Cyclodiathermy or Cyclo cryopexy for aphakic glaucoma.

Paracentesis

Indications
1. Secondary glaucoma due to acute iridocyclitis.
2. Secondary glaucoma due to burst Morgagnian cataract.
3. Secondary glaucoma due to corneal ulcer with hypopyon.
4. Threatened perforation of a corneal ulcer.
5. Severe hyphaema with secondary glaucoma.

Paracentesis is a temporary measure to lower the intra-ocular pressure.

Preparation and anaesthesia—As in cataract operation except ciliary block.

Instruments
1. Eye speculum.
2. Fixation forceps.
3. Broad needle or cataract knife or keratome.
4. Iris repositor.

Operation—The eyeball is fixed with the fixation forceps and either the point of a broad needle or a cataract knife or a keratome is introduced in the anterior chamber, for a short distance, in front of the iris, through the limbus from the temporal side. The puncturing instrument is then withdrawn. The posterior lip of the wound is depressed by the tip of an iris repositor and aqueous is drained out. Antibiotic ointment and atropine are applied and the eye is bandaged with pad. The procedure may have to be repeated, if there is again a rise of tension in the post-operative period.

Elliot's Sclero-Corneal Trephining Operation is almost replaced by the trabeculectomy and iridencleisis.

Iridencleisis

In this operation, a small piece of iris is kept entangled in a scleral wound near the limbus. the result is that the endothelial cells of iris proliferate and line the wound and the atrophied iris stroma acts like a filtering wick, along which aqueous sips out into the subconjunctival space, from where it is absorbed.

Indications—They are the same as for trephining operation. This operation can also be done for acute congestive glaucoma.

Preliminary investigations, preparations and anaesthesia are similar to those for trephining operation.

Instruments
   1. Eye speculum.
   2. Fixation forceps.
   3. Sharp-pointed straight iris scissors.
   4. Keratome.
   5. Iris forceps.
   6. Iris repositor.
   7. Needle holder, suturing needle and black silk.

Operation—A triangular flap of bulbar conjunctiva is raised as in case of trephining operation and the flap is dissected upto the limbus with sharp-pointed straight scissors. Bleeding points are checked by a thermo-cautery.

By fixing the eyeball with a fixation forceps, a keratome is introduced through the sclera, 2 mm. above the limbus at 12 o'clock position, into the anterior chamber in front of the iris. The scleral incision should be about 5 mm. long.

With iris forceps introduced into the anterior chamber through the keratome incision, the iris is caught at the pupillary margin and is drawn out. With iris scissors, the iris is cut in the 12 o'clock meridian from the pupillary margin to its root. The nasal pillar of the iris is left in the scleral wound, while the temporal pillar of the iris is reintroduced in the anterior chamber with an iris repositor.

The conjunctival flap is replaced and sutured. Atropine drop and antibiotic ointment are applied and both the eyes are bandaged, with pad.

Daily dressing with atropine and steroid antibiotic drop is supplemented with massage of the eyeball. There appears a bleb due to drainage of aqueous.

Complications

(a) Hyphaema.
(b) Infection.
(c) Rarely sympathetic ophthalmia in the other eye.

Anterior Sclerectomy

It is also a fistulizing operation for a temporary period only.

Cyclodialysis

By this operation a communication is made between the anterior chamber and the suprachoroidal space by detaching the ciliary body from its attachment to the scleral spur. The aqueous is absorbed from this space and so the tension remains under control.

Indication—Aphakic glaucoma.

Preliminary investigation, preparation of the patient and anaesthesia are the same as for trephining operation.

Instruments

1. Eye speculum.
2. Fixation forceps.
3. Straight sharp-pointed iris scissors.
4. Cataract knife.
5. Sinclair's cyclodialysis spatula.
6. Needle holder, black silk and suturing needle.

Operation—The bulbar conjunctiva is incised for 1 centimetre parallel to the limbus at a distance of 9 mm. from the limbus on the upper temporal side. The sclera is then incised for 2 to 3 mm. parallel to limbus at the same distance from the limbus, i.e., 9 mm. with the point of a cataract knife, taking care not to puncture the underlying choroid. The tip of a Sinclair's cyclodialysis spatula (*see* under instruments) is then introduced through the scleral wound and the spatula is pushed anteriorly through the space between the choroid and the sclera—the suprachoroidal space. As the spatula reaches the scleral spur, a resistance is felt. The spatula is pushed further forwards when the tip of the instrument, tearing the attachment of the ciliary body to the scleral spur, enters into the anterior chamber and becomes visible. The spatula is then moved from side to side, when the ciliary body becomes further detached for a distance of about 5 mm.

The spatula is then withdrawn and the scleral and conjunctival wounds are sutured. 1% pilocarpine nitras solution is dropped and antibiotic oinment is applied. Both the eyes are bandaged with pad.

Post-operative treatment—Application of miotic drop daily for 1 month. By miotic drop the pupil remains constricted and so the iris cannot block the new communication made between the anterior chamber and the suprachoroidal space.

Complications

   (a) Hyphaema.
   (b) Closure of the communication.
   (c) Infection.

Enucleation at the Eyeball

It means excision of the eyeball.

Indications

A. Absolute indications i.e., conditions in which if the eye is not enucleated, there is either risk for life or risk for the other eye.

1. Malignant tumour of the eyeball, e.g., retinoblastoma arising from the retina in children and malignant melanoma of the uveal tract in adults.

2. Severely injured and irritable eye with a risk of sympathetic ophthalmia developing in the other eye.

B. Relative indications, i.e., conditions in which there is no risk if the eye is not enucleated.

1. Anterior staphyloma.
2. Ciliary staphyloma.
3. Phthisis bulbi.—with ossification or calcification.
4. Any painful blind eye without sepsis.

C. Removal of eyes from dead body within 3 hours of death. This is for the collection of cornea for keratoplasty purpose.

Surgical procedure for Retina and Vitreous.

Short historical review of the operation reveals that the sealing of the retinal break was first done with aseptic inflammation with heat.

Later on diathermy was used in place of crude heat. Soon came the shortening of the globe with full thickness, scleral resection. Later it was totally replaced with lamellar scleral resection. In early 1960 there was buckling procedure with various synthetic and human tissues namely sclera, fascia lata etc. At present the buckling is usually done with silicon sponge and silicon rubber material. The buckling is done either over localised tear or all around encircling the globe between the equator and ora serrata. Buckling may also be done over the radial area. All depending upon the nature, and number of holes and the extent of retinal degeneration.

Most accepted method of operation is narrated below.

Anaesthesia : Retroublhar and facial block is given. Infiltration of all the recti muscles is done (General anaesthesia if available is certainly better).

Incision : Conjunctiva is cut with perilimbal incision with horizontal extension at 3 & 9 O' clock. The fornix based flaps are reflected. All the four recti muscles are identified and are lifted up within loops of suture. Sclera is cleaned. Four vortex veins are identified. With the measuring caliper 12 mm. to 14 mm. area from the limbus is identified and subjected to cryopexy. Loops of suture are passed through the layers of sclera at 10', 2', 5' and 7 O' clock position. Through the loops of the sutures and below the recti the silastic sponge is passed. The ends of the sponge are tied such that it produces an indentation of the sclera. Before fixing identing sponge the subretinal fluid is drained. Intra vitreal air is introduced through pars plana. Intra occular pressure is no case should be high, otherwise here in chance of collapse of the central retinal artery. Conjuctival flaps are sutured in position. Some surgeon do not prefer to drain the S.R. Fluid.

Vitrectomy

Detachment surgery in true sense is a vitreoretinal surgery. As the underlined defect is due to vitreoretinal pathology. Recently a phenomenal change has been noticed in the vitrectomy procedure.

Pars plana vitrectomy is not only safe but also very effective in conditions like vitreous haemorrhage or opacities.

The instrument used in Machemer VISC/Vitreous infusion suction cutter/or Peyman's vitrophage unit.

The tip of the VISC is introduced through the region of pars plana between 4 mm to 7 mm from the libmus. Tip of the instrument is observed through the dilated pupil with the operating microscope or indirect ophthalmoscope or co-axial illumination, through opposite side of pars plana.

Indications :
  i) Vitreous haemorrhages which is not absorved in 10 to 12 months time.
  ii) Vitreous opacities other than haemorrhage, Viz. post inflammatory.

iii) Traction detachment–diabetic retinopathy, Eales˄ disease, retinitis proliferens.

Many a time the vitrectomy over the proliferating vessels may cause fresh bleeding.

CHAPTER XXV

BLINDNESS PROFILE AND ITS CONTROL

Blindness in India: Its Prevention Cure and Rehabilitation

Though the term "Blindness" implies to loss of perception of light, from the practical point of view a person is said to be "blind" or better still "Visually handicapped" when he cannot carry on his day to day work. A person will be declared blind if he is unable to count the out stretched fingers from distance of 10 feet or if the vision is less than 3/60 in the better eye or his visual field is grossly reduced to 10° around fixation point.

Pattern of blindness in the country has changed a lot in the last 50 years. Ophthalmia neonatorum is seldom seen now a days. Small pox has been erradicated. Interstitial keratitis and tabetic optic atrophy are no longer seen. Trachoma blindness is on the decrease. Epidemic dropsy glaucoma is a matter of the past. However the blindness from cataract is on the increase today as the longivity of the population has increased. Due to the phenomenal growth of industry the ocular injuries have increased. As the diabetics are living longer so the blindness from diabetic retinopathy is also increasing. Frequent episodes of blindness are seen now a days from liquor poisoning. The iatrogenic blindness is also increasing and many useful drugs like sulphonamides, ethumbutol, chloroquine, contraceptive pills are responsible for several cases of blindness.

The last survey carried out by the I.C.M.R. is accepted as the present statistics of blind in our country. There are 9 million blinds and 45 million people are having impaired vision.
Main causes of blindness today are as follows :

Cataract	55%
Glaucoma	3%
Nutritional blindness	2%
Corneal blindness	20%
Posterior segment	
blindness	20%

80% of the total blindness is curable and good may of them are preventable. However there is gross inadequacy of trained ophthalmic personnel and infrastructure. As such the problem of the blindness is gigantic. Greemly aware of the sad situation Govt. of India has launched National Plan for the Control of Blindness (NPCB) in 1976. The aim of the plan is to provide immediate relief measure and establish permanent eye care facilities with graded experitse at different levels all over the country. As a result many primary health centres, district hospitals, medical colleges have been upgraded to render more services in the form of eye health care and manpower training. Overal supervision is done by the eight Regional Institute of Ophthalmology and the apex Institute in Delhi. Under this. National Programme for the Control of Blindness the blindness figure of 1.3% will be hopefully reduced to 0.2% by the year 2000.

Rehabilitation of the Incurable Blinds

About 15–20 per cent of 9 million blinds need rehabilitation in a special way so that they can earn their livelihood and live as useful citizens. For this gigantic task the facilities are few. There are about 100 odd blind schools in the country where there are facilities for Braille system of education. Besides this, they are trained in music, handicrafts, cane binding, book binding, candle making, chalk making, light engineering, telephone operating etc. They are also given training in poultry farming, cow keeping, and agriculture of various types. It has been experienced that the blind workers are in no way inferior to the sighted persons. As such more schools of such nature are badly needed to give the initial training necessary for rehabilitation.

CHAPTER XXVI

PSYCHOSOMATIC DISORDERS

OCULAR NEUROSES

Since most occupations are essentially visual or visuocerebral in nature the function of vision is of great importance in everyday life. Hence it is not surprising that symptoms relating to vision are common amongst those who, on account of some mental conflict, develop a psycho-neurotic disturbance.

It is, therefore, to be expected that many cases of psychoneurosis are first seen by an ophthalmologist. Correct diagnosis, advice and treatment in the early stage may avoid unnecessary radiological, pathological and other investigations, and save much valuable time.

It has been estimated that neurosis of one sort or another accounts for approximately 33 per cent of incapacity to work. It is, therefore, necessary for every ophthalmic practitioner to be familiar with the commoner neuroses and psychoneuroses. Not that it will be his job to treat the more complicated cases, because that lies within the realm of the expert psychiatrist, but it will be his duty to diagnose such condition and indeed to treat the slighter forms of anomaly, especially those of the mild 'anxiety' type.

A psychoneurosis may be defined as a manifestation of a faulty response to the difficulties which life may present. Such a faulty response may be due to inherited factors, defective training, or bad environment. There are three commoner types of abnormal reactions :

- The *anxiety reaction* (*overaction*), consisting of unreasonable fear and anxiety. Fear of blindness is commonly met with. Symptoms due to this reaction may include any or all of the sensations felt by the human body.
- The *obsessional* or *compulsive reaction*, in which the symptoms are a legion and usually grotesque, and in which there is a morbid interest taken by the patient in the working of his body. The obsessional patient does not really wish to be cured.
- The *hysterical reaction* (*underaction*), in which a subconscious wish is achieved by the production of a symptom. There is typically only one symptom presented and it consists essentially of a 'loss or defect of function'. The patient having acquired his symptom is happy and resigned.

There is no hard and fast dividing line between symptoms due to mental ill health, and those due to bodily ill health. It must therefore be constantly borne in mind that

- Symptoms due to an organic lesion may simulate those due to psychoneurosis and vice versa.
- Symptoms due to a slight organic ocular defect may be masked and distorted by other symptoms caused by a 'neurotic overlay'. Indeed a patient who suffers from an organic disease and who is of unstable nervous temperament may, if treated unsympathetically, acquire neurotic symptoms.
- Symptoms without obvious organic explanation may have some physical or physiological defect. Such symptoms must not be regarded as psychoneurotic cause without evidence of a definite psychogenic factor.

The anxiety reaction

Ocular symptoms. It should be borne in mind that symptoms such as 'blurred vision' or 'tired eyes' may be merely evidence of general bodily or mental fatigue. It is a mistake to diagnose the presence of a neurotic condition if the symptoms are readily explained on a purely physical basis. It is equally undesirable to attribute symptoms of ocular fatigue to some slight error of refraction or ocular muscle imbalance which cannot possibly bear any proportional relationship to the symptoms, or which although present, are not such as to give rise to the symptoms of which the patient complains.

Fatigue may, in a predisposed person, lead to a definite neurosis. If, in addition, such a person possesses a certain degree of ocular muscle imbalance, weakness of convergence, or some other defect of binocular vision, he is all the more likely to acquire symptoms due to the exacerbation of these conditions, especially if he is subjected to prolonged visual activity to the extent of causing gross fatigue.

Suspicion should always be aroused that a patient is probably suffering from ocular or visual symptoms of a neurotic nature if he walks into the semi-gloom of the ophthalmic consulting-room wearing a pair of dark glasses.

History. When taking the history of a case of suspected ocular neurosis (or, indeed, any ophthalmic case that presents symptoms which are not straight forward in nature) it is essential to spend considerable time, and to explore every possible channel that may help one towards one's objective—that of diagnosis and treatment.

Careful and detailed history-taking is essential. It is not necessary for the ophthalmologist, unless he has special experience, to undertake a full psychiatric history, but in order to assess the value of the signs and symptoms he should at least make a general survey of other aspects of the case besides those related to the eyes, including the domestic background, the nature of the patient's work or his general activities, whether his appetite is good and if he usually sleeps well and the presence or absence of worries. Case with obvious symptoms of psycho-neurosis and in which the ocular findings do not in any way account for the symptoms should be referred to a neuropsychiatrist for expert opinion.

Presenting symptoms. It must be remembered that the main symptom of which the patient complains may not be the most important symptom. Therefore, it is essential to interrogate the patient as to the occurrence of any other symptom. Patients who produce an interminable list of symptoms, especially if such symptoms are written on a piece of paper, should be regarded as potential hypochondriacs. On the other hand, a patient may produce only one or two trivial symptoms when in reality he has many others of a more profound nature, which for some reason he prefers not to declare, i.e., he may 'play a low card of a suit'!

Enquiry should be made as to the previous use of glasses, with details relating thereto (the 'spectacle history') and the previous ocular symptoms (if any).

If a patient gives a history of having worn glasses in early childhood, it at once makes one suspicious of the presence of either a manifest or a latent squint, which may be associated with hypermetropia or hyper-metropic astigmatism, and frequently with anisometropia, and possibly amblyopia.

Neurotic symptoms must be carefully analysed, and not confused with those due to physical or cerebral conditions.

In cases of brain tumour, especially when the tumour involves the frontal lobe, the early symptoms may be strongly suggestive of a psycho-neurosis. In some cases repeated clinical examination may be necessary before the correct diagnosis is established.

The actual visual complaints of patients suffering from an ocular neurosis vary considerably, but the following may be said to be among the more usual :

Periodic blurring of vision. The physiological explanation of this symptom occurring in a psychoneurotic individual is probably due to a relaxation of the ciliary muscle causing loss of its normal tone or its power to cause accommodation. It may be associated with weakness of convergence, in which case the presence of the following signs are strongly suggestive that the trouble is of psychoneurotic origin :

- An associated gross weakness of accommodation.
- Equal failure of both eyes to converge (as opposed to the condition in which one, or the other, eye 'fails' on the convergence test).

Blurring of vision is, however, a symptom which may be due to certain organic ocular abnormalities which must be excluded first, namely :

- Hypermetropia and hypermetropic astigmatism which has been previously uncorrected.
- Heterophoria in a state of partial decompensation, or simple convergence insufficiency.

- Cycloparalysis or cycloparesis which may occur in cases of diphtheria, or less commonly following or during the course of certain other febrile illness.
- Migraine, in which the symptoms occur in recurrent attacks typically associated with headache.

Constant blurring of vision. This, however, may be due to certain of the ocular abnormalities enumerated above, or it may be due to a localised lesion of the fundus, such as macular or paramacular retinopathy. Such lesions are usually uniocular, and a relative or absolute field defect is invariably demonstrable in the central part of the visual field.

'Watering of the eyes'. This, however, may be due to slight obstruction of the nasolacrimal ducts, or stenosis of the lower punctum or canaliculus. If the condition is unilateral, it is more likely to have an organic cause than a neurotic one.

True lacrimation is not usually a psychoneurotic symptom although a complaint of watering of the eyes, with little to show for it, is not uncommon especially in elderly people.

Photophobia. This is frequently a neurotic symptom, although it is one that may have an inherent individual cause. For instance, it is well-known that a person with fair skin and complexion not only has less pigment in his skin, but also less in his iris, choroid, and retina; hence bright light will irritate him to a greater extent than it will a normally or highly pigmented person. Furthermore patients suffering from high myopia, corneal or lens opacities, or from posterior synechia usually suffer from photophobia.

Defective night vision. During period of general stress it can be safely assumed that the vast majority of those complaining of defective night vision are either psychoneurotic persons or malingerers, especially if the alleged defect is of recent origin.

It should, however, be borne in mind that in a small percentage of cases there may be an organic explanation, e.g., pigmentary degeneration of the retina, chronic glaucoma, constricted pupils though rarely of recent origin. It may be associated with vitamin A deficiency.

Other symptoms often of psychoneurotic origin.
- Itching of the eyes
- A feeling of heat in and around the eyes
- A feeling of the necessity to close the eyes
- Constant blinking
- Aching of the eyeballs
- A feeling as if the eyes were 'on stalks'
- A feeling as if there is a film moving over the eyes
- Pain behind the eyes 'like red-hot coal'
- A feeling as if red-hot needles were being pushed into the eyes
- A sensation that, after looking at anything for a short time, it shakes up and down.

The physiological explanation of such symptoms as these is probably that they are caused by the tense and relaxed state of the musculo-skeletal system of a neurotic individual, but exaggerated to a degree consistent with his mental outlook.

Examination. No attempt is made in this chapter to deal with the purely ophthalmic examination of cases presenting symptoms of ocular neurosis, because this has been dealt with elsewhere. Suffice it to say that these cases require a careful and detailed routine examination including refraction, muscle balance tests, and tests for binocular vision. Examination of the visual fields both central and peripheral may also be required. Thorough examination in such cases is the reassurance (after such examination) that there is no sign of organic disease.

Diagnosis and treatment. As the result of a carefully taken history and a clinical examination the ophthalmologist should in the majority of cases be able to declare confidently either :

- that the symptoms are of ocular origin in which case appropriate ophthalmic treatment is recommended, or
- that there is no ocular cause for the symptoms, in which case,
  - they are due to ordinary fatigue with which there may be a mild anxiety factor (this may be brought on by excessive use of the eyes, or by bad working conditions), or
  - they are probably of psychoneurotic origin, or
- that there is a basic ocular cause for these symptoms with a 'top-dressing' of psychoneurosis.

In the second group [except in some cases in (b)] and also in the third group, provided the ocular defect is appropriately treated, treatment of the neurosis consists essentially of explanation and sympathetic reassurance. By this means the symptoms may entirely disappear. In other cases reference to a neuropsychiatrist may be necessary. It is quite useless to adopt the 'don't worry—pull yourself together' attitude towards a psychoneurotic patient, just as it is quite useless to tell him that 'there's nothing wrong with you'.

In the last group one may also include those who may be described as the 'cashers-in'. These are people who are well aware that they have an ocular defect of some sort but one which really gives rise to no inconveniencing symptoms, and which has been regarded as insufficient to render them unfit for their particular jobs. These people, when confronted with an unpleasant situation, an undesirable task, or some mental conflict, may suffer from complaints referable to, but out of all proportion to their known defect, and attempt to 'cash-in' on it and get excused the duty in question.

It should be emphasised that just as there must be adequate grounds to diagnose a case of organic disease both from the point of view of symptomatology and physical sings, so there must be adequate grounds psychogenically to diagnose a case of psychoneurosis. It must not be assumed because no organic disease is present that the symptoms described are due to psychoneurosis. It is only too commonly found that patients are diagnosed as psychoneurotic just because the doctor concerned with the case is unable to find an organic cause for the symptoms. Such cases may fall into group described as 'functional', that is to say, suffering from a 'disorder of function'. It is, however, a mistake to use the term 'functional' (as is so often done) as synonymous with 'psychoneurotic'. A 'disorder of function' may or may not have some slight underlying organic cause too subtle for detection by the ordinary clinical methods.

The following points are suggestive of a diagnosis of psychoneurosis of the anxiety type :

* Innumerable symptoms
* Grotesque symptoms
* Symptoms out of all proportions to the physical signs discovered
* The demeanour of the patient, e.g., overhelpful, openly antagonistic, or non-cooperative
* Likely motivation.

The obsessional reaction

The symptoms of patients suffering from obsessional neurosis are similar but more exaggerated than those who suffer from a purely anxiety neurosis. Obsessional patients often write all their symptoms down on a paper or arrive with innumerable pairs of glasses or with a sheaf of prescriptions from different ophthalmologists (the multiple-prescription wallah). Their chief interest in life is merely to come and recount their numerous symptoms to anyone who cares to listen. They do not really wish to be cured. They enjoy hospital outpatient departments; even sitting for hours on hard benches waiting to see the doctor has its advantage, for they can spend their time telling their waiting neighbours the full details of every illness they have ever had! Such cases are rarely curable and if their symptoms are of sufficient severity they should be referred to a psychiatrist.

The hysterical reaction

Aetiology. The patient is usually a girl or young woman, although the condition is sometimes met with in boys and men. There is usually some subconscious motivation, although this may not be obvious at first. The condition may follow an injury to one or both eyes or an injury elsewhere in the body.

Symptoms. The patient's demeanour is typically detached and indifferent and there appears to be a lack of appreciation of the apparent gravity of the symptoms. Having stated her symptoms she does not attempt to enlarge upon them or exaggerate them.

The commonest symptom is defective visual acuity, which may consists only of inability to read small print, or it may amount to complete blindness. The symptoms may be unilateral or bilateral.

Alternatively, or in addition, other symptoms may occur, such as diplopia of the uniocular type, photophobia, and blepharospasm.

Sometimes the defective vision takes the form of inability to see to read, due to dysfunction of the accommodation-convergence process (see below).

Signs.

• *Ocular signs.* The pupillary light reflex is brisk in each eye and there is no ophthalmoscopic abnormality. There may be hysterical corneal anaesthesia.

• *Other signs.* There may be other signs of hysterical hemi-anaesthesia or paralysis.

Treatment. In mild cases, when there is just a loss of visual acuity, the ophthalmologist may be able to cure the condition in one or two short sessions, provided he can prove to the patient subsequently that she can see perfectly well with the affected eye. The various tests and subterfuges employed are the same as those for malingering. In more complicated cases the advice of a psychiatrist is essential. In some cases it is difficult to be certain whether the symptoms are due to hysteria or to malingering, i.e., whether the symptoms are due to a subconscious or to a conscious effort to escape from reality. The only clear-cut difference between the two conditions is in the patient's attitude to his visual defect and his general demeanour. In doubtful cases it may be permissible to use the non-committal term 'hysteromalingering'.

Hysterical reactions involving dysfunction of the accommodation-convergence process

Two different types of hysterical reaction may involve the accommodational-convergence process. They are :

• Spasm of accommodation, associated with spasm of convergence.
• Relaxation of accommodation, associated with relaxation of convergence.

Spasm of accommodation and spasm of convergence

This condition occurs sometimes in school children (usually girls) and sometimes in young adults (usually females). However, it may occur in males—in fact many cases were met with during period of war and great stress as holocaust of 1947.

There is always an underlying psychiatric cause, which may be fairly obvious or may require detailed investigation before it can be discovered. For instance, it may occur in a schoolgirl who is being unduly pressed by her parents or teachers to work harder to pass an examination. As a defence mechanism against this pressure she produces an accommodative spasm and finds herself 'unable to see the blackboard'.

In young adult women the spasm of accommodation may occur as a defence mechanism against domestic worries.

Symptoms. Headaches, inability to see clear in the distance, and inability to read small print unless it is held close up to the eyes, are the three usual symptoms. Diplopia may occur, although it is rare since if a manifest strabismus occurs suppression usually takes place.

Clinical examination. The patient usually has a somewhat detached manner, and although obviously handicapped by her symptoms she does not appear to be unduly perturbed about them. There is lack of cooperation and when obtaining the history one gains the impression that the patient is not really trying to help.

Clinical examination is difficult because the patient appears to lack the incentive to make an effort.

Ocular posture. There may be a manifest convergent strabismus.

Cover test. This may show a latent convergent strabismus with slow recovery or it may demonstrate latent strabismus.

Ocular movements are usually rather jerky in character, and there may appear to be a defect of abduction (due to the spasm of the medial recti).

There may be a disinclination on the part of the patient to move her eyes at all and much persuasion may be required to investigate her ocular motility.

Pupils. These are usually small and may be observed to become progressively smaller when the patient is attempting to read (due to the accompanying spasm of the constrictor pupillae which contracts in association with the ciliary muscle).

Visual acuity

Snellen's test type at 6 metres. The patient is usually incapable of reading more than about 6/18 binoculary. When the vision of each eye is taken separately the vision may become progressively worse as the test proceeds, in which case if the occluded eye is observed from one side it will be seen to be in a convergent position. Uniocular visual acuity may be improved up to a point by minus spherical lenses, but even then it rarely can be corrected beyond 6/9. Binocular single vision may or may not be possible for the patient when each eye is corrected with such lenses on account of the fact that an esotropia is thereby produced causing horizontal homonymous diplopia.

Jaeger test type. The patient is usually able to read N6, but in order to do this he holds the print close up to the eyes.

Relaxation of accommodation associated with relaxation of convergence

The condition occurs sometimes in young adult women and always has a psychiatric cause. It is less common than spasm of accommodation. The chief symptoms are headache and blurred vision when reading or doing other close work. There is sometimes horizontal diplopia when viewing near objects.

The patient's demeanour is usually detached and uncooperative and there is lack of insight. Distance vision is usually normal or only slightly defective, but the patient cannot read small print without the addition of a +3.0 D spherical lens and then usually with only one eye at a time on account of the fact that one or other eye diverges when a near object is fixed.

Treatment. The treatment of these hysterical reactions consists of finding out the underlying mental conflict which is causing the trouble, and dealing with it. In many cases the help of a psychiatrist is needed. Spasm of accommodation, if not severe, may be overcome by full atropinisation and sometimes by correction of relevant refractive errors.

Malingering

When considering ocular neurosis in all its manifestations, one must include malingering. Although the definition of a malingerer is 'one who consciously and purposely (in order to deceive, to evade responsibility, or to derive gain) feigns illness and voluntarily tries to produce signs and symptoms which he really does not have' (invention), the term 'malingering' must be extended to include exaggeration, perseverance (in which symptoms are alleged to persist although the genuine symptoms have disappeared and the lesion has healed) and transference in which symptoms are fraudulently attributed to some cause which entitles the patient to benefit, although he knows that they are due to some other cause). The patient is usually a man and it is usual to find that there is a history of an injury received at work for which the patient considers he should receive compensation. His manner is usually rude, blustering, argumentative, and antagonistic.

The commonest ocular symptom is that of blindness or of gross defect of vision.

It is, therefore, necessary to consider the various tests that may be employed to prove that the patient has good vision.

Detection of malingering. The detection of simulated uniocular blindness is usually easy. One of the following tests may be employed :

- Place a light or other object 4.5 or 6 metres in front of the patient, and put a prism of 60, base upward or downward, before the sound eye; if the patient admits seeing double, it is an indication that vision is present in both eyes.
- With the light in the same position, cover up the supposed blind eye. Then produce uni-ocular diplopia by moving 6-degree prism, base upward or downward, until the apex corresponds to the centre of the pupil. Next uncover the blind eye, and at the same time move the prism until it covers the entire pupil. If then there is still double vision (which must obviously now be binocular diplopia) it is evident that both eyes see.
- Place a strong convex lens (+12 D) before the good eye and a weak concave lens (−0.25 D) in front of the supposed blind eye, and

direct the patient to read the distant test types; if he succeeds, it is proof of malingering, since it is impossible for him to see with the sound eye when it is covered by the strong lens.

• Show the patient picture or letters on the Bishop Harman diaphragm apparatus taking care that he keeps both eyes open. Patients frequently do not recognise that they are seeing the left-hand letter with the right eye and vice versa, and may well read only the letter seen by the pretended blind eye and refuse to acknowledge that they see the letter seen with the sound eye.

• Show the patient a pair of fusion pictures in the amblyoscope or synoptophore, e.g., the rabbits. If he sees both the 'controls' (the tail and the bunch of flowers) he clearly has good vision in each eye. There are also special slides—the flag series with sentences on them which in order to make sense, have to be read partly by one eye and partly by the other. The size of the accurate measurement of visual acuity can be made.

• Using the Javal series of stereograms in the Holmes stereoscope the patient is asked to read the print in front of his eyes. The sentences can only be completed if both eyes are employed.

• FRIEND test consists of the letters F R I E N D printed in alternate green and red letters and illuminated from behind. The patient wearing red and green glasses (red glass in front of the right eye and green glass in front of the left eye) is asked to read the letters. The red and green glasses and the red and green letters must be of complementary colour. If he reads all the letters he is obviously using both eyes. If he only reads the letters F I N he is only using his left eye and if he reads only R E D he is only using his right eye.

It is rare for a patient to simulate blindness in both eyes, and such a condition is more difficult to select to detect. In some cases malingering is suspected when there is an absence of agreement in the result of the functional and objective examination of the eyes, contradictory statements regarding the different steps in the functional examination, and brisk reaction of the pupils to light in cases of the absolute blindness, the lesion in such cases being situated in the visual cortex or in the visual tract between the lateral geniculate bodies and the visual cortex. In feigned binocular blindness a close watch must be kept on the patient when he thinks he is free from observation and the following test may be employed :

Place a light in front of the patient; hold a 6-degree prism, base outward, before one eye; if both eyes see, the one covered by the prism will move inward in order to avoid diplopia; on removing the prism, the eye will move outward, the other eye remaining fixed.

Defective vision of one eye may be due to a neglected squint, or to other causes of amblyopia exanopsia. Blindness of both eyes without ophthalmoscopic signs may occur immediately after a head injury.

In case of doubt examination may have to be repeated after a short interval of time before a definite diagnosis can be made.

It is more common for a patient to exaggerate some impairment of vision than to feign blindness, and such cases are often not easy to detect. One has to rely very largely on the consistency of the patient's answer in response to examination repeated under varying conditions, before coming to a decision as to his veracity. For example, he may only read 6/18 at the 6-metre distance; but later if asked to read the same types at a distance of 4 metres (when he should be able to read the 6/12 line) he may still only read the 6/18 line or read 6/6 line which indicates that his replies cannot be trusted.

Traumatic neurosis

This is really a misnomer, for trauma alone cannot be a cause of neurosis. The condition occurs following an injury or accident in circumstances which may render someone liable to pay monetary compensation to the sufferer. In civilian practice the condition may appear as a sequelae to a road, rail, or industrial accident in respect of which legislation has made compensation payable.

The patient's symptoms may be unrelated to the physical injury present or may consist of an exaggeration of the symptoms. The dominant features usually combine those of the anxiety neurosis and of the hysterical reaction.

A doctor can often do much to ward off the development of a psychoneurosis by allaying alarm and despondency and by maintaining a dispassionate attitude in his assessment of the patient's disability and the prognosis.

Once the legal claims are settled to the satisfaction of the patient rapid improvement of symptoms usually occur.

In the case of injury occurring at sports or games the sufferer usually minimises his symptoms. shows no grievance and neurosis rarely ensues.

CHAPTER XXVII

LASERS IN OPHTHALMOLOGY.

HISTORICAL

Laser (Light Amplification by Stimulated Emission of Radiation) was originally popularised as death ray in the warfare. It is actually a ray of hope in medical practice.

Einstein first described Laser in 1916 but it was in 1960 that the first practical solid state Ruby laser was constructed by Maimon.

The basic principle of Laser is that molecules of any substance oscillate and emit light at a certain frequency. A highly concentrated form of light can be coaxed out if the substance is stimulated with energy, be it mechanical heat, electric or even intense light of the same frequency. The coaxed light is called **Laser**. Most often the energy used is electric current.

Laser may simply be conceived as a device that converts electric energy to light energy emerging as a monochromatic coherent light that can be directed to a desired target. The emitted light is a radiational energy in the nature of monochromatic light, the colour and wavelength of which depends upon the substance in which the electric energy is passed. It can be so directed and targeted as to produce a selective destruction of the tissue by monochromatic laser light. Laser, a pin-point beam of light, in surgeon's skilled hands has revolutionised treatment techniques of medicine in general and ophthalmology in particular. In ophthalmology the state of the art is quite advanced.

Characteristics

The unique characteristics of lasers are :

- Various Laser wavelengths are selectively absorbed by different tissues resulting in different penetration, protection and destruction.
- The depth of penetration beam can be precisely regulated and varied.
- Laser surgery can be performed without the least traction on the target tissue.
- Systemically introduced dyes and chemotherapeutic agents can create enhanced absorption of the lasers in selective tissue.

Effective usage

The most effective use of a laser depends upon the proper selection of wavelength, power and pulse duration as well as the absorption characteristics of the tissue being treated. One of the most important factors is the way specific ocular tissue interacts with laser energy. This interaction dictates the type of tissue response, whether primarily thermal (coagulative or non-coagulative), disruptive (ionic) or photoablative.

Properties

The useful properties of laser light include its monochromism, its coherence, its collimation, its ability to be concentrated in short time intervals (Q-switching) and its ability to produce non-linear effects.

Theory

Classical Bohr theory on atomic energy elucidates that each electronic orbital is spaced by a definite energy interval. Substance which has the ability to lase has the unique property of transferring electrons from one orbital of lower energy to a second metastable orbit of higher energy (Fig. 27.1), they may suddenly jump to a lower energy level which was their original level energy. This jump from original orbital (lower energy level) to metastable orbital (higher energy level) and back to original level causes the emission of a new light energy (photon) of a particular wavelength and phase (laser light). This light energy has a singe wave-

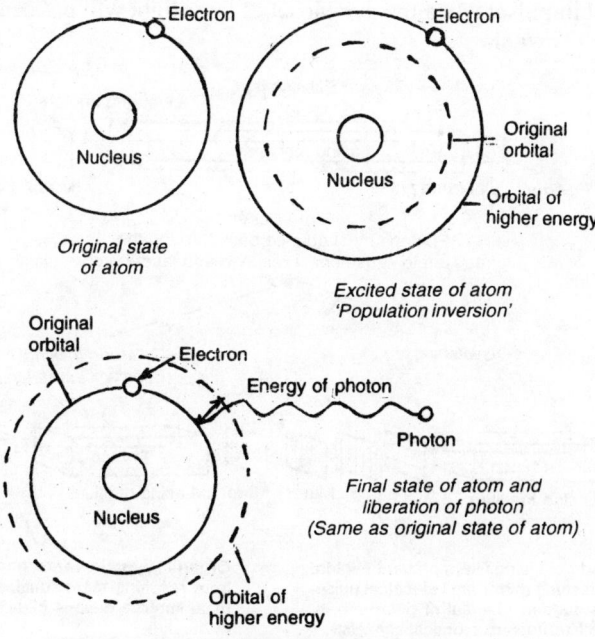

Fig. 27.1. Electronic orbitales.

length corresponding to the exact energy difference between the metastable orbital and the original orbital. It is *coherent* because all electrons jump at the same time and thus form a light wave which begins at the same time and is therefore, in the same place. The light then oscillates back and forth within the laser cavity (tube with a mirror at either end; one mirror is highly reflective and the other mirror allows source laser light to pass through for use in the eye). Because the light is oscillating back and forth within a long tube it tends to produce a beam of almost parallel rays of light with hardly any or a very low divergence and hence is said to be *collimated*.

Modes

The need in laser therapy is to further concentrate the laser light into a small time interval such as by quality switching (Q-switching) which may be active* (Q-switching) or passive (Mode-locking). The active quality switching (Q-switching) is performed by an acoustic-optical crystal (Fig. 27.2). The laser light is prohibited from further passage through the laser train by a polarizing filter oriented at 90° to a second polarizing filter. This second polarizing filter is an acoustic-optical crystal which suddenly changes its orientation by 90 degrees with the proper electrical impulse.

In passive Q-switching (mode-locking) the laser light is prohibited from passage due to a dye which has the property of bleaching with an electrical impulse; when the dye bleaches laser light will pass and it also acts as a Q switch.

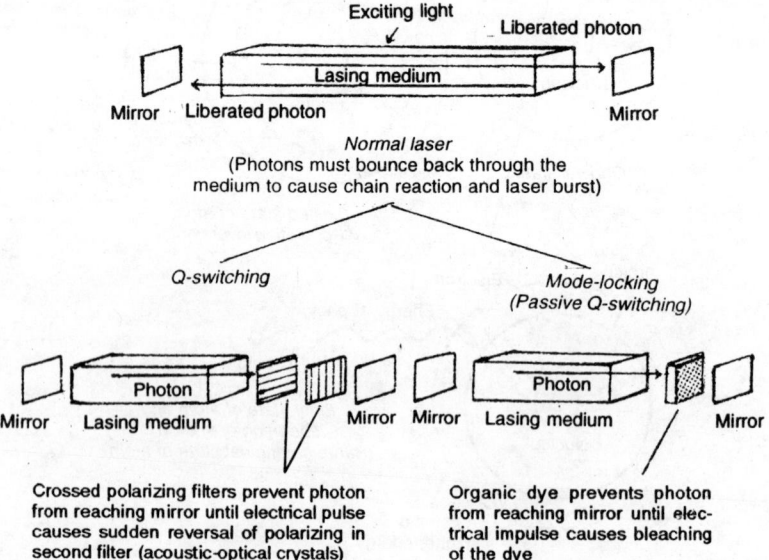

Fig. 27.2. Acoustic quality switching.

Mode locking can be performed much faster than active Q switching. Passive mode locking produces pulses of the order of 10^{-12} (picoseconds) while active Q switching does so in the order of 10^{-9} seconds (nanoseconds).

Nomenclature

The nomenclature of lasers depends upon the lasing medium, e.g., Argon, Krypton, Ruby, etc. The commonly used lasers are classified in Table 27.1.

Table 27.1. Commonly used ophthalmic lasers

Type	Maternal	Wavelength (nm)	Output	Clinical uses
I. Thermal	Argon	488-514	3.5 (W) to 1.5 (W)	Iridectomy Trabeculo-plasty Pan-retinal photo-coagulation Macular photo-coagulation Focal retinal photo-coagulation
	Argon/ Krypton Dye Lasers	Argon 488-514 Krypton 647	Argon 3.5 (W) to 1.5 (W) Krypton 1.5 (W) to 0.75 (W)	Pan-retinal photo-coagulation Macular photo-coagulation Focal photo-coagulation
II. Photo-disruptive	Nd-YAG	1064	0.50 to 15 (mJ)	Posterior capsulotomy Vitreous surgery Congenital glaucoma goniotomy Iridectomy
	Erbium-YAG	1540 nm		
III. Photo-ablators	Excimer	193 nm	160-180 mJ per sq. cm	Radial keratotomy Sclerostomy

Clinical application of thermal lasers

Aims

The aim of these lasers is to close blood vessels, to cause tissue necrosis and to create retino-choroidal adhesions.

To close blood vessels. The most important condition treated by this procedure is the diabetic retinopathy with pan-retinal photocoagulation. Argon laser blue-green range is employed for the purpose.

The neo-vascular attenuation from extensive panretinal photo-coagulation is probably due to decreased metabolic requirements, i.e., the ischaemic retina, with a subsequent decreased release of an angiogenic substance. Decreased requirement of oxygen seems to be the key factor. This mechanism by no means has been proved but is only a stipulation. The exact mechanism is still not fully understood.

Pan-retinal photocoagulation is an indirect method of treatment for retino-vitreal neovascularisation. It is achieved by using large sized spots of 500-1000 μ for 0.1 to 0.2 seconds.

Argon lasers

Argon blue and blue-green lasers are the most used of all the available lasers. A laser tube preferably beryllium oxide tube is filled with argon gas at a precise pressure level. When a current in the form of electrons passes across the tube, the argon gas emits blue-green light. The exact mechanism of achieving this has been described earlier. The emitted light is collected by mirrors at the either end of the tubes and delivered to a slit lamp through a fibre optic cord. Argon green laser are less harmful than argon blue or argon blue-green ones. Photochemical (non-thermal) absorption is higher with shorter wavelengths (blue) which is absorbed by yellow pigment of macula and is thus likely to produce damage to inner layers of the retina (Figs. 27.3 and 27.4).

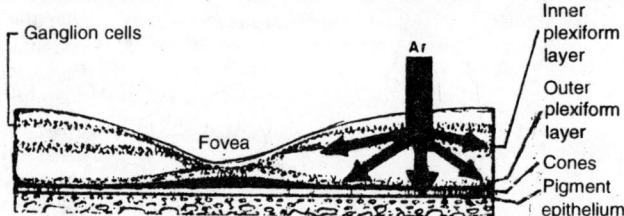

Fig. 27.3. Scattering of argon beam in tissues.

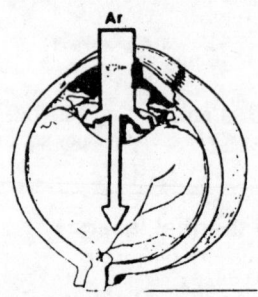

Fig. 27.4. Scattering of argon beam in the eye.

Pan-retinal coagulation. The aim of pan-retinal coagulation is to cover a defined area of retina with burns placed half a burn width apart. The treatment covers the retina extending 2 disc diameters from the centre of the macula superiorly, temporally and inferiorly. On the nasal side from one-half disc diameter nasal to the optic nerve head to or just beyond the equator. It is preferable to perform pan-retinal photo-coagulation in not less than 2 settings. In diabetic retinal study conducted the procedure was carried out in 3 settings with spot size of 500 microns and exposure time of 0.1 seconds. The power should be regulated to produce mild intensity burns. It will vary between 400 milliwatts to 2000 milliwatts and the exposure of 0.1 to 0.2 seconds depending upon the clarity of the media, the amount of retinal oedema and the density of the pigment in pigment epithelium. The number of spots required to cover the projected area is about 1200 to 1600. It is probably better to initiate the burns in nasal half of the retina (Figs. 27.5 and 27.6) and the treatment at each sitting should be confined to the areas between the major blood vessels, i.e., the upper and lower branches of the nasal branch of the central arterial and retinal veins. In the second sitting the remainder of the retina is treated starting posteriorly and adding burns progressively more peripherally out at least to the equator.

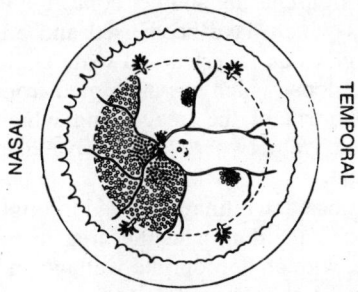 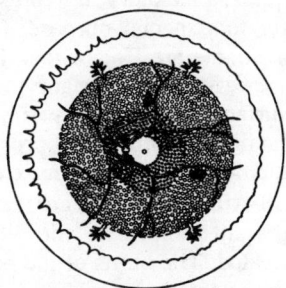

Fig. 27.5. Burns in the nasal half.   **Fig. 27.6.** Burns covering rest of retina.

To avoid blood vessels it would be better to use smaller size of burns say 200 microns or so posteriorly and to increase the size going up to 1000 microns towards the periphery. One can start the laser in the lower half first and then in the upper half.

The technique is very useful in diabetic retinopathy and central vein occlusion. For a branch vein thrombosis sectorial retinal coagulation be done in the area of drainage of the vessel.

Feeding vessels and fronds on the other hand are treated by direct treatment.

Techniques. After good local and regional anaesthesia (retrobulbar) the patient is seated on the slit lamp of laser (Fig. 27.7). Initial settings

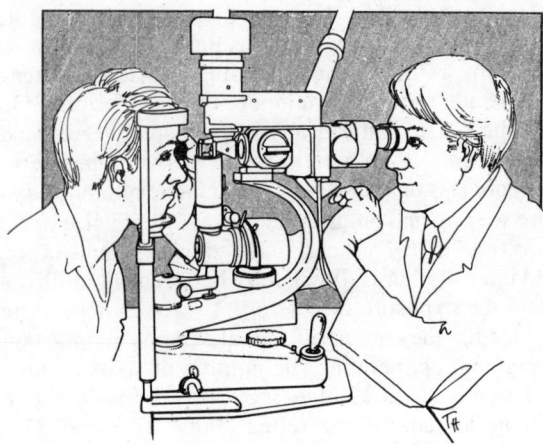

Fig. 27.7. Patient seated on the slit-lamp of the laser. (*Courtesy* : Dr. N.K. Pattnaik)

as programmed for initial spot size, burn duration and power are made. A contact lens is applied to the cornea. Goldmann's three mirror lens is quite satisfactory. It avoids the need for purchasing another contact lens for this special purpose. Other lenses which have been used and are available are Rodenstock lens which gives an inverted and wide angle view; Mclean prismatic fundus contact lens, which has an angled front surface providing a prismatic displacement of the image, and which facilitates applying burns to the area from two to about five disc diameters from the centre of the macula.

After the fundus contact lens is in place, the retina is viewed through the slit lamp. The slit beam is adjusted to illuminate the area to be treated. The burns of the required size, with an appropriate wattage and the selected time are applied as described earlier (size 200-1000 microns, power 400 to 2000 milliwatts and time 0.1 to 0.2 seconds).

It may be necessary to treat the feeding vessels and fronds. The spot size varies from 400 µ to 600 µ and the duration of spot is 0.2 seconds which may be extended to as much as 0.5 seconds when retrobulbar anaesthesia is used. High intensity lesions are applied first to occlude the artery then the vein. If the vessels are not occluded, they may be retreated after two to three weeks. The treatment should be avoided if the feeders are too large.

Macular photocoagulation can also be done in cases of neo-vascular sub-retinal membranes which are producing symptoms such as metamorphopsia. Krypton laser is chosen when the sub-retinal neo-vascular membrane is closer than 200 microns to the fovea. The krypton red laser is set at 0.5 seconds with a 200-500 µ spot and the energy level of 200 to 500 milliwatts depending upon the clarity of the media and the biologic nature of the fundus.

A slight degree of pressure on the contact lens is exerted in order to slow down the choroidal circulation and to stabilise the eye.

In all those cases a preoperative fluorescein angiography is necessary to detect a discrete source of neovascularisation (sub-retinal neovascularization—SRN). If such a situation exists the choice of laser should be argon green and the sub-retinal neovascularization should be taken care of first.

Localized macular oedema. Focal treatment of localized macular oedema is applied to the sites of specific leakage associated with macular oedema. The aim is to place moderate intensity burns over sites of discrete leakage demonstrated on a fluorescein angiogram and to at least whiten the background behind these leaks but preferably to darken the blood if there is a leaking microaneurysm. It may be desirable to at least whiten the walls of the microaneurysms. The blue-green or green argon laser should be chosen for the purpose. Some people prefer to use yellow light produced by the tunable dye laser (575 nm).

Krypton red light is unsuitable for this purpose. The size of spot can vary from 50-200 microns with a power varying from 250-600 milliwatts and for the duration of 0.1 seconds.

It is better to initiate by applying the 200 micron spot to clusters of aneurysms away from the centre of the macula producing mild to moderate white burn behind the lesion. The size is gradually reduced to 100-50 microns as the macula is being approached and near the walls of microaneurysms which have not been whitened. There is no need to treat the microaneurysms which are not filled with fluorescein dye. All red spots and haemorrhages need not be photocoagulated and laser treatment should be given only to those microaneurysms which are filled with fluorescein dye.

The lesions that need particular attention are :
* Discrete points of retinal hyperfluorescence or focal leakage 500 microns or more from the centre of macula.
* Focal leakage of 300 to 500 microns from the centres if visual acuity is 6/12 or worse and their leakage has persisted in spite of treatment further from the centre.
* Areas of diffuse leakage (either due to microaneurysms or diffuse leaking capillary bed).
* Thickened zones of capillary bed drop out.

Diffuse macular oedema. In cases of diffuse leakage from the retina or sites of thickening in zones of capillary bed drop out, a macular grid treatment is desirable. The aim of the treatment is to place small, mild intensity burns in an evenly spaced pattern one burn-width apart extending from 500 microns to 3000 microns from the centre of the macula.

The lasers used can be argon green laser, krypton red laser or yellow colour of tunable dye laser.

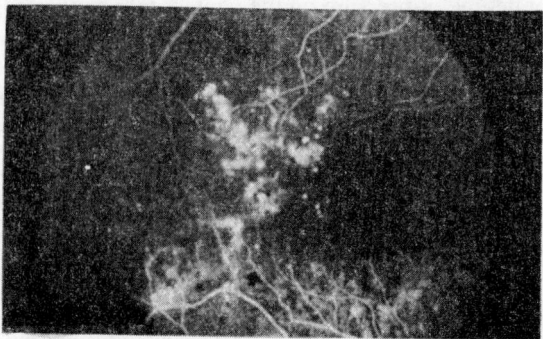

Fig. 27.8. Fluorescein angiographic picture.

A fluorescein angiography should be performed and an enlarged fluorescein angiographic picture (Fig. 27.8) is put on display during the time of treatment for ready reference.

Spot size varies from 50-200 microns, the smaller the better. The power should vary from 75 to 300 milliwatts and the exposure time should not exceed 0.1 seconds.

Burns are applied to a portion of the area selected for treatment that is farthest from the centre of macula. The power is adjusted until the desired end point of a pale white burn is achieved. Having adjusted the power, the size and the time of exposure such burns are placed over the entire affected area at intervals of one burn apart. The macular area 500 microns from its centre in all directions is spared. The farthest area is about 2 disc diameters or 3000 microns from the centre of the macula (Fig. 27.9).

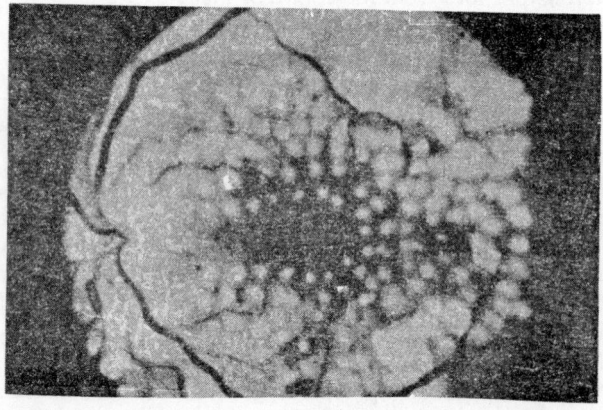

Fig. 27.9. Area of macula treated.

Other retinal conditions which are amenable to laser treatment and the lasers effective against them are given in Table 27.2.

These lasers particularly the argon-green laser can be used to seal retinal holes and tears in the retinal detachment.

The lasers are used to cause tissue necrosis in certain retinal diseases and they are summarised in Table 27.3.

The conditions in which lasers are used to close the blood vessels are tabulated in Table 27.4.

LASER IN GLAUCOMA SURGERY

Peripheral iridectomy

In acute angle closure glaucoma a peripheral button hole iridectomy releases the pupillary block and allows free flow of aqueous humour from posterior to the anterior chamber. The angle is opened up and the tension is stabilised.

Photo-disruptive process

On the same principle a peripheral iridectomy is performed in these cases using Nd-YAG laser through a photodisruptive process. Some laser experts use initially a thermal process to evaporate the selected site of iris by half its thickness and then complete the perforation of iris by a photodisruptive process.

The patient's eye is anaesthetised locally by xylocaine. If the patient is apprehensive of pain a retrobulbar injection may be given.

The patient after anaesthesia sits on the laser with chin on the chin rest. An Abraham contract lens (Fig. 27.10) is then inserted (many other contact lenses are available).

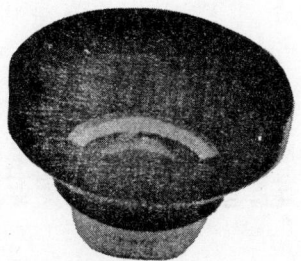

Fig. 27.10. Abraham contact lens.

Laser iridectomy should always be performed beneath the upper lid if possible. Often the patient may be required to look down in order to centre the area for iridectomy in the contact lens. Centering the iridectomy in the contact lens is essential to avoid astigmatic aberration and distortion of laser beam sometime leading to zones of optical breakdown at each end of the Sturm's conoidal interval. Iridectomy

Table 27.2.

Lesion	Laser	Parameters of lasers	Sittings
1. Diabetic retinopathy	Argon green laser, Krypton, Tunable dye	Pan-retinal coagulation. Spot size 500 microns. Power : 300-500 milliwatts if media is clear; 400-1600 milliwatts if media is hazy. 0.1 to 0.2 seconds but may be 0.2 to 0.5 seconds if media is very hazy.	2 to 3 sittings at the interval of at least one week.
2. Macular lesions	Argon green, Yellow tuned dye laser	Focal. Spot size 50-200 microns. Power 250-600 milliwatts. Time 0.1 seconds or less. Diffuse. Spot 50-200 microns. Power 75-300 milliwatts. Time not to exceed 0.1 seconds.	Initiate by 50 microns and decrease the size as one proceeds towards centre of macula. Display of fluorescein angiogram is a must.
3. Central retinal vein occlusion	Argon green, Krypton red, Tunable dye yellow	Spot 500 to 1000 microns. Time 0.1 seconds. Power 400-1600 milliwatts.	Same as for pan-retinal coagulation in diabetic retinopathy.
4. Branch retinal vein occlusion	Argon green, Krypton red, Tunable dye yellow	Parameters are the same as for central vein occlusion except that it is limited to the sector of involvement.	
5. Eales's diseases	Argon green, Krypton red, Tunable dye yellow	Same as for pan-retinal coagulation.	Limited to the periphery of the retina.
6. Miscellaneous causes of neo-vascularization (non-diabetic)	Green argon, Krypton red, Tunable dye laser	Spot size 500 μ one half burn apart. Power 400-800 milliwatts. Time 0.1 to 0.2 seconds	Better to treat them as is done in diabetic photocoagulation except the burns given in the previous column.

Table 27.3. Lasers in retinal diseases to produce tissue necrosis and chorio-retinal adhesions

Lesions	Spot size	Duration	Power
To cause tissue necrosis			
1. Central serous retinopathy	100 μ or so	Short 0.05 seconds	75-200 milliwatts
2. Retinal pigment epithelial detachment	200 μ or so	0.05-0.1 sec.	300-500 milliwatts
3. Retinoschisis	500 μ	0.1 sec.	300-500 milliwatts
4. Retinal tumours	500-2000 μ	0.5 to 2 sec.	150-1000 milliwatts
5. Choroidal tumours	500-2000 μ	0.5 to 2 sec.	150-1000 milliwatts
To create retinochoroidal adhesions	500-2000 μ	0.1-0.2 sec.	300-500 milliwatts

Table 27.4.

Lesions	Suggested spot size	Suggested duration	Suggested power
1. Sub-retinal neo-vascularization			
(a) Thin	200 μ	0.05-0.1 sec.	400-1000 milliwatts
(b) Thick	200 μ	0.2 sec.	400-1000 milliwatts
2. Retino-vitreal neo-vascularization			
(a) Pan-retinal photocoagulation	500-1000 μ	0.1 to 0.2 sec.	300-500 milliwatts
(b) Direct			
(i) Feeding vessels	500 μ	0.2 to 1.0 sec.	400-1000 milliwatts
(ii) Fronds	50 μ	0.1 sec.	400-1000 milliwatts
3. Large abnormal blood vessels as in Coat's disease	500-1000 μ	0.2-1.0 sec.	Variable
4. Small abnormal vessels macular oedema exudates	100 μ	0.1-0.2 sec.	250-1000 milliwatts
5. Vascular tumours			
(a) Direct	500 μ	0.2-0.5 sec.	25-150 milliwatts
(b) Feeding vessels	500 μ	0.2-0.5 sec.	400-1000 milliwatts

should not be performed in the palpebral opening area to avoid diplopia. The iridectomy should be placed as peripherally as possible preferably under the arcus senilis area.

The laser beam is focused on the appropriate area of the iris with energy level of 6 mJ or more but certainly below 10 mJ and a single shot is placed. Usually this is sufficient to cause through and through perforation.

If a multimode is available it should be employed to produce the largest hole possible. The minimum pulses should be 4 and a Q switch should be used.

The iridectomy thus performed by Nd-YAG laser is superior to one performed by argon green laser which is not being described.

The following complications are likely but not quite common if proper choice of power, size and pulse bursts are employed.

Haemorrhage, cataract, persistent iritis with posterior synechiae, corneal decompensation and incomplete or inadequate iridectomy especially in pigmented individuals.

Trabeculoplasty

Mechanism of action

Laser treatment causes localized zones of scarring in the trabecular meshwork rather than create permanent holes.

Technique

Anaesthesia. Topical anaesthesia is sufficient in most cases but retro-bulbar anaesthesia may be supplemented in nervous and non-cooperative patients.

Contact lens. Coated single mirror Goldmann's contact lens is used. The anterior surface of the lens is coated to reduce the possibility of laser beam reflection to the observer's eye and its damage.

Laser beam. The laser beam should be precisely aimed and it should be focused using smallest spot size and checking to see that it appears round and not ovoid. The treatment should only be started when both the view of the angle structures and the focus of the laser beam are perfect. In the presence of cloudy cornea and aqueous it is not possible to utilise this mode of treatment. The spot size is usually 50 μ and the exposure time of 0.1 seconds. The power setting will however differ according to the pigmentation of the angle structures. The power setting in our country should be around 300-500 milliwatts (mW) but in lightly pigmented areas of trabecular meshwork it could go up to 750 mW or even higher if the goal is to produce a visible effect without large bubbles or explosion. The initial spot is made and the energy level is assessed. The pigment is partially destroyed. If the patient complains of pain the power is reduced. The power setting will require to be changed as the pigmentation in different parts of the angle is not constant. One should constantly monitor the effect of the energy delivered.

Spot size and interval. Usually a spot size of 50 μ is sufficient and the interval between the shots is 5-6 times the width of the spot. The aim is to deliver about 100 spots in 360°.

In eyes with very high tension the treatment should be carried out in 2 to 3 settings delivering spots in an area extending to 180°-120° as post-operative rise of tension may otherwise abolish the small visual field of the patient. For the shift to the next sitting or even to rotate the goniolens in the same sitting one should end at an anatomically distinguishable mark, i.e., where the spot may lead to a depigmentation or where an area of high pigmentation is beginning. The same should be recorded on the case sheet for the next sitting if the treatment is being given in more than one sitting.

The angle view should always be good which can be achieved by constantly changing the angle of the light or if the patient is cooperative and intelligent by asking the patient to move his eye a little to the right or left, up or down as the need be.

In narrow angle glaucoma cases one should always perform peripheral iridectomy in the first sitting to open up the angle and perform trabeculoplasty in the next sittings.

As far as possible two eyes should not be treated at the same sitting. The treatment should always be started in the inferior portion of the angle as otherwise if some bleeding occurs, which is very unlikely, the blood will trickle down and obscure the angle view inferiorly necessitating the postponement of part of treatment till the angle view becomes clear which is undesirable.

Post-operative follow-up. The preoperative regime of medical treatment should continue in order to keep the pressure stabilised. Tension should be recorded 3 hrs, 24 hrs, 3 days and a week later by which time the reactionary tension should subside.

Pre-operative and post-operative corticosteroids are given to reduce the inflammatory reaction which inevitably follows. This has the effect of raising the intraocular pressure in the post-operative period particularly in patients who are corticosteroid responders. To prevent this from happening carbonic anhydrase inhibitors should be given (Acetazolamide 250 mg two to three times a day) in the immediate post-operative period besides continuing the preoperative medical regime as described above.

Post-operative complications. The complications may be early or late as under :

Early complications are :

• Elevation of intraocular pressure.

• Progressive visual field loss.

• Iritis.

• Transient blurred vision.

• Peripheral anterior synechiae.

• Haemorrhage.

- Transient corneal burns.
- Pupillary distortion.
- Angle closure glaucoma.
- Cystoid macular oedema.

Late complications are :

- Worsening of existing glaucoma.
- Corneal endothelialization of the trabecular meshwork of angle of anterior chamber.
- Iris atrophy.
- Late rise of intraocular pressure.

Early complications

Elevation of intraocular pressure. It is a transient rise in the intraocular pressure which may cause visual field loss where the fields are quite small in the beginning. There exists a possibility of retinal vein occlusion due to this rise of intraocular pressure though this has been rarely seen. This rise occurs in the first three hours. The tension should therefore be recorded after 3 hours as stated earlier. The tension should be monitored after 24 hours, after 3 days and then after a week. The preoperative medical treatment should be continued for about a month by which time the full effects of tension lowering get stabilised. No surgery should be contemplated or performed during this period.

Progressive visual field loss. Though usually the progressive field loss occurs in some cases and is probably due to elevation of intraocular pressure in the post-operative period yet even in the presence of a stabilised lowered intraocular pressure field loss may progressively occur. The management is by way of the medical treatment as for any other glaucoma. The tension should be monitored and controlled if there is a rise as described above.

Iritis. The iritic reaction usually lasts for about a week and can be controlled by local corticosteroids along with medical treatment of glaucoma.

Rarely it may be severe yet it can be managed by usual therapy for iritis without the use of atropine and on the principles of mobile pupil.

Transient blurred vision. It is of transient nature and needs no treatment. It may be due to gonioscopy solution used, corneal irregularity, pigment dispersal, anterior uveitis or in some cases injury to retinal photo receptors (bleaching which recovers).

Peripheral anterior synechiae. If the laser beam is properly focused the complication is uncommon. As elaborated earlier laser beam should be directed at the junction of the nonpigmented and the pigmented trabecular bands at low energy settings of 300-500 mW but not more than 750 mW. Above this power setting and with spot size larger than 50 μ the peripheral anterior synechiae are likely. These synechiae also commonly occur if laser treatment is given to structures posterior to trabecular meshwork or the posterior portion of trabecular meshwork is treated.

Haemorrhage. It occasionally occurs as an ooze from the canal of Schlemm but presents no problem if the pressure applied by gonioprism is increased or by lowering the power of photocoagulation setting and increasing the spot size at that particular area to 200 μ.

Transient corneal epithelial burns. These are often seen and present no problem as they resolve without scarring in nearly a week or so.

Pupillary distortion. At the settings commonly used, the complication is rather infrequent. It may occur if the iris root or the peripheral iris are inadvertently treated. It requires no treatment.

Angle closure glaucoma. It is rather infrequent and the only treatment required is continued medical therapy over a longer period.

Cystoid macular oedema. It is very rare and why it should occur belies any explanation. Continued medical therapy with addition of carbonic anhydrase inhibitors is advised.

Late complications

Worsening of existing glaucoma. It is rare and should be controlled with surgical trabeculectomy.

Corneal endothelialization of the trabecular meshwork of the angle of anterior chamber is probably due to anteriorly placed laser. It is difficult to diagnose from worsening or non-control of existing glaucoma and should be treated by trabeculectomy.

Iris atrophy. It is mild and is situated at the peripheral iris probably due to iris ischaemia. No treatment is needed.

Late rise in intraocular pressure. Sometimes seen particularly in glaucoma associated with pseudoexfoliation syndrome or in pigmentary glaucoma. It is best treated by trabeculectomy.

In the end it may be noted that laser trabeculoplasty is both safe and convenient and has low risk in the management of open angle glaucoma. It is preferable to a life long medical therapy and is as successful as surgical trabeculectomy. It, however, requires careful execution by an experienced laser therapist.

Other procedures

For the purpose of this book, a listing of other procedures of laser treatment of glaucoma is sufficient. They are :

Internal laser trabeculosclerostomy

External laser trabeculostomy with carbon dioxide lasers

CYCLODESTRUCTIVE PROCEDURES

Transpupillary argon laser cyclophotocoagulation

The procedure is useful for aphakic glaucoma and the aim is to reduce the formation of aqueous humour and requires careful choice of the level of energy required and the number of ciliary processes coagulated. It has the following advantages :

- A selective action on ciliary processes without damaging other ocular structures.
- More precise as far as degree of coagulation and the number of ciliary processes are coagulated.

The procedure, however, may need repetition and the results are not totally predictable.

The procedure is *indicated* and recommended in :

- Intractable glaucoma particularly if medical and surgical therapy have failed.
- Neovascular glaucoma.
- Epithelialization of anterior chamber leading to secondary glaucoma.
- Where sectorial iridectomy affords a good view of ciliary processes.

The procedure is *contraindicated* in :

- Hazy or opacified cornea.
- Presence of blood, pigment and other debris in the angle.
- If ciliary processes cannot be adequately viewed.
- In non-painful blind eye.

Technique. Widely dilate the pupil to enable a good view of the ciliary process. Coated Goldmann single mirror contact lens with indentation mechanism is used (Fig. 27.11). Ciliary process destruction rather than blanching should be preferred. The following parameters are useful.

- Size—50 to 100 μ
- Power—600-1000 mW
- Time of exposure—0.1 to 0.2 seconds.

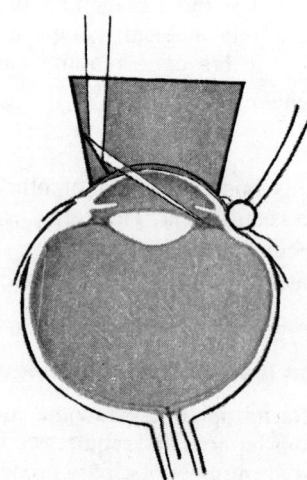

Fig. 27.11. Goldmann's contact lens (coated) with indentation provision.

The desired end point is concave, crater-like brown burn with pigment dispersion and gas bubble formation. 2 to 3 burns on the tip of each ciliary process should be inflicted. The aim should be to destroy about 25% of the ciliary processes distributed over the entire circumference.

The treatment may be complicated by post-operative increase in intraocular pressure. There may occur post-operative severe iridocyclitis which can be managed by usual cycloplegics and steroids.

Transcleral cyclophotocoagulation

Nd-YAG laser is used. Topical anaesthesia with a retrobulbar block is the anaesthesia of choice. A drop of neosynephrine is instilled to take away the congestion. The operation is performed under an operating microscope. The burns are given 3.5 mm away from the limbus and through 360°. The energy used is 8.5 J. The depth of focus is 1 mm and the number of spots given is 32. This gives enough destruction for the stabilisation of the intraocular pressure which occurs in 48 to 72 hours.

OTHER OPERATIONS

Other laser operations are *laser goniophotocoagulation, laser photo-mydriasis* through *pupilloplasty* and *sphincterotomy, reopening of filtration fistulas.* For the details of these operations the reader is referred to comprehensive textbook on lasers.

Nd-YAG LASER CAPSULOTOMY

Nd-YAG laser capsulotomy is the most common treatment for the thickened capsules in the extracapsular mode of cataract extraction with or without intraocular lens implantation. The results are achieved by a photodisruptive action and is not a direct thermal effect.

The most common mode of switching is the Q-switch procedure. The beam is delivered through a CGP (contact glass posterior) contact lens commonly known as Abraham YAG Contact Lens or Peyman YAG Contact Lens (Fig. 27.12).

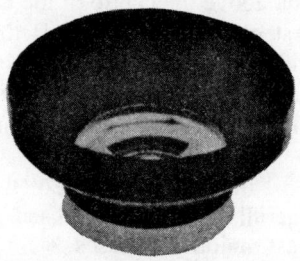

Fig. 27.12. Peyman's YAG contact lens.

The goal of the operation is to restore or improve visual acuity by cutting a small to medium-sized aperture out of the membrane. If a smaller aperture is used, specially so in cases where posterior chamber intraocular lens is not implanted, the probabilities of vitreous prolapse into the anterior chamber is reduced. Medium-sized aperture is otherwise programmed. It has the added advantage of facilitating the evaluation and treatment of retinal diseases though it increases the chances of vitreous prolapse in the anterior chamber.

The indications of Nd-YAG laser in capsular diseases are :

• Overgrowth of anterior hyaloid membrane by pigment epithelium.

• Extremely hard, hyaline and calcified cataract membrane.

• Post-cataract membrane after failed intracapsular cataract extraction.

• Thick post-cataract membrane after extracapsular cataract extraction, especially

• Thick pupillary membrane consisting of lens cortex and organised haemorrhage after perforating injury.

• Extremely thick and hard after-cataract as a complicating factor consisting of cortex and capsular material.

• Thick posterior capsule after aspiration of traumatic cataract.

• After cataract restricting vision.

The power used is 1-5 mJ in 0.1 mJ steps.

Number of bursts up to 5.

Size of focus 40 µ.

By this technique 3.5 to 4 mm capsular opening is obtained.

Because Nd-YAG laser beam is invisible red helium neon (HeNe) laser beams coincident to the YAG are used for aiming. Under ordinary circumstances, the Nd-YAG beam and HeNe aiming beam are almost in focus and there are no chromatic aberrations. If however, vitreous bands are to be cut the YAG beam is focused 0.3, 0.6 or 0.9 mm behind the HeNe beam as the resultant shock wave is displaced anteriorly and in these cases may damage the intraocular lens. The tower of the slit lamp may be angulated to achieve better visibility. The mechanism of focus is illustrated in Fig. 27.13.

The first shot is made above the centre of the non-dilated pupil with a burst using the lowest energy (about 1 mJ) through the Peyman's contact lens. One should be careful as with excessive energy and poor focus, especially in eyes where posterior chamber lenses have been implanted the lens itself may be hit. More than 1 burst but not exceeding 5 are usually necessary.

The results are almost immediate and the patient may begin to see well. The results are generally good and stabilised. It may reach the level of 6/12 or better in a vast majority of cases.

The Nd-YAG laser treatment is not without complications. These are listed in Table 27.5.

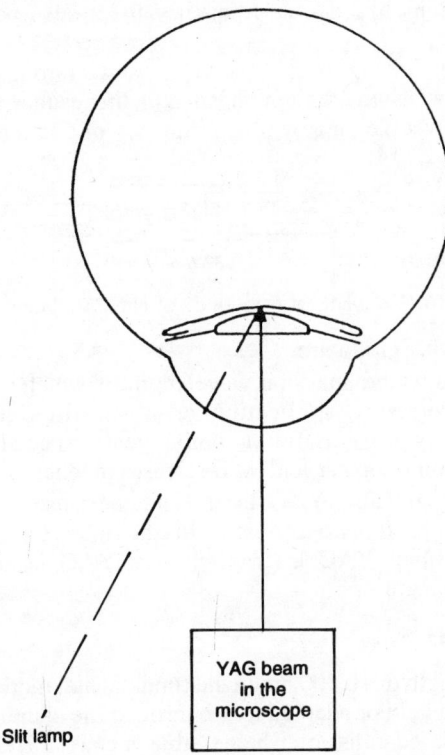

Fig. 27.13. Angulating the tower of the slit-lamp.

YAG beam
in the
microscope

Slit lamp

Table 27.5. Complications after Nd-YAG laser capsulotomy

Complication	Percentage
1. Intraocular pressure rise	30%
2. Damage to IOL	25%
3. Rupture of anterior face of vitreous	25%
4. Pupillary block glaucoma	Insignificant
5. Cystoid macular oedema	1 to 2%
6. Corneal oedema	0.5%
7. Retinal detachment	0.75 to 1%

Nd-YAG laser consists of the lasing medium neodymium ion, an ion of rare earth element which is doped into a YAG (Yttrium, Aluminium and Garnet crystal). We compare the Nd-YAG, for that purpose any other YAG laser, with a gun into its holster. The lasing medium being the gun and the YAG is the holster. The laser wavelength of Neodymium laser is 1064 nm. Essentially this laser is a photo tissue disrupter laser but with modifications like double frequency it can also be used as a thermal laser.

When laser beam arising from Nd-YAG is passed through a medium containing KTP (Potassium titanium phosphate), the resultant laser beam is in the ultraviolet-visible range with a frequency of 532, i.e., doubling the frequency (Fig. 27.14).

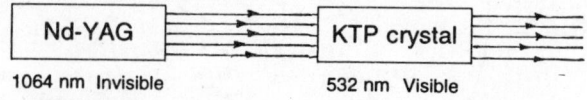

1064 nm Invisible   532 nm Visible

Fig. 27.14. Doubling of frequency of Nd-YAG laser.

Other lasers in this group are :

Erbium YAG laser, the emission wavelength of which is 1540 nm. This laser has promising application as a substitute for phaco-emulsification. It may prove useful in coming years especially with the advent of injectable intraocular lenses. It releases an energy of 100 mJ.

Holmium lasers are also YAG lasers and their use in refractive surgery is emerging. It also operates in the infrared zone. Like neodymium and erbium YAG lasers, holmium YAG lasers are also photodisruptive in nature.

Carbon dioxide laser

It emits at a wavelength of 10,600 nm in the fundamental mode. Delivery systems can be hand held or adapted to use through the operating micro-scope since the infra red emission is not visible, a coaxial Helium-Neon laser is usually incorporated for aiming and visualisation. They operate at 2060 nanometres. The energy output is 35 mJ. It is the water content of tissues and not their pigmentation that determines the effect produced by the CO_2 laser.

The water from the tissues is rapidly vapourized by energy from carbon dioxide laser thereby creating a wound in an explosive fashion. The thermal side effects of this vapourization are conducted to adjacent tissues and produce cauterization of small vessels as well as thermal damage. The excellent haemostasis produced by this cauterization is the major intraoperative advantage of CO_2 laser produced incisions.

Uses. The laser is useful in the intraocular photocautery, filtering procedures, sclerostomy for neovascular glaucoma, removal of capillary haemangiomas, lymphangiomas, papillomas and blepharoplasties.

The techniques for the above operations are not being described and the readers are referred to detailed texts on lasers and their uses in ophthalmic practice.

Dye lasers

The principle of dye lasers is that energy is 'pumped' by an incandescent xenon flash lamp or by another laser like Argon or YAG on a specific liquid dye. Lasing is then produced within this dye and a new range of wavelengths results. It is possible, theoretically, to cover the entire spectrum with a series of dyes but the constraint is that of today an easy method of changing dyes has not been found and the dyes cannot mix. The wavelength/lengths of dye laser have become specific.

As of today thermal or long duration dye lasers and pulsed or short duration dye lasers are available for clinical use.

Thermal dye lasers are primarily used for photocoagulating lesions in the posterior pole of the eye particularly microaneurysms and neo-vascularization beneath the macula or choroidal melanomas. The yellow dye laser may be considered to be as effective as Krypton red laser. The thermal dye lasers are pumped by high powered argon lasers hence they can act as dual lasers, i.e., Argon lasers at high power as well as yellow dye lasers at yellow wavelengths. Thermal dye lasers can also be used for photodynamic therapy. It has been found to be useful in the treatment of malignant melanomas of choroid and the retino-blastomas. The duration of dye laser treatment is in micro-seconds. The shorter the duration the higher the power attained by the laser.

Pulsed dye lasers are pumped directly by an incandescent xenon flash lamp. These lasers are used more specifically and better than Argon lasers in treating port wine stains in Sturge-Weber syndrome. The pulsed laser can also be used for sclerostomy though so far only a small series has been reported. At the present moment indications for sclerostomy by this laser are minimal.

In a manner similar to YAG laser the dye laser can be used for performing iridectomy but it is seldom employed as it does not give any advantages over YAG lasers.

Dye laser is also employed for age related macular disorders.

At the moment dye lasers, though theoretically attractive, have not attracted much practical use.

Diode lasers. In ophthalmology lasers are widely used and gaining more and more acceptance. All lasers whether thermal, photodisruptive or photoablative suffer from the severe drawback as a result of their very low electrical to optical efficiency. This is responsible for the extremely high power consumption, large size, high cost and troublesome maintenance of these lasers.

Recently, however, semi-conductor diode lasers have been in use. These lasers as of present emit in the far-red or near-infra-red spectral range. The lasing wavelengths of the highest power diode laser are presently limited to a narrow spectral of region from 750 to 950 nm because of the use of most developed gallium-aluminium-arsenide (GaAlAs) crystal technology.

An interesting approach to generating high-laser power is represented by the 'phased diode laser array'. It consists of several tens of single active diode structures built in the same clip and separated by a very short distance. Coupling between the adjacent active zones makes the overall laser emission spatially coherent and power as high as 3 W continuous wave at room temperature. A diode laser with 810 nm wave range and energy range from 0.5 to 500 mW and size spot up to 250 μm at probe is available for use.

It is anticipated that rapid development in diode laser technology will take place and production of highly effective lasers with Q switching and mode locking techniques will become available. Their applicability to Nd-YAG and Er-YAG will greatly enhance laser technology and its applicability.

Erbium YAG laser : This laser is developing very fast and through its use capsulotomy, phacoemulsification and all others functions of photodisruption are emerging.

Even *Nd-YAG laser* is becoming more effective and versatile with the availability of double frequency.

PHOTOABLATIVE LASERS

The most common example is the Excimer Laser.

Excimer laser

The most effective use of laser depends on the proper selection of wavelength, power and pulse duration. It is also necessary to know the absorption characteristics of the tissue being treated. It also depends upon the way the specific ocular tissue interacts with the laser energy which determines whether the response is primarily thermal, ionic (disruptive) or photoablative.

Photoablation is the non-linear photon-induced removal of matter. It enables extremely precise removal of tissue without much thermal interaction. It, therefore, offers considerable advantages in corneal surgery where minimal thermal effect and scarring is desirable.

This is available only if the output is in the ultraviolet zone.

Excimer actually means an excited dimer. Dimer is the association of two gasses to create a laser in the ultraviolet range. The most commonly used laser is where argon and fluorine gases are employed for lasing to produce an output of 193 nm. Theoretically the combination and their proportions can produce a series of excimer lasers (like krypton-fluorine).

Laser tissue interactions. The effect may be thermal. It allows for precise tissue heating. With local rise of temperature and vapourising of water it is possible to remove tissues. Laser radiation can be focused to a very small spot size, there occurs a deeper penetration into the tissue and diffusion of heat out of the focal region. This reaction can result in thermal damage to the tissue around the focal spot. This reaction can be useful but sometimes it causes tissue damage and inadvertent tissue destruction in the adjacent area.

The second effect is photoacoustic which is due to high energies delivered over very short durations. This causes ionization of target tissue and plasma formation leading to mechanical shock wave propagation (photoacoustic action). This is utilised to photo-disrupt the tissue.

The third effect is the photo-chemical effect which enables the removal of tissue with sub-micron precision (photoablation). It is this potential which is being used in excimer lasers.

Photoablation therefore is the non-linear photon-induced removal of matter as stated above. It is possible to excise tissues precisely with sharply defined margins without any thermal effects in the surrounding area particularly of the very short time exposure of the tissues.

Excimer laser, which emits light in the ultraviolet region, is used because of the fact that (1) photon energy increases at shorter wavelengths; (2) single ultraviolet photon energies exceed both peptide and carbon-carbon bond energies and are, therefore, (3) organic polymers are chromophores containing molecules capable of selective light absorption the peak being in the ultraviolet region.

Excimer lasers are sources of high power density, pulsed ultraviolet radiation. The atoms of a rare gas (argon/krypton/xenon) mostly argon combined with halogen (fluorine/chlorine) mostly fluorine to form a short-lived excited rare gas-halide dimer. As these highly unstable molecules decay in returning to the ground state, they emit ultraviolet photons. The combination of gas mixture or argon and fluorine emits at 193 nm which produces minimal absorption, precision of tissue excision is enhanced at this wavelength. The depth of tissue removed per pulse is determined by the wavelength and pulse-energy limited by the penetration depth.

A hard PMMA contact lens in which 150 micron slits are cut and which are coated with a reflective film to prevent its thermal loading while being exposed to laser beam (Fig. 27.15) is used as a mask. A beam of excimer laser (193 nm) is focused at a 6 mm optical zone, centred on the cornea. With this method the excision depth in the cornea

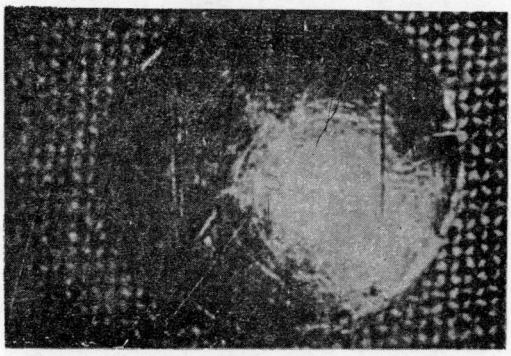

Fig. 27.15. PMMA contact lens mask.

varies by less than 4.5% which is not achievable by steel blades or even with diamond blades. It is now well established that it is the accuracy of the depth of incisions in radial keratotomy which determines the final outcome, excimer laser photo keratectomy is more predictable than any other method of correcting the refractive error.

The myopic errors can be corrected by linear or biconcave excisions. The laser can also be used for correction of astigmatic and hyper-metropic errors through biconvex incisions.

Photoablative keratectomy corrects the refractive errors not only by curvilinear or linear excisions but also through areal ablation which aims at refashioning the refractive surface of the cornea where tissues are precisely excised.

Excimer lasers are now well established tools for refractive surgery and may overtake the radial keratotomy procedures currently in use.

LASER USES IN SUMMARY

As described above lasers are used as thermal (photocoagulation), photo-disruption (capsulotomy, etc.) and photoablators (refractive surgery, etc.). Briefly recapitulating various lasers one can come to the following :

Thermal lasers

The most commonly used lasers in this group are :

Argon lasers

These lasers usually work in the green area in the wavelength of 488-514 nm of the spectrum. The most common uses of this laser are :

Pan-retinal coagulation which is indicated in eyes of diabetic retinopathy, central vein occlusion, Eales's disease, neo-vascular glaucoma, extensive retinal neovascularisation and diabetic vitreal haemorrhage.

The spot size varies from 500-1000 microns scattered confluently over the retina except near the optic disc and the posterior pole. The exposure time is 0.1 second. The power setting does not exceed 3.5 W. The aim is fulfilled in several sittings rather than in one sitting.

Focal photocoagulation. The principles are the same as for pan-retinal coagulation except that the area to be photocoagulated is extremely limited and confined to the site of the lesion.

Macular photocoagulation. It is indicated in neovascular sub-retinal membranes. The spot size used is 100-500 microns for a duration of 0.2 to 1 second and the energy output is titrated by observing the white chalky spots produced. Macular grid treatment as described earlier is desirable if the macular oedema is diffuse. In the grid treatment small size, mild intensity burns are used evenly placed extending from 500 microns to 3000 microns from the centre of macula.

Iridectomy. The indications are the same as for any surgical iridectomy.

An Abraham or Peyman's lens is used to sharply focus the laser energy on the iris. Stretch burns of 200 milliwatts of 500 micron size are focused on the iris crypts for a duration of 0.1 second. Alternatively 2 watt intensity 500 micron size spots are focused on the iris tissue for 0.2 to 0.1 seconds to achieve penetration. It is less effective than Nd-YAG laser.

It may cause corneal burns. Corneal oedema and hyphaema are other complications though they are less than after Nd-YAG laser therapy.

Trabeculoplasty. It can be used for any eye with uncontrolled glaucoma as medical therapy.

50-100 spots of 50 microns are placed in the anterior trabecular meshwork with exposure time of 0.1 seconds with about 300-500 milliwatt power.

The details of these procedures have been given earlier in this chapter.

Krypton laser

This laser operates in the region of 647 nm (red). The energy used is 1.5 watts to 0.75 watts. The micron size varies and is in the neighbourhood of 200 microns and the exposure time is 0.1 second.

It is indicated in :

Macular photocoagulation. It is particularly used when sub-retinal neo-vascular membrane is closer than 200 microns to the fovea otherwise argon laser is quite suitable.

The lesions produced need not be chalk white but a grey whitening is sufficient.

It may lead to choroidal haemorrhage, destruction of foveal photo receptors and decreased vision.

Pan-retinal photocoagulation. It can be used as an alternative to argon laser photocoagulation only in cases where massive vitreous haemorrhage precludes argon laser photocoagulation because of its ineffectivity.

Dye laser

The laser operates at 668 nm and is used for :

Sclerostomy. Methylene blue is iontophoresed at the limbus. A special gonio-lens (March gonio-lens) is applied to maintain the proper angle.

Iridectomy. Dye lasers can also be used for iridectomy the indications for which are the same as for Nd-YAG lasers.

Malignant melanoma. Haemotoporphyrin derivative is injected 36 hours before radiation and the wavelength used is 633 nm. Follow-up ultrasonography and fluorescein angiography is employed to complete destruction of the tumour otherwise the treatment is repeated.

Age-related macular degeneration. Thermal dye lasers are primarily used for photocoagulating lesions in the posterior pole of the eye particularly microaneurysms and neo-vascularization beneath the macula.

Diode lasers

These are promising lasers but suffer from the drawback of causing pain and discomfort during therapy even in the presence of local topical and regional anaesthesia. The indications are the same as far any thermal laser.

CO_2 lasers

These lasers work at about 10,600 nm and are dependent for their action on the water content of the tissues. Their extinction length is 0.03 mm. They can be safely used in *blepharoplasty, sclerostomy* in *neo-vascular glaucoma* and *Sturge-Weber syndrome* in need of surgical intervention. It achieves excellent *intraoperative haemostasis* and is therefore useful in patients with *bleeding diathesis.* They are also useful in the treatment of *basal cell carcinomas* and *papillomas.*

Photodisruptive lasers

These are essentially those in which YAG (Yttrium-Aluminium-Garnet) crystals are doped with lasing agent which is a rare earth metal. For these lasers HeNe (a gas laser containing a mixture of helium and neon) is used as the red aiming beam.

Nd-YAG laser

In this neodymium ion is doped into a YAG crystal. It is most commonly used at 1064 nm. It is clinically used in :

Posterior capsulotomy. It is useful in any opacified posterior capsule reducing vision. The beam is accurately focused on the posterior capsule or just behind the posterior capsule and minimum power is used ranging from 1-5 mJ in 0.1 mJ steps, the size of spot is about 40 microns. An intervention of a coated contact lens is necessary.

Vitreous surgery. It is used for cutting the vitreous membranes, strands or traction bands. It flattens retinal flap tears, frees encapsulated foreign bodies. It relieves cystoid macular degeneration induced by vitreous traction.

Congenital glaucoma. The indications are the same as for goniotomy and trabeculum is visualised through a special gonio-lens. The membrane seen is cut in as much of the angle as possible.

Iridectomy. It is performed in narrow angle glaucoma, pupillary block glaucoma and iris blocking of the visual axis. The iridectomy should be performed in the peripheral area where iris caves away from the lens.

Holmium YAG laser

Like Nd-YAG laser, in this laser the holmium metal is doped in YAG crystal as lasing medium. It is mostly used in refractive surgery particularly in hypermetropia. It also acts in the infra-red zone of over 1064 nm as a pulsed laser.

Erbium YAG laser

Its emission wavelength is 1540 nm. This laser is being extensively tried and one of the important applications is as a substitute phacoemulsifier.

Photoablative lasers

The most common example is the excimer laser. It is used at 193 nm or 364 nm wavelength.

It is used in radial keratotomy, refractive keratectomy and sometimes in sclerostomy.

Some of the lasers in clinical use have been summarised but more and more lasers are likely to be developed for clinical use and the existing ones refined.

CHAPTER XXVIII

THERAPEUTICS

INTRODUCTION

Therapeutic measures in the eye have certain peculiar problems and advantages of their own. Most of the infections are superficial lesions and can be easily tackled by surface medications. The response can be directly monitored under a biomicroscope. The inflammations of the eye are usually inside the globe, their etiology is unknown and speculative hence the therapy is empirical and symptomatic. The systemic administrations have difficulty in crossing the blood-aqueous and blood-vitreous barriers. Direct injection into the globe has its own hazards. One, therefore, has not only to choose a proper drug but also an appropriate route of administration.

The drugs used in ophthalmology may be broadly classified as (1) drugs acting on the autonomic nervous system—mostly the mydriatics, cycloplegics and miotics; (2) hormones, usually the corticosteroids and other non-steroidal anti-inflammatory drugs; (3) heavy metal components; (4) anti-microbial therapy, i.e., the chemotherapeutic drugs, the antibiotics, the antifungal agents, the anti-viral agents and the antiprotozoal agents; (5) carbonic anhydrase inhibitors; (6) pyrexia producing agents; (7) tissue implants; (8) diagnostic agents like fluorescein, endrophonium chloride, methacholine; (9) vitamins; (10) other agents like alpha-chymotrypsin, hyaluronidase, ethylenediamine tetra-acetate (EDTA) deferoxamine; and (11) antimetabolites which are essentially immuno-suppressive agents.

DYNAMICS OF DRUG DISTRIBUTION IN OCULAR FLUIDS

Before embarking on discussing the dynamics of drug distribution in ocular fluids, a well-known, yet fully ignored, statement may be recalled that all drugs are poisons, drugs alone and in combination affect the body (young, old, well or sick) and the body, well or sick, affects the drugs. One, therefore, should project in one's mind whether one is using them for curative, suppressive or preventive purposes and whether the benefits outweigh the risks—and can one choose a drug which will have hardly any side-effects while giving maximum benefits.

The dynamics of drugs administration in ocular fluids is directly governed by the route of administration, penetration and the tissue action on drug, therefore, permeability of ocular tissues plays an important part.

The penetration of drugs through the intact cornea is not a simple process of diffusion but is due to differential solubility. The solutions have to be biphasic being both water and fat soluble. Corneal structure is such that cornea is fat-water-fat sandwich. Both the endothelium and epithelium have very high lipid content which is about 100 times more than the stroma. They are relatively impermeable to electrolytes but can be readily passed by fat soluble substances. The stroma is readily penetrated by electrolytes but is relatively impermeable to lipid soluble substances. Lipids are the non-ionized and electrolytes are the ionized forms. If one can recall the developmental, structural and physiological similarities of the conjunctival and corneal epithelium, it can be easily surmised that the characteristics displayed by the corneal epithelium are also displayed by the conjunctival epithelium.

Barriers with a differential solubility resistance comparable to that of cornea also surround the entire eye particularly the retinal and choroidal structures.

Sclera though structurally tough does not exhibit any differential solubility barrier. The iris circulation exhibits this barrier and the choriocapillaris do not. The ciliary epithelium is rather unique in as much as that it actively secretes some ions and permits free passage of others.

The pigment epithelium of the retina is impermeable to dyes and the retinal vasculature in general exhibits the same barrier.

Such is the affair in normal eyes but inflammatory processes grossly alter this state and many of the barriers are broken down. What is permeable on small molecular basis may permit large molecules to penetrate and the differential solubility barriers are grossly altered if not totally abolished. However, in choosing a particular medication and its route of administration these basic facts have to be kept in mind.

Another matter which must come in reckoning while determining the therapeutic concentrations is the factors and rate of removal of the drugs from the ocular tissues. The two main sources of the drug loss are (1) diffusion into the circulating blood; and (2) escape via the aqueous humour into the canal of Schlemm. Again at the angle of the anterior chamber the mechanism is not as simple as one would like to believe.

Drugs which need to enter the eye have to cross important barriers even when given intravenously. The ciliary epithelium, the barriers at the level of pigment epithelium of the eye and the retinal vasculature. These barriers block the entry of proteins and antibiotics of high molecular weight into the aqueous, vitreous or even the retinal layers. In the inflammatory state or even after injury—mechanical, thermal, chemical or biological—there are evidences to show the breakdown of these barriers yet some differential is retained. Based on these considerations several routes of administration are utilized for therapeutic purposes depending upon the target organs.

Routes of administration

These routes are (1) topical; (2) subconjunctival, sub-Tenon's and retrobulbar injections; (3) intraocular injections; (4) intramuscular injections; (5) intravenous injections; (6) oral preparations and retrograde arterial perfusion. Each one of these requires careful consideration.

Topical. Several innovations have been used to make this route more effective. A single drop instilled in the eye does not remain within the eye but spreads all over the body tissues. There is, no doubt, a rapid escape of the drugs from the eye but therapeutic levels persist for clinically effective duration of time. In some cases topical application is more useful than intravenous or subcutaneous route.

Tetracaine when given topically in 2% solution gives adequate concentrations. In experiments with dogs it has been seen that when it is given in 30 mg dose by rapid intravenous injection (in 30 seconds) slow intravenous injection (20 minutes) and subconjunctival injection the blood level were lower than tracheal and pharyngeal instillation with 2% solution.

Local instillation is sufficient, for high levels of drug in the cornea can be judged by the fact that instillation of 2-3 drops of 0.1% solution of dexamethasone drug can be demonstrated in the cornea for more than 2 hours and that it can be demonstrated, though in much lower concentrations, in the aqueous humour and the iris.

It seems that for better penetration and higher maintenance levels the attention should be concentrated on the mode of delivery and the vehicle used to deliver.

In topical administration the vehicle in which a drug is applied needs careful attention. More viscous fluids prolong ocular contact thereby increasing drug absorption. In drug design many considerations should apply to the vehicle, chiefly pH, toxicity, electrolyte composition stability and wetting effect. To these may be added preservatives and antioxidants.

Combination of drugs are not usually good but if they have to be used incompatibilities should be avoided.

Pilocarpine can be taken as an example. When used at pH 4.0 its penetration into aqueous is about half as used at pH 7.5 but alkaline solution is unstable and deteriorates rapidly.

Ointment. The ointment base must take two factors into account. Firstly the allergic reaction. Many atropine allergies are essentially due to the atropine ointment base. Secondly the easy release of drug when instilled into the eye. No doubt that increased contact can lead to enhanced penetration but it may be offset by a slow release of drug. If improper vehicle is used it may even slow the corneal epithelium healing rate.

Commonly used ophthalmic ointment bases and liquid oily vehicles (petrolatum, lanolin and peanut oil) are toxic to interior of the eye. They cause endothelial damage, corneal oedema, vascularization and scarring. Using post-operatively after intraocular surgery one may accidentally cause entry of these ointments in the anterior chamber and it may result in severe irritation and secondary glaucoma. Some surgeons feel practice of routine use of ointments after intraocular surgery should be discontinued at least for 48 hours. The author, however, has not seen such adverse reactions even in an era when sutures were not used.

Continuous irrigation. The second mode of administration can be continuous irrigation. It, no doubt, delivers high concentration of drug continuously to the surface structures of the eye and perhaps greater concentration in intraocular fluids. It is, however, cumbersome and has the defect of washing away the natural defences of leucocytes and enzymes in the tears. The only condition where it may be used is dry eye syndrome through a pump delivering 3-8 ml of fluid per day. The method is still questionable.

Iontephoresis. Yet another method for better concentration of drug is iontephoresis, i.e., using electromotive force. Theoretically it sounds good but practically it has never been popular.

Massage. Vigorous massage after giving medication may be useful but is better avoided. This may cause sufficient corneal epithelial damage and permit better penetration of even poorly soluble substances and very low concentration of penetrable solution may give equally effective results.

Hydrophilic contact lens drug application

Soft contact lenses or hydrophilic contact lenses have the capability to absorb and slowly release chemical in solution but not in suspension. The second point of importance is that in order to use drugs with soft contact lenses as the applicator, the drugs should not contain preservatives as otherwise they will act as metabolic poisons to the corneal epithelium and damage it, sometimes with grave consequences. The use of pre-soaked soft lens to deliver medication to the eye prolongs delivery time and results in longer presence (4 hours or so) of small molecular weight drugs within the eye. The author has not found this mode of delivery as a useful adjunct in clinical practice as the lens has to be taken out at quite regular intervals and reinserted after resoaking. This, if proper hygiene is not maintained, may even cause ocular infection.

Ocuserts. A much better method of delivery is by ocuserts which are essentially membrane controlled diffusional systems. Such systems can be prepared and they can release drugs at predetermined contact rate up to a period of about a week. To comprehend it fully it may be said that the rate of release is dependent upon the permeability of the membrane to the drug and the area of the membrane in contact with the eye. It will remain effective if the osmotic and permeability relationships do not draw water into the delivery system.

Devices are in use where about 20 μg of pilocarpine per hour within a 10% tolerance continue for as long as a week. The author is not much enamoured of these devices because he feels the same results can be obtained by more frequent use of drops.

The advantages of the systems claimed are prolonged release of drug, better patient compliance with therapy since both ration of repeated instillation is avoided and the accommodative myopia seen in children after instillation of pilocarpine is minimized if not avoided. Some ophthalmologists consider this form of therapy as very useful in dry eye syndromes and also in drugs delivery like IDU where its continuous presence greatly helps.

Ocuserts are notorious for their unnoticed escape especially in children. The disadvantage of unnoticed missing of therapy far outweighs any advantages claimed.

Subconjunctival, sub-Tenon's and retrobulbar injections

The ocular dynamics of drugs through these routes of injection needs the understanding of how the drugs reach the interior of the eye. It can pass through permeable sclera, or through orbital plexuses of veins or through the corneal stroma and endothelium.

There are conflicting claims with regard to the therapeutic concentrations of drugs inside the eye after administration through different routes. The claims are mostly made on the basis of animal studies and the model chosen is rabbit. Rabbit structures particularly the richness of orbital venous plexuses makes the result inapplicable to human beings. Secondly the evaluation is difficult because of the uncontrollable factor of injury to ocular barriers during injection, the arbitrary selection of dosage and frequency of administration. There are no doubts on two counts (1) single subconjunctival injections will achieve higher intraocular drug levels than will a few topical instillations; and (2) repeated topical applications will achieve intraocular levels that compare respectably with those of subconjunctival injections.

Subconjunctival injections should therefore be considered only in situations (1) if there is an emergency; (2) post-operatively because one may not like to open the eye frequently; (3) if the drug used is of low penetration quality (like antibiotics and not mydriatics) and finally a combination is desired to be used (as midricin).

The disadvantages are several and they usually nullify the advantages. Patient apprehensions, subsequent inflammation and pains, inconvenience, expense and possible intraocular perforation.

The author employs this route of administration only immediately after intraocular surgery or in an emergency to tackle the acute infection of the anterior segment.

When one gives subconjunctival injection is one sure that it is subconjunctival particularly when it is given 4-5 mm away from the limbus or is one penetrating the Tenon's capsule? It is anyway better to give it under the Tenon's capsule by holding both the conjunctiva and the Tenon's. It is penetrated by a needle bevel down to avoid injury to episcleral vessels.

The drug penetrates into the eye primarily by diffusion across the sclera, a small part through the systemic circulation after absorption from the subconjunctival/ sub-Tenon's space. Some of the drug leaks out of the subconjunctival space, mixes tear with fluid and then transmitted across the cornea.

Retrobulbar. Another route of administration is the retrobulbar route—a blind injection into the retrobulbar space. It is alright for regional anaesthesia but has it any advantages in other medications? The clinical value of retrobulbar routes of administration is doubtful. The most common preparation given by ophthalmologists is corticosteroids for inflammations of the posterior segment. Surprisingly the ocular levels in the inflamed eye is 1/2 of the one achieved in normal eye contrary to the expectations because natural barriers are usually broken down in inflamed eyes. Probably greater loss of drug occurs into the systemic circulation via the inflamed orbital vessels. A better route seems to be subconjunctival depot.

Intraocular injections. The dangers inherent in intraocular injections far outweigh possible benefits in almost all cases and in all circumstances. Perhaps in desperate endophthalmitis cases where vitrectomy is performed injection of Garamycin or Chloramphenicol in the centre of the vitreous cavity may be justified. There are surgeons who claimed good result after Garamycin injection intraocularly after cataract surgery particularly in the anterior chamber. The drugs which cannot penetrate into the eye are also usually too toxic and irritative to be given intraocularly.

Systemic administration. Systemic administration of drugs either parenterally or orally are as useful. No doubt retino-vitreal barriers, choroido-retinal barriers, barriers at the ciliary epithelium and the corneal barriers all work against most of the drugs but they still remain the most efficient route for controlling posterior segment disease except the vitreous infection when vitrectomy is the obvious choice.

Intramuscular and intravenous routes of administration

One cannot comprehend the value of these injections as systemically administered medications do not readily penetrate into the eye because of blood-aqueous and blood-vitreous barriers. Electrolytes do not readily penetrate. The various intraocular epithelial and endothelial membranes constitute these barriers. Antibiotics, except low molecular ones which partially penetrate, do not enter the eye. This is not entirely true of inflammations as a result of infection.

Continuous intravenous administration of antibiotics may certainly be a dramatic way of impressing the patients but it is ineffective in passing through the intraocular barriers. Ampicillin, chloramphenicol, erythromycin can to an extent penetrate the eye and be maintained perhaps at adequate therapeutic levels up to four hours but they need not be given as a continuous infusion. They may be administered as a repetitive 'pulse' to achieve the aims of this therapy.

The oral preparations called the delayed release oral pills, i.e., retards are effective as simple tablets given in divided doses. They can be usefully employed.

Last but not the least is retrograde arterial perfusion it may be quite impressive in experimental models but they do not seem to be practical. One cannot conceive of this route becoming an effective tool in the dynamics of drug distribution in intraocular fluids.

Summary

It may be summarised that the ocular tissues present several barriers, the epithelial and endothelial barriers for electrolyte ions and stroma for liquid soluble substances at the cornea level, the ciliary epithelium, the choroidal endothelial vessel wall, the retinal pigment epithelium and the endothelial walls of the retinal vasculature. They regulate the entry of the corticosteroids and high molecular weight antibiotics. Local medication as drops or as ointments in appropriate frequency is adequate. Subconjunctival and retrobulbar injections are hardly of much value. Subconjunctival injections may, however, be resorted to in acute emergencies for the infection of the anterior segments. Oral medication is adequate for enzymes inhibitors. Only in acute inflammations of the posterior segment due to infection should one resort to intravenous administration of antibiotics. Intraocular route is a measure of desperation.

DRUGS ACTING ON AUTONOMIC SYSTEM

Stimulation of sympathetic and depression of parasympathetic produce dilatation of pupil. Stimulation of parasympathetic and depression of sympathetic produce miosis. The parasympathetic and sympathetic nerve endings at the end of 1st neuron produce acetylcholine and nicotine. The parasympathetic at terminal nerve endings produces acetylcholine which acts on the motor end plates to produce its actions. The acetylcholine action is limited due to its destruction by cholinesterase or cholinesterase acts as a filter for acetylcholine. The sympathetic at terminal nerve endings produces sympathin which can be destroyed by aminoxidases. The sympathin acts on the end plates and produces its effects. In both parasympathetic and sympathetic nervous system some drugs act directly on the muscle cells to produce corresponding action. Their action is well represented in Fig. 28.1 and these drugs can accordingly be classified as under :

I. Parasympathomimetic drugs (cholinergic drugs)
   • Agents which protect acetylcholine by binding cholinesterase, e.g.,

physostigmine (eserine), prostigmin and DFP.
- Agents which directly stimulate the motor end plate, e.g., acetylcholine, mecholyl, doryl and pilocarpine.
- Agents which act directly on muscle cell, e.g., histamine.

II. Parasympatholytic drugs
- Drugs which prevent the action of acetylcholine, e.g., atropine, homatropine, scopolamine (hyoscine) and euphthalmine, cyclopentolate and tropicamide.

III. Sympathomimetic drugs
- Drugs which protect sympathin, being anti-monoaminooxidase in action, e.g., cocaine.
- Drugs which directly stimulate the end plate, e.g., epinephrine (adrenaline), neosynephrine, paredrine and hydroxyamphetamine.

IV. Sympatholytic drugs
- Drugs which act on the motor end plate, e.g., dibenamine and priscol.
- Drugs which act directly on muscle cell, e.g., ergot and its alkaloids.

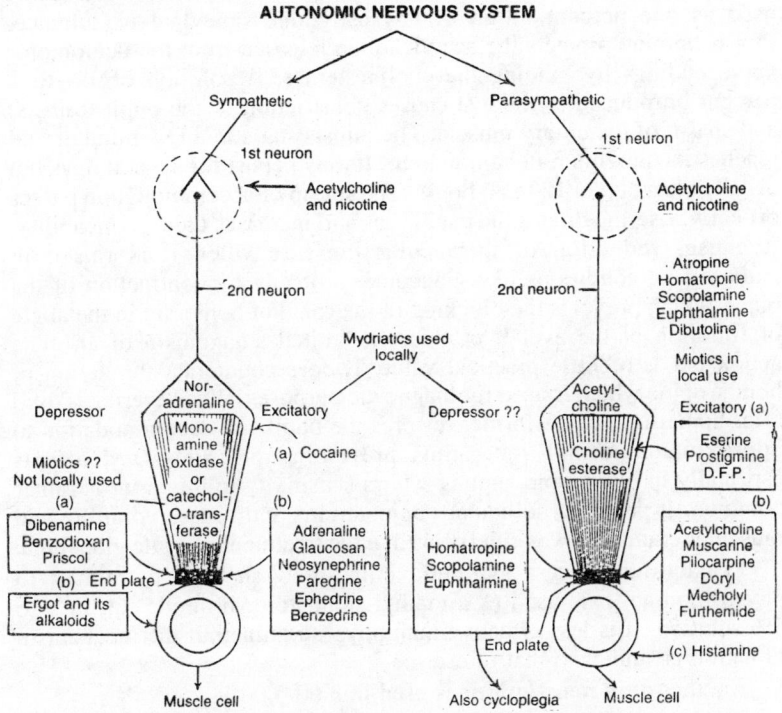

Fig. 28.1. Drugs acting on autonomic nervous system.

Parasympathomimetic drugs

Agents which protect acetylcholine by binding cholinesterase (anticholinesterases)—Table 28.1

The drugs can be grouped into reversible (physostigmine, neostigmine and prostigmin) and irreversible ones (DFP, echothiophate iodide and demecarium bromide).

Table 28.1. Anticholinesterases

U.S.P. or N.F. name	Concentration (%)	Duration of miotic action
Reversible		
Physostigmine (eserine)	0.25-1.0	
Neostigmine	3.0-5.0	12-36 hours
Prostigmine	3.0-5.0	
Irreversible		
Di-isopropylfluorophosphate	0.01-0.1	days to weeks
Echothiophate iodide	0.03-0.25	days to weeks
Demecarium bromide	0.25-0.5	days to weeks

Physostigmine (eserine). It is an alkaloid from calaber bean and is used as one percent lotion of physostigmine salicylate or sulphate. Physostigmine protects the acetylcholine released from the oculomotor nerve endings by binding the cholinesterase. A solution of 1/4 to 1 percent introduced in the eye causes constriction of the pupil (miosis) and spasm of the ciliary muscle. The miosis starts in a few minutes and reaches its maximum in half an hour. It may persist for several days but usually clears up in 12 to 36 hours. The spasm of accommodation passes off early. Eserine dilates the capillaries and increases their permeability. It causes reduction of intraocular pressure when it is raised in pathological conditions like glaucoma, probably by contraction of the pupil, which prevents the blocking of the canal of Schlemm in the angle of filtration of the eye. It produces a limited antagonism of atropine action but is of little practical value. It does counteract the action of homatropine which is used for diagnostic purposes. When eserine is used after homatropine, the former restores the pupil and accommodation to approximate normal state, thus preventing any untoward affects especially in old people, among whom sensitivity to this drug is rather common. It produces follicular conjunctivitis and causes vomiting and muscular cramps. It was chiefly used in the treatment of acute glaucoma.

Prostigmin. It is a synthetic compound chemically related to physostigmine. It is used as a methyl-sulphate or bromide salt in 3 to 5% solution. It is less effective than physostigmine but the mechanism of action is similar to that of eserine.

Another drug **neostigmine** is used in 3.00-5.00%.

Di-isopropyl-fluorophosphate (DFP). It inhibits the action of cholinesterase. It is more effective than eserine or prostigmin or neostigmine, having more prolonged and a more powerful effect producing a miosis which may last for about as many as 27 days. There is ciliary spasm lasting for about 48 hours or so. It produces dilatation of the capillaries of the iris and ciliary body and an increase in their permeability. It has been known to produce dangerous effects in chronic congestive glaucoma. Its use has almost been given up. It used to be employed in 0.01 to 0.1% solution in peanut oil and was particularly considered to be useful in aphakic glaucoma.

Echothiophate iodide in 0.03 to 0.25% and **demecarium bromide** from 0.125 to 0.25% are other drugs employed in this group. Their action lasts from days to weeks and can be counteracted by atropine.

Agents directly stimulating the motor end plate (Table 28.2)

Pilocarpine. It is an alkaloid obtained from the leaves of pilocarpus jaborandi. It directly acts on motor end plate. It constricts the pupil and produces spasm of ciliary muscle which persists for several hours. It is poor in counteracting the mydriatic effect produced by homatropine and atropine. Its action takes longer time to appear but also lasts longer.

Table 28.2. Cholinergic drugs

U.S.P. or N.F. name	Concentration (%)	Duration of miotic action
Pilocarpine	0.5-10	4-8 hours
Carbachol	0.75-3	2 hours
Methacholine drugs	0.75	Same day but usually not used
Doryl (carbamylcholine)	0.75	commercially.
Furmethide	10	Quite useful but not generally employed.

Acetylcholine. It physiologically stimulates muscle cells by acting directly upon the motor end plate but it is so rapidly destroyed by the cholinesterase of the tissues that it produces no miosis when instilled into the conjunctival sac, and is, therefore, not used.

Mecholyl (metacholine chloride). It is more resistant than acetylcholine. It stimulates the sphincter pupillae. It causes marked dilatation of the conjunctival blood vessels and probably also of the vessels of the uveal tract. It is used in aqueous solution which is very unstable. It can be used in combination with eserine or drugs of that group but it is not in general use.

Doryl (carbamylcholine). It is a powerful miotic, is more stable than mecholyl and has a more prolonged action. It has a double action of stimulating the motor end plate and to some extent inhibiting the action of cholinesterase. It increases the permeability of the blood-aqueous barrier but to a lesser extent than eserine or mecholyl. It is used in 0.75% aqueous solution. Its absorption is poor and is, therefore, used in combination of 2% pilocarpine and 1% eserine. It is usually not commercially employed.

Furmethide in 10% solution is also used.

Drugs acting on muscle cells directly

Histamine is thought to be the most powerful miotic and is supposed to counteract mydriasis produced by atropine. It produces considerable capillary dilatation and increase in capillary permeability leading to escape of fluid and protein. It may thus precipitate acute attack of glaucoma. The drug is therefore, not in therapeutic use.

Parasympatholytic drugs (Table 28.3)

They depress the action of the parasympathetic nervous system by a direct action on the motor end plate. Most of the drugs are related to each other and are alkaloids of belladonna. A few of them are synthetic drugs.

Table 28.3. Parasympatholytic drugs

U.S.P. or N.F. name	Percent	Max. mydriasis Max. cycloplegia	Duration of mydriasis Duration of cycloplegia
Atropine	0.25-4	30-40 minutes	12 days
		Several hours	2 weeks
Homatropine	1-2	10-30 minutes	6 hours - 4 days
		30-90 minutes	10-48 hours
Scopolamine	0.25-0.5	15-30 minutes	Several days
		30-45 minutes	5-7 days
Cyclopentolate	0.5-2	15-30 minutes	24 hours
		15-45 minutes	24 hours
Tropicamide	1-2	20-30 minutes	4 hours
		20-25 minutes	6 hours
Oxyphenonium (antrenyl)	1-5	Comparable to atropine	4 days 12 days
Eucatropine	5-10	30 minutes	4 hours
Euphthalmine	5-10	Poor cycloplegia	
Lachesine	1	30 minutes	10 hours

Atropine. This is a widely used drug in ophthalmology and is an alkaloid of belladonna. It is generally used in 1% strength as solution, ointment or lamella. When applied to the conjunctival sac its maximum mydriatic action takes 30-40 minutes and lasts for 10-12 days and the cycloplegic action takes several hours lasting for about 2 weeks. It paralyses the sphincter muscle of the iris and the ciliary muscle by preventing the action of acetylcholine on the motor end plate of the muscle cell. It may have a direct action on the blood vessels of the eye causing a decrease in their permeability to proteins. Large doses of atropine cause immobilization of the ciliary muscle and iris ensuring rest in an inflamed eye. The drug is therefore useful in acute inflammations. Atropine causes a rise of intraocular pressure, probably due to blockage of filtration angle in the anterior chamber of the eye by the iris. The action is almost insignificant in a normal eye but if intraocular pressure is already high then atropine will raise it more and may produce an acute attack. This action once started is difficult to inhibit. It may result in destruction of the function of the eye. Its action cannot be reversed by eserine. This drug should only be used in children and in cases where complete paralysis of the iris sphincter and ciliary muscle is desired.

Homatropine. It is a synthetic compound closely allied to atropine in chemical structure and is used as homatropine hydrobromide in 1 to 2% solution. Its action is short-lived and can be counteracted by eserine. This makes it an excellent drug to be used for refraction in adults and for diagnostic examination of the fundus. Its action is similar to that of atropine. Maximum mydriasis is produced in 10-30 minutes and lasts for 6 hours to days while the cycloplegic action takes 30-90 minutes and lasts for 10-40 hours.

Hyoscine (scopolamine). It produces the same effect as atropine, i.e., it produces mydriasis and paralysis of ciliary muscles. It may be used as 0.5% solution. Its effect lasts for several days. Care must be taken in its prolonged use. It is likely to produce hallucinations and psychic disturbances.

The belladonna alkaloids may produce allergic reactions. The earliest sign of these reactions is the oily look of the conjunctiva followed by folliculosis and conjunctivitis. If a person is allergic to one drug in this group, he is usually allergic to others. In such cases synthetic drugs may be used.

Lachesine. It is also a synthetic drug possessing atropine-like actions; 1% solution causes mydriasis and cycloplegia but the effects seldom last for more than 10 hours.

Euphthalmine. It is synthetic member of the group and has considerably weaker action than other drugs. It has little effect on the ciliary muscle. It is a good drug for funduscopy and is usually employed in 5 to 10% drops.

Cylopentolate. It is used in 0.5 to 2% solution. It produces maximum mydriasis in 15 to 30 minutes which lasts for about 24 hours. The maximum cycloplegia is produced in 15 to 45 minutes and lasts for about 24 hours.

Tropicamide. It is used as 1-2% solution. The mydriatic and cycloplegic action is produced in 20-30 minutes and lasts for 4-6 hours. It is an ideal mydriatic for refraction and examination of fundus.

Eucatropine. It is used in 5-10% solution. The mydriasis develops in about 1/2 an hour. It is a poor cycloplegic and is, therefore, not much in use.

There are several other compounds which are still to be fully evaluated.

Sympathomimetic drugs (Table 28.4)

Drugs protecting sympathin from aminoxidase

Cocaine. It produces mydriasis probably by protecting sympathin from being destroyed by aminoxidase. It is used as 2 to 10% solution. It produces mydriasis which begins within a few minutes and reaches the maximum in 15 minutes. The action persists for about four hours. It produces local anaesthesia of the conjunctiva and cornea (4%, 4 drops every 4 minutes and 4 times). It also produces vasoconstriction of the conjunctival vessels. The drug is toxic to the corneal epithelium and causes its desquammation.

Table 28.4. Sympathomimetic drugs

U.S.P. or N.F. name	Percent	Maximum mydriasis	Duration of mydriasis
Cocaine	2-4	20 minutes	2 hours
Adrenaline	1/1000		
Phenylephrine	2.5 and 10	20 minutes	3 hours
Hydroxyamphetamine	1	40 minutes	
Ephedrine	5	30 minutes	3 hours
Neosynephrine	10	20 minutes	Lasting effect
Paredrine	1% in 2% boric acid	30 minutes	1-2 hours

Agents which stimulate the motor end plate

Adrenaline (epinephrine). Dilutions of 1/1000 do not produce any effect on the pupil in normal individuals but a solution of 1/1000 is also a mydriatic agent in inflammatory disorders and is used to break up posterior synechia. Small doses dilate the capillaries of the uveal tract but large doses cause marked constriction of the arterioles and capillaries of the eye. It causes little change in the permeability of the blood-aqueous barrier. If injected subconjunctivally it produces a small rise in intraocular pressure which is followed by a fall. Initial vasoconstriction is followed by a reactionary vasodilatation and hyperaemia.

Neosynephrine. It is a synthetic substance chemically related to adrenaline. It is more stable and has a more lasting effect. It is a powerful mydriatic and vasoconstrictor drug and is similar to adrenaline in action. It is useful in breaking posterior synechia. It is commonly used as a 10% solution or emulsion. A weak 1% solution can also be used.

Paredrine. It is a synthetic compound which is more stable than neosynephrine. It is used as a 1% solution in 2% boric acid lotion. It causes mydriasis which lasts for 1 to 2 hours and its effects are easily countered by pilocarpine or eserine.

Phenylephrine. It is used in 2.5 to 10% solution. Its maximum mydriatic effect takes 20 minutes or so and lasts for about 3 hours. It is a direct action sympathomimetic drug. It should not be used in patients with cardiac problems who are taking monoamino-oxidase inhibitors. Indirectly acting drugs are hydroxyamphetamine and ephedrine.

Sympatholytic drugs

Drugs acting on motor end plate

Dibenamine. It is a synthetic compound which acts on the motor end plates. It has no local action but it produces its effects when given systemically. The drug besides lowering the ocular tension and producing miosis causes a considerable fall in blood pressure. Orthostatic hypotension with this drug is always a source of anxiety and has precluded its wider application. In selected cases the drug lowers intra-ocular pressure.

Priscol. It is a drug which acts directly on the motor end plates. It is not used locally in the eye. The drug has been employed sub-conjunctivally to produce vasodilatation and increase in intraocular pressure. Its utility is in the diagnosis of glaucoma as a provocative test. The drug has also been employed with some success in vasospastic conditions of the macula. In these conditions it has been given as a retrobulbar injection.

Drugs acting on the muscle cell itself

Ergot and its alkaloids. These drugs prevent the effector organs from responding to sympathetic nervous stimuli or adrenaline. The ergot alkaloids also possess certain central actions (i) they produce peripheral vasodilatation by their influence on the vasomotor centre; (ii) the proprioceptive mechanism regulating the blood pressure is inhibited to a certain extent.

The drugs are employed in herpes zoster ophthalmicus, herpes cornea, acute and chronic glaucoma, migraine-like cephalgias.

HORMONES

During recent years hormones secreted by the adrenal cortex have been extensively used in ophthalmology. The first such hormone was cortisone. Its special advantages in ophthalmology are that the toxic effects resulting from its systemic use are not encountered in its topical use. Hydrocortisone is more potent when it is applied locally. Prednisone, dexamethasone and betamethasone are even more effective. They can be used systemically since toxic effects of cortisone are not seen to the same degree, with these drugs. It has now been fully established that in genetically susceptible persons these drugs can cause glaucoma. The tension of the eye should, therefore, be regularly checked when these drugs are given. Adrenocorticotrophic hormone of the pituitary gland (anterior lobe) stimulates the secretion of cortisone by the adrenals and is thus effective only on systemic administration. Before administering this it should be made sure that the adrenal functions are normal.

These drugs act by temporarily blocking the exudative phases of inflammation and inhibiting the fibroblast formation in the process of tissue repair, notwithstanding the cause of damage which may be bacterial, anaphylactic, allergic or traumatic. Cortisone does not affect the cause of the damage. It merely affords mesenchymal tissues temporary protection against an irritation. The result is that the tissue cells become resistant to an injury and are capable of functioning normally in a grossly abnormal environment. Thus the effect of the drug is the blocking of the pathological evidence so long as the drug is administered. On withdrawal of the drug, the disease resumes its normal and natural course. It follows, therefore, that cortisone is effective in controlling the acute disease and is altogether ineffective in removing the structural damage caused by chronic inflammation. It is also not of any value in treating degenerative conditions. Relative therapeutic potencies of corticosteroids are given in Table 28.5. Ophthalmic corticosteroid preparations are given in Table 28.6.

Table 28.5. Relative therapeutic potencies of corticosteroids

Drug	Approximate systemic equivalent dose (mg)	Approximate anti-inflammatory potency factor
Hydrocortisone	20	1
Cortisone	25	0.8
Prednisolone	5	4
Prednisone	5	4
Dexamethasone	0.75	25
Methylprednisolone	4	5
Triamcinolone	4	5
Betamethasone	0.6	25
Fluorometholone	NA	NA

It is thus clear that cortisone is not curative. It only checks the acute phases of inflammation, leaving other measures or body resistance to effect the necessary cure. The advantage of cortisone therapy in ophthalmology is that the ocular tissue, due to its extreme delicacy requires this inhibition of the inflammatory reaction. In fact if this inhibition is maintained till the disease is treated by other suitable means, the eye will ultimately escape permanent damage. The disadvantage of cortisone therapy is that if the cause is not eliminated by other means, the disease resumes its course on withdrawal of cortisone in a more violent form. In fact the temporary inhibition of the inflammatory reaction may really constitute a danger. It would thus appear that cortisone is of limited value only. While it can control the deleterious aspects of the inflammatory manifestations of the disease, the pathological cause should be eliminated by some other means and until this cause is removed cortisone treatment should not be withdrawn. It

Table 28.6. Ophthalmic corticosteroid preparations

Generic name	Trade name	Strength (%)
I. Hydrocortisone		
Acetate suspension	Hydrocortone acetate	2.5
Acetate ointment	Hydrocortone acetate	1.5
Solution	Optef drops	0.2
II. Prednisolone		
Acetate suspension	Pred Mild/Pred Forte	0.12/1.0
Acetate suspension	Econopred/Econopred plus	0.125/1.0
Sodium phosphate solution	Inflamase/Inflamase Forte	0.12/1.0
B-H^{TM}	Prednisolone	0.125/1.0
Phosphate solution	Hydeltrasol	0.5
Phosphate solution	Metreton	0.5
Phosphate ointment	Hydeltrasol	0.25
III. Dexamethasone		
Phosphate solution	Decadron	0.1
Phosphate ointment	Decadron	0.05
Suspension	Maxidex	0.1
IV. Progesterone-like compounds		
Medrysone	HMS	1.0
Fluorometholone suspension	FML	0.1

many a time gives a feeling of complacency and one may be deceived into believing that one has cured the disease while all that has been attained is a check of the inflammatory process.

In ophthalmology, cortisone and related compounds can be administered locally or systemically. Most diseases of the outer eye can be effectively treated by local application but for treatment of diseases of the inner eye, subconjunctival injections of the hormones or systemic administration may be resorted to. Usual routes of steroid administration in ocular inflammation are given in Table 28.7. Various eye drops and ointments containing cortisone, hydrocortisone and prednisolone are available. The drops are prepared in saline or buffered phosphate vehicle. They should be used every 2 to 3 hours. The ointment contains 24 mg in a bland base, is well absorbed into the eye and has a longer action. More prolonged action lasting two or three days may be produced by subconjunctival injection (0.2 to 0.4 ml), the injection being given after local anaesthesia. These drugs may be administered systemically either orally or parenterally. The importance of such treatment is in an acute inflammatory disease of the posterior segment of the globe which is not readily and easily affected by local treatment. In severe and acute cases intravenous injection of ACTH has been known to produce dramatic effect. The indications for these preparations are conjunctivitis, infective superficial keratitis, syphilitic interstitial keratitis, spring catarrh, episcleritis, acute iridocyclitis, active elements of chronic iridocyclitis and particularly sympathetic ophthalmitis.

In acute or subacute generalised uveitis or local choroiditis systemic therapy is of value. Post-operative corticosteroid therapy is of immense value.

Table 28.7. Usual route of steroid administration in ocular inflammation

Condition	Route
Blepharitis	Topical
Conjunctivitis	Topical
Episcleritis	Topical
Scleritis	Topical and/or systemic
Keratitis	Topical
Anterior uveitis	Topical and/or depot
Posterior uveitis	Systemic and/or depot
Endophthalmitis	Systemic/depot, intravitreal
Optic neuritis	Systemic or depot
Cranial arteritis	Systemic
Sympathetic ophthalmia	Systemic and topical

DRUGS USED AS ANTIMICROBIAL AGENTS

Disinfection of the eye is brought about by employing (a) classical disinfectants, especially heavy metal compounds and microbes can be effectively treated by (b) chemotherapeutic agents like the sulphonamides and (c) antibiotics.

Among heavy metal compounds silver salts have been largely used for treating eye infections. Silver nitrate, when brought in contact with living tissue, coagulates proteins and forms a film of silver albuminate which becomes black owing to reduction of the silver. Concentrated solutions of silver nitrate are caustic and can be used to remove warts; dilute solutions have an astringent action. An instillation of 1/2 to 1% silver nitrate into the eye of a newborn baby has been used for many years as a prophylactic against ophthalmia neonatorum. For applications to the mucous membrane silver nitrate has the double disadvantage of being irritant and of being precipitated by the chlorides in the secretions of mucous membranes; the same objections apply to all silver preparations containing free silver ions. Silver preparations have been used to produce epithelial scarring in trachoma; 2% silver nitrate cautery is quite effective.

There are certain types of silver preparations which are relatively non-irritant because in these the greater part of silver is in a non-ionised form. These are chiefly used as disinfectants of the eye. Colloidal preparations consist of silver or silver oxide in a colloidal state combined with some protective such as casein or albumin. Silver proteinate are of two types : (1) The argyrol type which contains about 25 per cent of silver, very little of which is ionised. These preparations are non-irritant and do not give a precipitate with chlorides. (2) The protargol type which contains about ten per cent of silver. These preparations are more irritant and yield a precipitate with chloride. Their prolonged use gives rise to argyrosis of various structures of the eye. They are better avoided.

Chemotherapeutic drugs. These drugs have an advantage over antiseptics in general in that they have the property of doing more harm to the invading organisms than to the tissues of the host, while the antiseptics act by killing both indiscriminately. Chemotherapeutic drugs and antibiotics, however, are largely bacteriostatic rather than bactericidal, competing probably for the essential metabolites of the organisms. The result is that since the organisms are inhibited from growing and multiplying, the natural defence of the body can deal with those already present. As soon as the drug is withdrawn, the surviving organisms can resume growth and can multiply. Hence the rationale of treatment with chemotherapeutic agents is to keep the drug continuously in contact with the infected tissue until the infection is overcome. Since these drugs are rapidly excreted or diffuse quickly from any site of local administration, repeated or continuous administration of these during the period of acute infection is essential. The value of these drugs lies in the treatment of acute infections; in chronic cases they are relatively in-effective or relapses follow their use. The most important chemotherapeutic compounds concerned with the common ophthalmological infection are the sulphonamides, the sulphones, PAS and isoniazid.

Sulphonamides. The more commonly used sulphonamides are (1) Sulphatriad (2) Sulphadiazine (3) Sulphacetamide (4) Sulphamezathine (5) Sulphadimidine (6) Sulphamerazine and the long acting (7) Sulphamethoxy-pyridazine and (8) Sulphaperazole. These drugs can be used for treating a number of ocular infections. They are effective against haemolytic streptococci, pneumococci, *Staphylococcus aureus*, meningococci, diplobacilli, the influenza bacillus, coliform bacilli, Freidlander's bacillus and the gas gangrene organisms. They show great activity against the beta-haemolytic streptococcus, while they have low activity against the staphylococcus. These drugs do not elicit response from tuberculous, leprous, syphilitic brucellar or tularaemic infections and are also ineffective against infections due to non-haemolytic or anaerobic streptococci. Trachoma, inclusion blennorrhoea and lympho-granuloma venereum are sensitive to sulphonamides. In all these cases resistant strains of organisms have been encountered.

These drugs may be administered systemically or applied locally, as they are lipoid-soluble, they cross the blood-aqueous barrier rather easily. Consequently systemic administration is effective in acute ocular diseases as well as in infections of the conjunctiva, lids and orbit. During systemic administration it is required to have effective blood concentrations for long periods. Hence the dose for an adult should be initial dose of 1.0 g. To an infant one-tenth of this dose is considered adequate.

Both the sulphonamides and antibiotics are used topically. The most popular sulphonamide in this respect is sodium sulphacetamide, which is almost non-irritant and is free from untoward reactions. It is employed either as 10 to 30 percent solution or as 6 to 10 percent ointment. This provides the most effective treatment for trachoma.

Sulphones. In experimental tuberculosis in rabbits certain diamino-diphenyl sulphones (Dapsons, Solapsons and Promin) have been shown to have beneficial effect when administered with streptomycin. Clinical results have been disappointing. These drugs are therefore not employed for tubercular infections. Sulphones are particularly useful against leprosy and are in wide use.

Para-amino-salicylic acid (PAS). It has been found that PAS given systemically by mouth in four daily doses of 3.0 g each with strepto-mycin form a much more effective combination than the sulphones do with streptomycin for combating tuberculosis. The combination of PAS and streptomycin is effective in treating both intra and extraocular tuberculosis of an infective nature.

Isoniazid. With the introduction of INH (iso-nicotinic acid hydra-zide) it has been found that a combination of this (25 mg per kg body weight) drug with streptomycin is the most effective combination against tuberculosis. The drug is also capable of acting alone. The choice in treatment of extra and intraocular tubercular lesions should be the combination of INH and streptomycin with or without the addition of PAS.

Antibiotics. It is known that certain micro-organisms can liberate substances which inhibit the growth of micro-organisms. Such substances are called antibiotics and are elaborated by a wide range of bacteria, fungi and actinomycetes. The important antibiotics that are in use are Ampicillin, Penicillin G, Streptomycin, Soframycin, Neomycin, Carbencillin, Bacitracin, Cephaloricidine, Erythromycin, Gentamicin, Polymyxin, Cephalothin, Chloramphenicol, Cindamycin, Colistin, Methicillin, Idnomycin, Tetracyclines, Tobramycin, Vancomycin, etc. Penicillin is largely effective against Gram-positive organisms and certain spirochaetes. Streptomycin is effective against Gram-negative organisms and certain acid-fast bacilli. The broad-spectrum antibiotics, viz., chloramphenicol, tetracyclines, and neomycin have been shown clinically to be effective against Gram-positive as well as Gram-negative organisms, rickettsiae, some large viruses and certain spirochaetes and protozoa. These antibiotics are inactivated by heavy metals hence lotions containing zinc or mercury should not be used along with them.

Penicillin. It is obtained from the mould *Penicillium*. It is very commonly used in ophthalmology, because of its cheapness, availability, the wide range of organisms over which it is effective and relative absence of toxicity (apart from the hypersensitivity which some patients show towards it). It is an effective bacteriostatic agent covering Gram-positive organisms and Gram-negative cocci. Being a large molecule substance, it cannot diffuse into the eye in effective quantities unless administered in high doses. In this respect the sulphonamides having smaller molecules score over penicillin. Thus penicillin is largely useful in extraocular infections while the sulphonamides are useful in intraocular infections. In deep-seated inflammations of the orbit or lids, penicillin is administered parenterally. In superficial conjunctival or corneal inflammations it is administered locally as drops, ointments, subconjunctival injection (most effective) or powder. In intraocular infections it is injected subconjunctivally or very rarely directly into the eye. A large number of variants of penicillin are in use.

The penicillins in use may be classified as under :

1. Penicillins which are not acid stable and can only be given parenterally **(Benzyl penicillin)**.

2. **Penicillinase resistant penicillins.** They are quite useful against penicillin-resistant organisms specially staphylococci. They are cloxacillin sodium, floxacillin sodium, methicillin sodium, etc. They can be used both locally and parenterally.

3. **Ampicillin.** It is a broad-spectrum antibiotic and is active against penicillinase-producing staphylococci. The drug can be used both orally and parenterally.

4. **Carbencillin sodium.** This is active against *Pseudomonas auruginose* and is given parenterally.

5. **Norfloxacillin.** This is quite effective locally and parenterally.

Systemic administration. A daily dose varying from 10 to 20 lac units of the less soluble and more strongly absorbed preparations of penicillin can be administered for some days. The preparations are not considered suitable because they are not effective and because of their effects on the mucosa of the mouth and bowel. Oral therapy is required to be combined with large doses of vitamin B complex.

Local application. The topical preparations of penicillin or its allied products comprise of drops, ointment powder or subconjunctival injections. In all these preparations the sodium salt is always employed, drops generally contain 100,000 units per ml depending upon the acuteness of infection. The eye should not be washed in boric acid if penicillin has to be used. The action of penicillin is destroyed in the presence of weak acids.

Intraocular administration. Subconjunctival injections of 500,000 to a million units of penicillin with epinephrine (1 in 1,000) in 0.5 ml repeated every three hours form the most convenient and effective method of administering the drug. The drug should be preferably dissolved in xylocaine or even in mydricaine if mydriasis (as is usually required) is desired.

Streptomycin. This antibiotic is effective against a number of penicillin-resistant organisms, the most important being tubercle bacillus. On prolonged use, the drug sometimes shows toxic complications namely affection of the eighth nerve causing giddiness, deafness and sometimes nystagmus. This complication is, however, not common. Another disadvantage of the drug is that organisms frequently tend to acquire resistance to streptomycin. Consequently in ophthalmology the drug is used systemically in combination with PAS largely in the treatment of tuberculosis.

The drug is found to be quite effective when instilled locally or when injected subconjunctivally. For local drops it is better to use a combination of penicillin and streptomycin. 0.5 g of streptomycin and 50,000 units of penicillin are dissolved in 10 cc of normal saline. A few drops every 2 hours give satisfactory results. For subconjunctival injection streptomycin is given in daily doses of 50-100 mg.

Tetracycline group of antibiotics. These possess considerable antibacterial action against both Gram-positive and Gram-negative organisms as well as fungi, rickettsia, the larger viruses and Tric agent. They have a lesser penetrating power than penicillin with respect to the ocular tissues, either from the conjunctival sac or after systemic administration. Consequently they are largely employed as ointments for superficial ocular infections. Their irritability limits their use as subconjunctival injections. Due to their instability they are not marketed as drops.

Neomycin. In therapeutics it is used as neomycin sulphate. It exhibits activity against a variety of Gram-positive and Gram-negative bacteria. It has a wider antibacterial spectrum than bacitracin, penicillin or streptomycin, and it is sometimes effective against pseudomonas and proteus infections. It is not active against fungi. In ophthalmology neomycin sulphate is useful for topical application as a solution or ointment in the treatment of conjunctivitis, blepharitis and stye (hordeolum externum). An ointment containing 0.5 percent hydrocortisone and 0.35 percent neomycin sulphate (or a mixture of neomycin sulphate and bacitracin) is used for local application in ophthalmology. Recently it has been suggested that neomycin may be suitable for subconjunctival injection in 250-500 mg doses. Sorsby and Ungar (1958) have shown that 500 mg of neomycin dissolved in 1 ml of 1/4000 adrenaline solution may be given safely by subconjunctival injection. Also one such injection produces a therapeutic level of neomycin in the aqueous humour lasting for 24 hours. As regards the effectiveness of neomycin in intraocular infection, it seems that it is fairly useful. Intraocular infections progress very rapidly and early effective treatment is essential if sight is to be saved. As neomycin is active against both cocci and Gram-negative bacilli it may well prove valuable when the nature of infecting organism is not immediately apparent. Additional advantage in the use of neomycin is that sensitive organisms do not develop resistance readily.

Polymyxins. They are obtained from different strains of *B. polymyxa*. They are very effective against Gram-negative bacteria. The special advantage of this group is its usefulness against extra- or intraocular infections by *Pseudomonas pyocynaea*, which is not affected by most other antibiotics. They are used as drops in extraocular infections and can be used as subconjunctival injections.

Soframycin. It is highly effective against Gram-positive cocci and Gram-negative bacilli (including *Pseudomonas pyocynaea*). It is non-irritant and hence suitable for subconjunctival injection. It can be given in the anterior chamber in doses of 15 mg per ml without any untoward reaction. In fact it is a very promising antibiotic in ophthalmology.

Gentamicin. It is a newer antibiotic which is effective against a large number of organisms including those resistant to penicillin especially the staphycoccus and *Ps. pyocyanes*. It can be given as drops or subconjunctival injection, or injection into Tenon's space. It can also be given intravitreally.

Every day newer drugs as successive generations of antibiotics are being added to the test. Norfloxacin is such a drug.

Penetration of antibiotics in the eye and comparative assessment in ophthalmology

The penetration of antibiotics in the eye depends upon the condition of the eye and the route of administration. In general an inflamed eye absorbs the drug more rapidly than a non-inflamed eye. Many drugs do not penetrate an intact cornea, however, if the cornea has been abraded almost all the antibiotics will penetrate it well. Penetration into the posterior segment of the eye is best accomplished with systemic administration. Chloramphenicol penetrates the non-inflamed eye better than any other antibiotic regardless of the route of administration. Oxytetracycline, chlortetracycline and tetracycline penetrate poorly. Topically they enter the eye in effective doses only if corneal epithelium is damaged, even then very little penetration occurs in structures beyond cornea. There is some evidence that systemic administration of 3.0 g per day will give the required intraocular concentration levels for tetracycline but not of oxytetracyclines or chlortetracycline. The sulphonamides fall between the tetracyclines and chloramphenicol in their ability to penetrate the eye, the sulphapyridines being the most effective and causing less untoward reactions. Penicillin is moderately effective. It does not penetrate the posterior segment well. Therapeutic doses of four million units (intramuscular) per day give therapeutic intraocular levels; streptomycin requires high dose to be effective.

It should, however, be borne in mind that in the treatment of the infections of the eye itself, systemic or topical applications do not provide the therapeutic intraocular concentrations. For this purpose subconjunctival injection of a drug is the only satisfactory course. It has been observed that penicillin, streptomycin and polymyxin are suitable for subconjunctival injection because they are water soluble and also less irritant. Chloramphenicol, aureomycin, terramycin and erythromycin are unsuitable for subconjunctival injection because of their low solubility in water. Tetracycline, though more soluble than other similar antibiotics, is not sufficiently so to be thoroughly satisfactory for subconjunctival use. As regards streptomycin, subconjunctival injections of 200 mg, four times a day have been suggested. This produces higher concentration of drug in the tissue if administered with epinephrine. However untoward reactions are not unknown and its use should be judicious. The suitability of neomycin by subconjunctival injection has recently been shown. It has been shown that one injection of 500 mg of neomycin dissolved in 1 ml of 1 in 4,000 adrenaline solution is sufficient to produce therapeutic levels of neomycin in the aqueous humour lasting for 24 hours. Neomycin may prove invaluable in cases where the nature of the invading organisms is not immediately apparent.

Soframycin is a promising antibiotic. It can be used in panophthalmitis as an intracamreal injection with little damage to the ocular tissues.

Ampicillin, carbenicillin, cephaloroidine, chloramphenicol, erythromycin, gentamicin, methicillin and vancomycin all can be used intravitreally. The concentration and dosage are given in Table 28.8.

Antiviral agents

The antiviral drugs essentially act by preventing viral replication. The most recent development is the production of interferon which damps down the oxidative processes which are necessary for viral synthesis and replication. For some time past 5-iodo-2-deoxyuridine (IDU) has been used as 0.5% ointment 4 hourly or 0.1% drops at least once in 2 hours throughout the day and night. The drug acts by inhibiting the synthesis of DNA thus interfering in the viral replication. It is a good agent against herpes virus. Another drug adenine arabinoside (Ara-A or Vira-A) is used as ointment every 4 hours. It is a purine nucleotide. It also interferes with viral DNA synthesis. The principal metabolite is arabinosyl-hypoxanthine (Ara-Hz). Unfortunately both IDU and Ara-A are not selective in their inhibition of DNA and therefore effect both the virus and the host cell. They cause superficial punctate erosions of the epithelium. IDU in addition causes punctal stenosis. Acyclognanosine (acyclovir) is a compound which probably has a selective effect on viral thymidine kinase. This knowledge may ultimately result in a new era in antiviral therapy. A similar action is attained by cytosine arabinoside hydrochloride (CA) by blocking the synthesis of nucleic acids. Yet another antiviral agent is trifluorothymidine (T₃F) which is a water-soluble compound and is effective in the treatment of herpes epithelial disease. It is said that the drug is toxic to corneal epithelium. The drug is used as drops every two hours and the frequency is reduced as the condition ameliorates. The concentration and dosage of some of them are given in Table 28.9.

Antifungal agents (Table 28.10)

Unfortunately fungal infections of the eye are on the increase in India primarily because of indiscriminate use of antibiotics and corticosteroids

Table 28.8. Concentrations and dosages of principal antibiotics

Antibiotic	Topical	Subconjunctival	Intravitreal	Intravenous
Ampicillin	—	50-250 mg	5000 µg	2.0-4.0 gm/4 hr.
Bacitracin	10,000 units/ml	10,000 units	—	—
Carbenicillin	4.0 mg/ml	100 mg	250 µg-2.0 mg	2.0 gm/4 hr.
Cephaloroidine	—	100 mg	250 µg	0.5-1.0 gm/6 hr.
Cephalothin	—	50-100 mg	—	1.0 gm/4 hr.
Chloramphenicol	5 mg/ml	500-1000 mg	2 mg	50 mg/kg/day
Clindamycin	—	15-40 mg	—	300-600 mg/8 hr.
Colistin	5-10 mg/ml	15-37.5 mg	—	5.0 mg/kg/day
Erythromycin	—	100 mg	500 µg	—
Gentamicin	8-15 mg/ml	20-40 mg	100-400 µg	5.0 mg/kg/day
Lincomycin	—	150 mg	1.5 mg	600 mg/8 hr.
Methicillin	—	150-200 mg	2.0 mg	2.0 gm/4 hr.
Neomycin	5-8 mg/ml	250-500 µg	—	—
Penicillin G	100,000 units/ml	0.5-1.0 million units	—	2.0-6.0 mega units/4 hr.
Polymyxin	16,250 units/ml	10 mg	—	—
Streptomycin	—	50-100 mg	—	15-25 mg/kg/day
Tobramycin	3 mg/ml	—	—	—
Vancomycin	50 mg/ml	25 mg	1.0 mg	1.0 gm/12 hr.

Table 28.9. Antiviral agents

U.S.P. or N.F. name	Dosage	Duration of treatment	Complications
1. 5-iodo-2-deoxyuridine (IDU)	(a) Ointment 0.5%, 5 times a day; (b) Solution 0.1%, at least every 2 hours day and night	Dendritic ulcer—5 days; If no improvement then mechanical debridement	Superficial Punctate erosions, punctal stenosis
2. Adenine arabinoside (Ara-A)	Ointment, 5 times daily		
3. Trifluorothymidine (T3F)	1 gtt Q2h until reepithelialization then Q4h/7 days		Epithelial erosions

Table 28.10. Antifungal agents

U.S.P. or N.F. name	Dosage	Spectrum	Toxicity

1. Amphotericin B
   Topical solution
   Subconjunctival injection
	2.5-10 mg/ml of diluent
	Distilled water or 5% dextrose solution
	750 mcg/ml of diluent (as above) every other day
		Blastomyces
		Candida coccidioides
		Histoplasma	

2. Amphotericin B (Intravenous)	Start with 0.25 mg/kg body weight and increase to 1-1.5 utilizing a preparation of 0.1 mg. Amphotericin B/ml solution obtained by diluting 50 ml of powder in 10 ml sterile water and then diluting final concentration 0.1 mg/dl		Chills, fever, nausea, vomiting, renal impairment hematuria, albuminuria, bone marrow depression, thrombo- phlebitis at site of injection
3. Amphotericin B (intravitreal)	5-10 µg		
4. Nystatin (topical)	Ointment 100,000 units/gm	Aspergillus candida	
5. Flucytosine	(a) PO : 200 mg/kg body weight (b) Topical : 1% solution	Candida cryptococcus	Diarrhoea, nausea Nausea
6. Natamycin (topical suspension)	5% suspension	Candida aspergillus Cephalosporium Fusarium penicillium	
7. Miconazole	(a) PO (IV) 0.3 gm/day (b) Topical, 1% solution	Candida aspergillus	Phlebitis, GI disturbance enhances coumadin effect

Table 28.11. Antiprotozoal agents

Organism	Drug	Indication for treatment	Oral medication
Toxoplasma gondii	Pyrimethamine	Vision-threatening uveitis	Initial dose 100 mg followed by 25 mg twice daily
	Trisulfapyrimidines	Uveitis	2-6 gm daily for 3-4 weeks
	Corticosteroid preparation	Uveitis	40 mg daily orally
	Clindamycin	Uveitis	Subconjunctival clindamycin phosphate (40 mg/ml) diluted 1 : 3 in normal saline. Dose 15-40 mg or oral clindamycin hydrochloride 300 mg q.i.d./4 weeks.

and frequent agricultural injuries. Drugs against the fungi are few and not as effective as one would like them to be. Search for newer antifungal agents is going on but much has not been achieved. Some of the antifungal agents used are (1) Amphotericin B (Fungizone) 2.5 to 10 mg per ml in water or 5% Dextrose for local drops or 750 microgram per ml for subconjunctival injection. It can be given intravitreally in 5-10 microgram doses. It has been used intravenously in desperate cases. It is very toxic by this route. Nystatin as 5-10% ointment, Flucytosine as 1% solution, Antamycin as 5% suspension and Miconazole as 1% solution are some of the other agents employed.

Antiprotozoal agents (Table 28.11)

Most of the drugs are used orally against toxoplasmosis in varying doses. They are Pyrimethamine, Trisulfapyrimidines and Cindamycin. Cindamycin can also be given subconjunctivally 10 mg per ml diluted in 1 to 3 solution of normal saline—15 to 40 mg of this can be given.

ANTI-GLAUCOMA DRUGS

The antiglaucoma therapy is mostly carried out with miotics, hyperosmotic agents, carbonic anhydrase inhibitors and adrenergic agents.

Carbonic anhydrase inhibitors

Acetazolamide (Diamox), Methazolamide (Neptazane), Dichlorphenamide and Ethoxozolamide are the drugs used in this group. These drugs (Table 28.12) essentially act by inhibition of carbonic anhydrase. Their compounds are allied to sulphonamides. In the eye carbonic anhydrase assists in the formation of aqueous humour while in the kidneys it is responsible for the reabsorption of fluid from the tubules. These drugs, therefore, cause diuresis in the kidney and diminished aqueous inflow in the ciliary head. The aqueous outflow is increased through the iris crypts but the drug in no way affects the outflow from the canal of Schlemm. These drugs are clinically used in glaucoma, singly or in combination with miotics, for restoration of post-operative flat chambers and as a pre-operative measure in cataract surgery where the operation may be completed without vitreous prolapse. They are also used pre-operatively in glaucoma and in hypertensive ocular states. The usual dose of diamox is 500 mg daily preferably given as a single dose but may be divided into two. Neptazane is more powerful drug and is given in 50 mg three times a day. It is effective in cases which prove refractory to diamox. Dichlorphenamide is also used as 100 mg twice daily and ethoxozolamide 125 mg 2-4 times in a day.

Nowadays Dorzolamide is under trial to be used as 2% ophthalmic solution for topical use in glaucoma to control aqueous inflow and reduce intraocular pressure.

Table 28.12. Carbonic anhydrase inhibitors

U.S.P. or N.F. name	Dosage	Action onset/duration	Complications or side-effect in long-term therapy
Acetazolamide (oral)	125-250 mg 1-4 times daily	2 hr./4-6 hr.	Paresthesias, GI discomfort, anorexia, ureteral colic and calculi potassium depletion, metabolic acidosis
Acetazolamide (intravenous)	250-500 mg in 5-10 ml distilled water	5-10 min./2 hr.	Acetazolamide is a sulfonamide derivative and similarly may cause skin reactions and bone marrow suppression
Dichlorphenamide (oral)	50 mg 1-4 times daily	30 min./6 hr.	Similar but potassium depletion more of a problem
Ethaxozolamide (oral)	125 mg 1-4 times daily	2 hr./5 hr.	Similar to acetazolamide
Methazolamide (oral)	50-100 mg 3 times a day	2 hr./4-6 hr.	Similar but generalized malaise, fatigue and drowsiness may develop
Dorzolamide (topical)	2% as drops	4-6 hr.	No side-effects reported so far

Table 28.13. Hyperosmotic agents

U.S.P. or N.F. name (solution)	Dosage	Route	Action onset/duration	Complications and side-effects
Glycerol (50%)	1-1.5 gm/kg body weight	Oral	10-30 min./4-5 hr.	Nausea and vomiting. May produce hyperglycemia and glycosuria
Mannitol (20%)	1-2 gm/kg body weight	I.V.	30-60 min./6 hr.	Warm solution if crystals present hypervolemia
Urea (30%)	1-2 gm/kg body weight	I.V.	30-45 min./5-6 hr.	Headache. Sloughing of underlying tissue after extravasation

OSMOTIC AGENTS

Hyperosmotic agents

Three preparations are commonly used (Table 28.13), i.e., glycerol (50%), mannitol (20%) and urea (30%).

Glycerol. It is usually given orally as 50% solution with orange juice over ice. Its maximum hypotensive effect occurs in 1-2 hours and lasts for 5-6 hours. It produces nausea and vomiting and may lead to hyperglycemia and glycosuria.

Mannitol. It is used as 20% solution in water. Its maximum hypotensive effect occurs in 30-60 minutes which lasts for about 6 hours. It is given as an intravenous drip. About 300 cc are infused.

Urea. It is used as a 30% solution. Its maximum hypotensive effect occurs in about 30-45 minutes and lasts for about 5-6 hours. It may cause headache. If extravasation occurs it may lead to sloughing of underlying tissue. It is hardly ever used now.

These agents are normally used in the management of acute angle closure glaucoma or acute secondary glaucoma especially the phakomorphic type or in such cases where the tension needs to be reduced either pre- or post-operatively.

All these drugs have a rebound phenomenon. The tension rises to initial level or even overshoots the mark once the administration is stopped.

Adrenergic agents

Under this group are directly acting agents and blocking agents. Epinephrine is a common drug which is both alpha- and beta-adrenergic. It is used as 2% bitartrate (Epitrate), 1/4 to 1% borate (Epinol) or 1/4 to 2% dipavalyl epinephrine hydrochloride (Glaucon). It acts by both decreasing aqueous formation and increasing its outflow. About 25% of patients develop local allergies. They also cause headache and heart palpitations.

Among the β-adrenergic blockers, timolol malleate is used twice a day. It is a betanergic blocker. It is used as a topical agent for the treatment of chronic open angle glaucoma as a 0.25% or 0.5% solution. It lowers the intraocular pressure without causing miosis or accommodation. The drug should be avoided in patients with asthma and cardiac problems. β-adrenergic blockers are listed in Table 28.14.

Table 28.14. Beta-adrenergic blockers

Name of blocking agent	Concentration	Number of times daily
Timolol	0.25% to 0.50%	Twice
Betaxolol	0.50%	Thrice but safest
Laevobunol	0.50%	Twice

They cause pain, burning and irritation. They can produce allergic blepharoconjunctivitis, keratitic hyperaemia, corneal anaesthesia and dry eyes.

They have systemic side-effects on cardiac and pulmonary symptoms. In the pulmonary system they produce bronchospasm, dyspnoea and respiratory disorders.

NON-STEROIDAL ANTI-INFLAMMATORY DRUGS

The drugs utilised in this group probably produce their action by stimulating the adrenal cortex which secretes corticosteroids. These, therefore, provide an indirect corticosteroid therapy. They are most beneficial in subacute and chronic ocular inflammations. The commonly employed ones are milk, T.A.B. vaccine (10 million organisms as initial dose but the dose can be taken to 100 million organisms) and autogenous blood.

Most of them are pyrazole derivatives either alone or in combination with paracetamol or amidopyrine group of drugs. Whatever be the mechanism of action they have the following actions : (1) anti-inflammatory, (2) anti-allergic, (3) analgesic when mixed with amidopyrine, (4) anti-rheumatic, (5) anti-platelet, and (6) anti-capillary permeability. They are useful in most ocular inflammations. These drugs are used orally, by systemic injections or as local drops. The drugs commonly used topically are (1) Diclofenac 0.1%, (2) Indomethacin 1%, (3) Suprofen 1% (4) Flurbiprofen 0.03%, and (5) Ketaralec 0.5%. Flurbiprofen (0.03%), Suprofen (1%) and Indomethacin (1%) as drops are useful in preventing intraoperative miosis particularly in cataract surgery. These drugs are also of value in treating various ocular inflammations and even vernal keratoconjunctivitis (spring catarrh). Indomethacin 1% also has intraocular pressure lowering effect.

Butazolidin. Some persons think that this pyrazole derivative acts as a nonspecific therapy but the claim is contested. Whatever be the mechanism of its action it is a useful drug having the following actions : (1) anti-inflammatory, (2) anti-allergic, (3) analgesic when mixed with amidopyrine, (4) anti-rheumatic, and (5) anti-capillary permeability. It is useful in most ocular inflammations.

Tissue therapy. Implants and injections of tissues or their extracts are said to act as biogenic stimulator substances and are said to be useful in degenerative conditions of the eye, e.g., retinitis pigmentosa, progressive myopia, optic atrophy, etc., but in most cases of these diseases the results are negligible. Commonly placental implants and placental extracts have been employed. The only condition where we have found this to be of some benefit is parenchymatous xerosis after trachoma.

VITAMINS

1. **Vitamin A.** Vitamin A has two main physiological functions :

(i) It combines with protein to form visual purple, a substance in the rods of the retina which is concerned with dark adaptation.

(ii) It is an essential factor for the normal metabolism of epithelial cells and is beneficially used in deficiency syndromes like xerophthalmia and night blindness.

2. **Vitamins of B group.** Vitamins B_1 and B_{12} are antineuritic vitamins. Their deficiency produces beri-beri and peripheral neuritis. They are usefully employed in the deficiency state and in the treatment of herpes zoster and optic neuritis.

3. **Nicotinic acid.** Nicotinamide, an amide of nicotinic acid is a constituent part of the coenzymes, diphosphopyridine nucleotide (DPN) and triphosphopyridine nucleotide (TPN), which are present in all living cells. These coenzymes, when attached to specific proteins function in oxidation-reduction systems by virtue of their ability to accept hydrogen from certain substrates and transfer them to other hydrogen accepting substrates such as the flavian enzymes. Nicotinic acid is thus required for a number of reactions which are essential for the survival of the cell. It is therapeutically used by some for corneal ulcers. It may be used systemically or preferably subconjunctivally. The only disadvantage of subconjunctival use is that the redness in the eye persists even after complete healing of the corneal ulcer.

4. **Vitamin B_2 (Riboflavin).** Riboflavin phosphate combines with a protein to form the yellow respiratory enzyme which Warburg has shown as constituting a portion of the normal oxidative mechanism of living cells.

It probably functions in conjunction with aneurine and nicotinamide, in the oxidation of carbohydrates. Several other enzyme systems in the body have been shown to contain riboflavin as a coenzyme. In the deficiency of this enzyme the eye is affected and photophobia, impairment of visual acuity, congestion of the sclera and interstitial keratitis occur; examination of the eye shows vascularization of the cornea. The drug is used in its deficiency; some people also use it in the treatment of phlyctenular disease and spring catarrh. They claim that it lessens the relapse.

5. **Vitamin C (ascorbic acid).** Ascorbic acid is a strong reducing agent and plays a part in cellular oxidation-reduction reactions. It appears to be particularly important for the formation of bone, teeth and collagen tissues. High concentrations of ascorbic acid are present in the adrenal cortex from which it can be released by the administration of ACTH. The deficiency of ascorbic acid leads to scurvy. In the eye it leads to kerato-conjunctivitis and conjunctival and retinal haemorrhages. Vitamin C is used to combat its deficiency, to increase resistance to infection and to help in the healing of corneal wounds.

6. **Vitamin P (rutin).** It is responsible for the health of the capillaries and is sometimes used in diabetes and epidemic dropsy glaucoma.

Table 28.15. Artificial tear solutions

Product and ingredients	Product and ingredients	Product and ingredients
Adapettes (Alcon, BP) Adsorbobase* Thimerosol 0.002% Disodium edetate 0.05%	**Isopto Tears (Alcon)** Hydroxypropyl methylcellulose 0.5% Benzalkonium chloride 0.01%	**Methulose (Softcon)** Methylcellulose 0.25% Buffered solution Benzalkonium chloride 0.004%
Adapt (Alcon, BP) Adsorbobase* Hydroxyethyl cellulose 0.55% Thimerosol 0.002% Disodium edetate 0.05%	**Lacril (Allergan)** Hydroxypropyl methylcellulose Polysorbate 80 Gelatin A Buffered isotonic solution Chlorobutanol 0.5%	**Tearisol (CooperVision)** Hydroxypropyl methylcellulose 0.5% Benzalkonium chloride 0.01% Edetate disodium Buffered isotonic solution
Adsorbotear (Alcon, BP) Adsorbobase* Hydroxyethyl cellulose Buffered isotonic solution Thimerosol 0.002% Disodium edetate 0.05%	**Liquifilm Forte (Allergan)** Polyvinyl alcohol 3% Thimerosol 0.002% Edetate disodium	**Tears Naturale (Alcon)** Duasorb* polymeric system with dextran Benzalkonium chloride 0.01% Edetate disodium 0.05%
Hypotears (CooperVision) Lipiden™ polymeric system Benzalkonium chloride 0.01% Edetate disodium 0.03% Nonionic tonicity adjusters Sterile hypotonic solution	**Liquifilm Tears (Allergan)** Polyvinyl alcohol 1.4% Chlorobutanol 0.5%	**Tears Plus (Allergan)** Polyvinyl alcohol 1.4% Povidone Chlorobutanol 0.5%
	Lyteers (Barnes-Hind) Hydroxyethyl cellulose 0.2% Buffered isotonic solution Benzalkonium chloride 0.01% Disodium edetate 0.05%	**Visculose (Softcon)** Methylcellulose 0.5 or 1.0% Buffered solution Benzalkonium chloride 0.004%

* Adsorbobase = polyvinyl pyrrolidone soluble polymers (PVP) 1.67% with water.

AGENTS FOR DRY EYES

Dry eye is essentially a condition of disturbances of pre-corneal tear film due to the deficiency of either the aqueous or the mucin contents. Three important conditions are the Stevens-Johnson syndrome, the kerato-conjunctivitis sicca and the xerosis (epithelial or parenchymatous type). A large number of products are available to give symptomatic relief: like Isoptotears (hydroxypropyl methyl cellulose), Adsorbobase (polyvinyl pyrrolidone soluble polymers, thimerosal and disodium edetate); Hypotears, Lacril, Methulose, Tearisol, Tears Naturale, Hypotears, Visculose, etc. Some of the drugs are listed in Table 28.15. The main components are methylcellulose and related chemicals, polyvinyl alcohol and related chemicals and gelatin.

CHAPTER XXIX

OPHTHALMIC PRESCRIPTIONS

Prescriptions for some of the common eye medications are :

Paints

For lids

The paints are only necessary for ulcerative blepharitis but hardly ever used now.

Silver nitrate

10% is the only one left which is occasionally used in recalcitrant cases.

For conjunctiva

1-2% silver nitrate is used sometimes for resistant trachoma cases to be painted on everted lids.

For cornea

Cauterization of cornea is not uncommonly resorted to. For this purpose pure alcohol, pure carbolic acid or iodine cautery is used. The iodine solution is made as under :

Iodine 7 parts, pot. iodide 5 part, add 90% alcohol to make it 100 parts.

Lotions

For lids

Lotions are required for dissolving the crusts in blepharitis and can be used in conjunction with salicylic acid or resorcin 1 to 2% strength. They are : sodium bicarbonate 2.00, add distilled water to make it 100. A 2% boric solution is also useful. Other lotions are amphoteric lotion and saline eye lotion.

Amphoteric lotion

Hydrated potassium acid phosphate	7.0
Hydrated sodium phosphate	18.0
Distilled water	to 100.0

Saline eye lotion

Sodium chloride	0.57
Potassium chloride	0.02

Calcium chloride anhydrous   0.016
Distilled water   to 100.00
This is equivalent to 2/3 strength of Ringer solution.

Sodium bicarbonate eye lotion

Sodium bicarbonate   2.0
Distilled water   to 100.0

For conjunctiva

The above lotions are equally good. All eye lotions act as mechanical irrigators only.

Boric acid lotion 2% solution

Boric acid   0.6
Soda bicarb   0.6
Rose water   5
Distilled water   to 30

Collyria

A large number of eye-drops are used and they are listed according to their actions.

Miotics

Pilocarpic eye-drops 1/4 to 4%

Pilocarpic hydrochloride   0.25 to 4.00
Benzalkonium chloride   0.01
Distilled water   to 100.00

Pilocarpic nitrate

Pilocarpic nitrate   1 to 4
Thiomersal   0.005
Distilled water   to 100

Pilocarpine and eserine eye-drops

Pilocarpine hydrochloride   2.0 to 4.0
Physostigmine sulphate   0.25 to 1.0
Sodium metabisulphite   0.2
Ascorbic acid   0.1
Benzalkonium chloride   0.01
Distilled water   to 100.0

Physostigmine eye-drops

Physostigmine sulphate   0.25 to 1.0
Sodium metabisulphite   0.2
Ascorbic acid   0.1
Benzalkonium chloride   0.01
Distilled water   to 100.0

Phospholine eye-drops (echothiophate eye-drops)

Phospholine iodide	0.06 to 0.25
Chlorbutol	0.5
Mannitol	1.2
Boric acid	0.06
Sodium phosphate hydrated	0.026
Distilled water	to 100.0

Carbachol eye-drops

Carbachol	0.75 to 3.0
Benzalkonium chloride	0.01
Distilled water	to 100.0

Eserine eye-drops

Physostigmine sulphate	0.25 to 1
Sodium metabisulphite	0.2
Ascorbic acid	0.1
Benzalkonium chloride	0.01
Distilled water	to 100.0

Bimiotic eye-drops

Pilocarpine hydrochloride	2 to 4
Physostigmine sulphate	0.25 to 1
Chlorbutol	0.5
Mannitol	1.2
Boric acid	0.06
Hydrated sodium phosphate	0.025
Distilled water	to 100.0

Neostigmine 2.5 to 5% solution

Demecarium bromide (Humorsol) 0.12 to 0.25%

Mydriatics

Phenylephrine eye-drops

Phenylephrine hydrochloride	10.0
Sodium citrate	0.3
Sodium metabisulphate	0.5
Benzalkonium chloride	0.02
Distilled water	to 100.0

Atropine eye-drops 1/4 to 1%

Atropine sulphate	0.25 to 1
Boric acid	2
Phenyl mercuric nitrate	0.002
Distilled water	to 100.0

Homatropine eye-drops 1-2%

Homatropine hydrobromide	1 to 2
Chlorhexidine acetate	0.01
Distilled water	to 100.0

Cyclopentolate eye-drops (0.5 to 1% w/v)

Cyclopentolate is available under the trade name of Cyclopentone.

Tropicamide eye-drops

Tropicamide	1 to 2
Thiomersal	0.05
Distilled water	to 100.0

Hyoscine eye-drops (0.25 to 0.5%)

Hyoscine hydrobromide	0.25-0.50
Chlorhexidine acetate	0.01
Distilled water	to 100.0

Should be used in children.

Hyoscine eye-drops (0.05%)

Hyoscine hydrobromide	0.05
Chlorhexidine acetate	0.01
Distilled water	to 100.0

For use in refraction of children. This drug is highly toxic, therefore, this strength should not be exceeded in children.

Lachesine eye-drops

Lachesine hydrochloride	1.0
Phenylmercuric nitrate	0.002
Distilled water	to 100.0

Chemotherapeutic drugs

Sulphacetamide eye-drops (10-30%)

Sodium sulphacetamide	10-30
Sodium metabisulphate	0.1
Thiomersal	0.005
Distilled water	to 100.0

Dispense in neutral bottles.

Zinco-sulpha eye-drops

Sodium sulphacetamide	5.0
Zinc sulphate	0.1
Sodium carbomethyl cellulose	1.0
Phenyl mercuric nitrate	0.004
Distilled water	to 100.0

Antibiotics

A large number of proprietary preparations are available and they should
be used as such.

Chloramphenicol eye-drops (1/2%)

Chloramphenicol	0.5
Borax	0.3
Boric acid	1.5
Phenyl mercuric acetate	0.002
Distilled water	to 100.0

Amphotericin B

Amphotericin B	0.5
Thiomersal	0.005
Distilled water	to 100.0

Cloxacillin

Cloxacillin	2.5
Thiomersal	0.005
Distilled water	to 100.0

Penicillin eye-drops

Benzyl penicillin	5,000 units
Sodium citrate	5 mg
Phenyl mercuric nitrate	20 µg
Distilled water	to 1 ml

Norfloxacin

Norfloxacin	0.3
Benzalkonium chloride	0.02
Distilled water	to 100.0

Penicillin cum streptomycin eye-drops

Benzyl penicillin	100,000 units
Streptomycin sulphate	0.1 g
Phenyl mercuric nitrate	20 µg
Distilled water	to 1 ml

Framycetin eye-drops (soframycin)

Framycetin sulphate	1.0
Phenyl mercuric nitrate	0.002
Distilled water	to 100.0

Neomycin eye-drops

Neomycin sulphate	0.5
Hydrated sodium phosphate	0.7

Hydrated sodium acid phosphate	0.7
Disodium edetate	0.01
Phenyl mercuric nitrate	0.002
Distilled water	to 100.0

Gentamicin eye-drops

Gentamicin sulphate	1.6
Thiomersal	0.005
Distilled water	to 100.0

Ciprofloxacin

Ciprofloxacin	0.3
Benzalkonium chloride	0.02
Distilled water	to 100.0

Polymyxin B

| Distilled water | to 100 ml |

Tobramycin

| Distilled water | to 100 ml |

Kanamycin eye-drops

Kanamycin	0.5
Boric acid	1.54
Borax	0.286
Phenylmercuric nitrate	0.002
Distilled water	to 100.0

Antiviral agents

Idoxuridine eye-drops

Idoxuridine	0.1
Sodium citrate	1.125
Citric acid	0.25
Benzalkonium chloride	0.01
Distilled water	to 100.0

Antifungal agents

Amphotericin B eye-drops

Amphotericin B	0.5
Dextrose	5
Thiomersal	0.004
Distilled water	to 100.0

5-Fluorocytosine eye-drops

| 5-fluorocytosine | 1.0 g |

| Thiomersal | 5 µg |
| Distilled water | to 100 ml |

Miconazole eye-drops

Miconazole	1.0
Thionazole	0.005
Distilled water	to 100.0

Silver sulfadiazine drops

Silver sulfadiazine	1
Methyl cellulose	0.5
Thiomersal	0.005
Distilled water'	to 100.0

ANTI-INFLAMMATORY DRUGS

Corticosteroids

Hydrocortisone

Hydrocortisone acetate suspension 1% w/v
Solution 0.2%

Prednisolone eye-drops

Prednisolone acetate suspension mild 0.12%
Prednisolone acetate suspension forte 1.00%
Prednisolone sodium phosphate mild 0.12%
Prednisolone sodium phosphate forte 1%
Prednisolone phosphate 0.5%
Dexamethasone phosphate solution (Decadron) 0.1%
Betamethasone in 0.3% solution
These solutions are also available in combination with 0.5% w/v neomycin sulphate.

Prednisolone eye-drops

Prednisolone sodium phosphate	0.31
Boric acid	0.3
Sodium borate	0.03
Disodium edetate	0.01
Phenylmercuric nitrate	0.004
Distilled water	to 100.0

Forte drops can also be made by increasing the quantity of prednisolone to 1.0 instead of 0.31.

The drops can also be combined with neomycin by adding neomycin 0.5 to the above drops.

Betamethasone in 0.3% solution

It would be better if various equivalents are taken with hydrocortisone as unit. It is given below :

	Approx. systemic equivalent dose (mg)	Approx. anti-inflammatory potency factor
Hydrocortisone	20	1.0
Cortisone	25	0.8
Prednisolone	5	4.0
Dexamethasone	0.75	25.0
Betamethasone	0.6	25.0

Indomethacin eye-drops

Indomethacin	1
Sodium hydride	2
Boric acid	8
Distilled water	to 100

In spring catarrh.

Artificial tear solutions

Adsorbabase

Thiomersal	0.002%
Disodium edetate	0.05%

Hypotears

Lipiden polymeric system	
Benzalkonium chloride	0.01%
Disodium edetate	0.03%

Along with are also mixed non-ionic tonicity adjusters and sterile hypotonic solution.

Tears Naturale

Duasorb polymeric system with dextran containing benzalkonium chloride and disodium edetate.

There are large number of other compounds available.

OINTMENTS

Atropine eye ointments

Atropine sulphate	0.50-2
Sterile base (white vaseline)	to 100

Chloramphenicol eye ointments

Chloramphenicol	1
White vaseline	to 100

Framycetin eye ointment

| Framycetin | 0.5 |
| White vaseline | to 100.0 |

Idoxuridine eye ointment (IDU)

| Micronized idoxuridine | 0.5 |
| White vaseline | to 100.0 |

Neomycin eye ointment

| Neomycin sulphate | 0.5 |
| White vaseline | 100.0 |

Sulphacetamide eye ointment

| Sodium sulphacetamide | 6-10 |
| White vaseline | to 100 |

A large number of other ointments can be prepared on the same principle.

Anaesthetics

Local

Cocaine hydrochloride drops (2-4%)

Cocaine hydrochloride	2-4
Chlorhexidine acetate	0.01
Distilled water	to 10

Tetracaine hydrochloride (0.5%) eye-drops

| Tetracaine hydrochloride | 0.5 |
| Distilled water | to 100.0 |

Proparacaine hydrochloride (0.5%) eye-drops

Proparacaine hydrochloride	0.5
Chlorhexidine acetate	0.01
Distilled water	to 100.0

Regional

Procaine (1-4%), Tetracaine (1/4%), Xylocaine (1-2%) are the common solutions used for regional infiltration.

Anti-glaucoma agents

Hyperosmotic agents

Glycerol solution in fruit juice through oral route (50%).
Mannitol (20-30%) solution by intravenous route.
Urea (30%) solution by intravenous route.

Carbonic anhydrase inhibitors

Acetazolamide both by oral and intravenous route.

Daranide
Cardase (ethoxzolimide)
Neptazane (methazolimide)

Diagnostic agents

Fluorescein (2%) as solution or strips for local staining of cornea.
Fluorescein (10% to 20%) solution for intravenous route for fluorescein angiography.
Bengal rose (1%) for staining.
Methacholine as a 2.5% solution for contracting pupils in Adie's pupil.

α-chymotrypsin hyaluronidase sodium hyaluronate

Heialon are other solutions used for various purposes.
Interferon, methotrexate, cyclophosphamide, 6-mer- captopurine and azathioprine are antimetabolites in common use.
Butazolidine group of drugs is used as anti- inflammatory agents.
Ergot alkaloids, preiscoline and others are the drugs used as sympathicolytics.

Vitamins

Vitamin A, vitamin B, vitamin B_2, nicotinic acid, vitamin C (ascorbic acid) and vitamin P are vitamins in common use in ophthalmology.

Acetylcysteine

Acetylcysteine	10
Thiomersal	0.005
Distilled water	to 100.0

For spring catarrh.

Acetylcysteine 2%, 5%, 10%, 20%

Prepare solution of 20% with hypromellose (alkaline) eye-drops and then dilute it to the required strength. Adjust pH to 9.0 with 4% solution of sodium hydroxide solution.

Xylocaine (1 to 4%) eye-drops

Lignocaine	1-4
Chlorhexidine acetate	0.01
Distilled water	to 100.0

Antazoline eye-drops

Antazoline hydrochloride	0.5
Naphazoline nitrate	0.025
Sodium chloride	0.84
Phenylmercuric nitrate	0.002
Distilled water	to 100.0

Oxyphenonium eye-drops (Antrenyl)

Oxyphenonium bromide	1.0 to 5.0
Chlorhexidine acetate	0.01
Distilled water	to 100.0

INDEX

CBS BOOKS ON OPHTHALMOLOGY

CBS MEDICAL TEXT

Agarwal L.P.   : Eye Diseases, 2nd ed.
Agarwal L.P.   : Principles of Optics & Refraction, 5th ed.
Agarwal L.P.   : Ophthalmic Assistant (in 5 vols.)
                  Vol I   : General and Ocular Anatomy
                  Vol II : Physiology, Pharmacology & Microbiology
Agarwal L.P.   : Essentials of Ophthalmology
Khurana A.K.   : Anatomy and Physiology of the Eye
Khurana A.K.   : Ophthalmology (Quick Text Revision & MCQs)
Khurana A.K.   : Ophthalmology Viva (Questions & Answers)
May & Worth's   : Diseases of the Eye, 13th ed.
Galloway / Vernon   : MCQs in Ophthalmology
Omkarnath   : Ophthalmology Pre-PG Test Review
Gupta L.C.   : Anatomy of Eye & Adnexa
Ahmed E.   : MCQs in Ophthalmology
Subash C. Gupta   : Ocular Syndromes
Gupta / Aggarwal   : Clinical Examination of Ophthalmic Cases, 2nd ed.
Gupta / Aggarwal   : Differential Diagnosis in Ophthalmology
Apley   : System of Orthopedics & Fracture
Athreya H.   : Clinical Methods in Paediatric Diagnosis
Babhulkar S.S.   : Orthopaedic Manifestations and Bone Changes in Sickle Cell Haemoglobinopathy
Benerjee S.   : Long Cases in Surgery
Barker   : Basic Child Psychiatry
Behl P.N.   : Practice of Dermatology, 8th ed.
Bernstein   : Obstetrics & Gynaecology (Problem-Oriented Approach)
Bhargava S.K.   : Textbook of Radiology for Technicians
Bhargava S.K.   : Textbook of Radiology Technicians **(Hindi)**
Bhargava S.K.   : Cancer Ke Tathya **(Hindi)**
Bhargava S.K.   : Colour Doppler Imaging
Bhatia M.S.   : Synopsis History of Psychiatry, Psychology
Bhatia M.S.   : Directory of Postgraduate (PG) Medical Courses and Services Examination (of India and Abroad)
Bhatia M.S.   : Essentials of Psychiatry, 2nd ed.
Bhatia M.S.   : Dictionary of Psychiatry, Psychology, Neurology
Bhatia M.S.   : Concised Textbook Quick Medical Text Review (in 3 vols.)
                  Vol. I   : Basic Sciences, 3rd ed.
                  Vol. II : Clinical Sciences, 3rd ed.
                  Vol. III : Surgical Sciences, 3rd ed.
Bhatia M.S.   : Quick Medical Examination Review (in 3 vols.)
                  Vol. I   : Basic Sciences, 7th ed.
                  Vol. II : Medical Sciences, 7th ed.
                  Vol. III : Surgical Sciences, 7th ed.
Bhatia / Dhar   : Comprehensive Textbook of Child Adolescent Psychiatry

Bhattacharya	:	Short Cases in Surgery, 4th ed.
Bhatty G.B.	:	Essentials of Neurosurgery
Bisen P.S.	:	Handbook of Microbiology
Camm / McCarthy	:	First Aid—Step by Step
Chamberlain's	:	Symptoms, Signs Clinical Medicine, 12th ed.
Chard-Lilford	:	Basic Sciences for Obstetrics & Gynaecology, 3rd ed.
Chatterjee B.M.	:	Handbook of Ophthalmology, 6th ed.
Chaurasia B.D.	:	Human Anatomy : Regional & Applied (in 3 vols.)
		Part I : Upper Limb & Thorax, 3rd ed.
		Part II : Lower Limb & Abdomen, 3rd ed.
		Part III : Head, Neck & Brain, 3rd ed.
Chaurasia B.D.	:	Handbook of General Anatomy, 3rd ed.
Chenoy R.	:	Manipal Manual of Surgery
Chesney D.N.	:	Radiographic Imaging, 4th ed.
Chesney D.N.	:	X-Ray Equipment for Radiographers, 3rd ed.
Chesney D.N.	:	Care of the Patient in Diagnostic Radiography, 5th ed.
Clark's	:	Positioning In Radiography, 7th ed.
Clayton's	:	Electrotherapy : Theory & Practice, 8th ed.
Craft / Upton	:	Key Topics in Anaesthesia
Craft / Upton	:	Key Questions in Anaesthesia
Crofton J. et al.	:	Clinical Tuberculosis
Dandiya P.C. et al.	:	The Pharmacist's Year Book
Dandiya P.C. et al.	:	Doctors' Therapeutic Manual
Dudley	:	Guide Practical Procedures Medicine and Surgery
Elliott	:	MCQs for General Practitioners
Feldman	:	Problems in Anaesthesia
Ganjoo C.L.	:	Leaking Secrets!
Gautam Allahbadia	:	Vaginosonography in Obstetrics & Gynaecology
Glickman	:	Phantom Notes : Medicine, 6th ed.
Glickman	:	Phantom Notes : Obstetrics & Gynaecology, 3rd ed.
Glickman	:	Phantom Notes : Surgery, 2nd ed.
Glickman	:	Phantom Notes : Wards, 2nd ed.
Glickman	:	Phantom Notes : Nursing Medical-Surgical
Goel T.C.	:	Cases in Clinical Practice (Vols. II & III)
Gothi Rajesh	:	Textbook Diagnostic Ultrasound & Imaging
Gothi Rajesh	:	Textbook of Abdominal Ultrasound
Gothi Rajesh	:	Textbook of Ultrasound in Obstetrics & Gynaecology
Grover Ashok et al.	:	Manual of Medical Emergencies
Gupta L.C.	:	Signs and Syndromes in Radiology
Gupta L.C.	:	Aids to Medicine
Gupta L.C. et al.	:	Medicine Update
Hamilton Bailey's	:	Physical Signs (Demonstrations of Physical Signs in Clinical Surgery), 18th ed.
Harrison	:	Pocket Medical Dictionary
Hoffbrand	:	Postgraduate Haematology, 3rd ed.

Contact your local bookseller
or
write to the publisher :

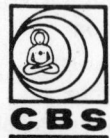

CBS PUBLISHERS & DISTRIBUTORS

4596/1A, 11 Daryaganj, New Delhi - 110 002